Biotechnology
Fifth edition

Biotechnology is the major technology of the twenty-first century – yet few people realise how much it impacts on many aspects of human society. The defining aim of this new fifth edition is to re-establish the correct understanding of the term biotechnology. Using the straightforward style that made the previous editions of his textbook so popular, John Smith once again helps students and general readers alike with the deciphering and use of biological knowledge. He explains the historical developments in biotechnology and the range of activities from brewing beer, the treatment of sewage and other wastes, and the creation of biofuels. He also discusses the innovations in molecular biology, genomics and proteomics, systems biology and their impact on new biotechnology. In this edition John Smith also re-examines the ethics and morality of aspects of biotechnology and puts new emphasis on stem cells and regenerative medicine and micro RNA.

JOHN E. SMITH is Emeritus Professor of Applied Microbiology in the Institute of Pharmacy and Biomedical Sciences, University of Strathclyde, Glasgow and Scientific Advisor to GlycaNova, Norway.

Biotechnology
Fifth edition

John E. Smith
University of Strathclyde

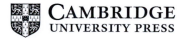
CAMBRIDGE
UNIVERSITY PRESS

CAMBRIDGE UNIVERSITY PRESS
Cambridge, New York, Melbourne, Madrid, Cape Town, Singapore, São Paulo, Delhi

Cambridge University Press
The Edinburgh Building, Cambridge CB2 8RU, UK

Published in the United States of America by Cambridge University Press, New York

www.cambridge.org
Information on this title: www.cambridge.org/9780521884945

First published by Edward Arnold 1981 (0 7131 2960 3)
Second edition 1988
Third edition 1996
Fourth edition 2004
Fifth edition 2009

Printed in the United Kingdom at the University Press, Cambridge

A catalogue record for this publication is available from the British Library

Library of Congress Cataloguing in Publication data
Smith, John E.
Biotechnology / John E. Smith. – 5th ed.
    p.   cm.
Includes index.
ISBN 978-0-521-88494-5 (hardback)
1. Biotechnology.   I. Title.
TP248.2.S66   2009
660.6 – dc22   2008030071

ISBN 978-0-521-88494-5 hardback
ISBN 978-0-521-71193-7 paperback

I dedicate this fifth edition to my grown-up children, Sheri, Jill and Fraser, who have been a constant source of inspiration.

Contents

Preface

A defining aim of this fifth edition of *Biotechnology* has been to re-establish the correct understanding of the true meaning of biotechnology.

Biotechnology is in essence the deciphering and use of biological knowledge. It is highly multidisciplinary since it has its foundations in many disciplines including biology, microbiology, biochemistry, molecular biology, genetics, chemistry and chemical and process engineering. It may also be viewed as a series of enabling technologies that involve the practical application of organisms (especially microorganisms) or their cellular components to manufacturing and service industries and environmental management. Historically, biotechnology was an artisanal skill rather than a science, exemplified in the manufacture of wines, beers, cheeses, etc. where the techniques of manufacture were well worked out and reproducible, while the biological mechanisms were not understood. As the scientific basis of these biotechnology processes has developed this has led to more efficient manufacturing of the traditional processes that still represent the major financial returns of biotechnology, i.e. bread, beers, wines, cheeses, etc. Modern biotechnological processes have generated a wide range of new and novel products including antibiotics, vaccines and monoclonal antibodies, the production of which has been optimised by improved fermentation practices. Biotechnology has been further revolutionised by a range of new molecular biology innovations, allowing unprecedented molecular changes to be made to living organisms. The increasing understanding of genomics and proteomics has led to the creation of a vast range of transgenic microorganisms, agricultural (genetically modified) crops and animals, and major new recombinant protein drugs, and has revolutionised activities in the traditional food and drinks industries. In the environment, biotechnology innovations are creating major advances in water and land management and also remediating the pollution generated by over-industrialisation.

There have been vast investments in molecular diagnostics, not only in medicine but in plant and animal agriculture and the environment. Will the huge potential of stem cells for remedial medicine soon be realised?

Until recently, much attention has been given to determining the 'nuts and bolts' of biological systems. Now, systems biology is aiming to describe and to understand the operation of complex biological systems and ultimately to develop predictive models of, for example, human disease and complex fermenter systems used in biotechnology.

Some of the new aspects of biotechnology, such as genetic engineering, have aroused certain social sensitivities of an ethical, moral and political character. Regulatory authorities throughout the world are now examining the implications of these new and revolutionary techniques. It is hoped that common sense will prevail.

Undoubtedly, modern biotechnology can only maximise its full potential to benefit mankind through achieving a basis of public understanding, awareness, and knowledge of the technologies. Participating scientists must learn to communicate openly with the public and attempt to demystify the complex nature of living systems. By doing so they will generate a greater level of confidence and trust between the scientific community and the public at large.

This expanded fifth edition of *Biotechnology* is again aimed to give an integrated overview of its complex, multifaceted and often ill-maligned subjects, and for some young readers to point the way forward to exciting, satisfying and rewarding careers. Biotechnology will undoubtedly be the major technology of the twenty-first century and should be so recognised by the lay public.

I am again deeply indebted to the long-suffering Elizabeth Clements for her skilful processing of the manuscript and her continued dedication.

Chapter 1

The nature of biotechnology

1.1 | Introduction

Major events in human history have, to a large extent, been driven by technology. Improved awareness of agriculture and metalworking brought mankind out of the Stone Age, while in the nineteenth century the Industrial Revolution created a multitude of machinery together with increasingly larger cities. The twentieth century was undoubtedly the age of chemistry and physics, spawning huge industrial activities such as petrochemicals, pharmaceuticals, fertilisers, the atom bomb, transmitters, the laser and microchips. However, there can be little doubt that the huge understanding of the fundamentals of life processes achieved in the latter part of the twentieth century will ensure that the twenty-first century will be dominated by biology and its associated technologies.

Societal changes are increasingly driven by science and technology. Currently, the impact of new biological developments must be absorbed not just by a minority (the scientists) but by large numbers of people (the general public). If this does not happen, the majority will be alienated. It is increasingly important to ensure a broad understanding of what bioscience and its related technologies will involve, and especially what the consequences will be of accepting or rejecting the new technical innovations.

The following chapters will examine how the new biotechnologists are developing new therapies and cures for many human and animal diseases; designing diagnostic tests for increasing disease prevention and pollution control; improving many aspects of plant and animal agriculture and food production; cleaning-up and improving the environment; designing clean industrial manufacturing processes; exploring the potential for biological fuel generation; and unravelling the power of stem cell technology. Undoubtedly, biotechnology can be seen to be the most innovative technology that mankind has witnessed. The development of biotechnological products is knowledge and resource intensive.

While biotechnology will undoubtedly offer major opportunities to human development (nutrition, medicine, industry) it cannot be denied that it is creating social–ethical apprehensions because of considered dangers to human rights that improper use could create. The advancement of genetic engineering, and especially the ramifications of the Human Genome Project, are achieving unique importance.

1.2 | What is biotechnology?

There is little doubt that modern biology is the most diversified of all the natural sciences, exhibiting a bewildering array of subdisciplines: microbiology, plant and animal anatomy, biochemistry, immunology, cell biology, molecular biology, plant and animal physiology, morphogenesis, systematics, ecology, genetics and many others. The increasing diversity of modern biology has been derived primarily from the largely post-war introduction into biology of other scientific disciplines such as physics, chemistry and mathematics, which have made possible the description of life processes at the cellular and molecular level. In the last two decades well over 20 Nobel prizes have been awarded for discoveries in these fields of study.

This newly acquired biological knowledge has already made vastly important contributions to the health and welfare of mankind. Yet few people fully recognise that the life sciences affect over 30% of global economic turnover by way of healthcare, food and energy, agriculture and forestry, and that this economic impact will grow as biotechnology provides new ways of influencing raw material processing. Biotechnology will increasingly affect the efficiency of all fields involving the life sciences, and it is now realistically accepted that by the early twenty-first century it will be contributing many trillions of pounds to world markets.

In the following chapters, biotechnology will be shown to cover a multitude of different applications ranging from the very simple and traditional, such as the production of beers, wines and cheeses, to highly complex molecular processes, such as the use of recombinant DNA technologies to yield new drugs or to introduce new traits into commercial crops and animals. The association of old traditional industries such as brewing with modern genetic engineering is gaining in momentum, and it is not for nothing that industrial giants such as Guinness, Carlsberg and Bass are heavily involved in biotechnology research. Biotechnology is developing at a phenomenal pace, and will increasingly be seen as a necessary part of the advance of modern life and not simply a way to make money!

While biotechnology has been defined in many forms (Table 1.1), in essence it implies the use of microbial, animal or plant cells or enzymes to synthesise, break down or transform materials.

The European Federation of Biotechnology (EFB) considers biotechnology as 'the integration of natural sciences and organisms, cells, parts thereof, and molecular analogues for products and services'. The aims of this federation are:

(1) to advance biotechnology for the public benefit
(2) to promote awareness, communication and collaboration in all fields of biotechnology

Table 1.1	Some selected definitions of biotechnology

A collective noun for the application of biological organisms, systems or processes to manufacturing and service industries.

The integrated use of biochemistry, microbiology and engineering sciences in order to achieve technological (industrial) application capabilities of microorganisms, cultured tissue cells and parts thereof.

A technology using biological phenomena for copying and manufacturing various kinds of useful substances.

The application of scientific and engineering principles to the processing of materials by biological agents to provide goods and services.

The science of the production processes based on the action of microorganisms and their active components and of production processes involving the use of cells and tissues from higher organisms. Medical technology, agriculture and traditional crop breeding are not generally regarded as biotechnology.

Really no more than a name given to a set of techniques and processes.

The use of living organisms and their components in agriculture, food and other industrial processes.

The deciphering and use of biological knowledge.

The application of our knowledge and understanding of biology to meet practical needs.

(3) to provide governmental and supranational bodies with information and informed opinions on biotechnology

(4) to promote public understanding of biotechnology.

The EFB definition is applicable to both 'traditional or old' and 'new or modern' biotechnology. Traditional biotechnology refers to the conventional techniques that have been used for many centuries to produce beer, wine, cheese and many other foods, while 'new' biotechnology embraces all methods of genetic modification by recombinant DNA and cell fusion techniques together with the modern developments of 'traditional' biotechnological processes.

It is unfortunate that the term 'biotechnology' has become, in some quarters, a substitute for genetic modification or genetic engineering. This originated in the USA many years ago to offset the activists who were demonising these new genetic procedures to the lay public. Using the term biotechnology when describing trans-species genetic modifications was considered to be more friendly sounding and to arouse less anxiety! The term was then picked up by the media and by politicians, and subsequently found its way into government documents and legislation. A defining aim of this book is to re-establish the correct understanding of biotechnology.

In truth, genetic modification has been used by mankind for over 10 000 years to improve plants and animals by selective breeding. Only within the last 50 years has this process used new methods, such as polyploidisation, mutagenesis and X-rays, to achieve changes in genetic composition.

Genetic manipulation/modification/engineering is the modern method of selectively moving genes within the same species or between species, using modern molecular biology techniques.

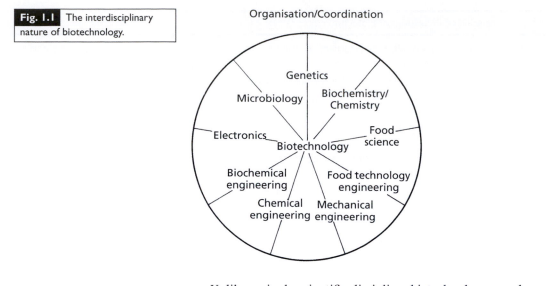

Fig. 1.1 The interdisciplinary nature of biotechnology.

Unlike a single scientific discipline, biotechnology can draw upon a wide array of relevant fields, such as microbiology, biochemistry, molecular biology, cell biology, immunology, protein engineering, enzymology, classified breeding techniques, and the full range of bioprocess technologies (Fig. 1.1). Biotechnology is not itself a product or range of products like microelectronics: rather it should be regarded as a range of enabling technologies that will find significant application in many industrial sectors. As will be seen in later chapters, it is a technology in search of new applications and the main benefits lie in the future.

As stated by McCormick (1996), a former editor of the *Journal Bio/Technology*: 'There is no such thing as biotechnology, there are biotechnologies. There is no biotechnology industry; there are industries that depend on biotechnologies for new products and competitive advantage.'

It should be recognised that biotechnology is not something new but represents a developing and expanding series of technologies dating back (in many cases) thousands of years, when humans first began unwittingly to use microbes to produce foods and beverages, such as bread and beer, and to modify plants and animals through progressive selection for desired traits. Biotechnology encompasses many traditional processes, such as brewing, baking, winemaking, cheese production, oriental foods (e.g. soy sauce and tempeh) and sewage treatment, where the use of microorganisms has been developed somewhat empirically over countless years (Table 1.2). It is only relatively recently that these processes have been subjected to rigorous scientific scrutiny and analysis; even so it will surely take some time, if at all possible, for modern scientifically based practices fully to replace traditional empiricism.

The new biotechnology revolution began in the 1970s and early 1980s when scientists learned to alter precisely the genetic constitution of living organisms by processes outside of traditional breeding practices. This 'genetic engineering' has had a profound impact on almost all areas of traditional biotechnology and further permitted breakthroughs in medicine and agriculture, in particular, that would be impossible by traditional

Table 1.2	Historical development of biotechnology

Biotechnological production of foods and beverages
Sumarians and Babylonians were drinking beer by 6000 BC, they were the first to apply direct fermentation to product development; Egyptians were baking leavened bread by 4000 BC; wine was known in the Near East by the time of the book of Genesis. Microorganisms were first seen in the seventeenth century by Anton van Leeuwenhoek who developed the simple microscope; the fermentative ability of microorganisms was demonstrated between 1857 and 1876 by Pasteur – *the father of biotechnology*; cheese production has ancient origins, as does mushroom cultivation.

Biotechnological processes initially developed under non-sterile conditions
Ethanol, acetic acid, butanol and acetone were produced by the end of the nineteenth century by open microbial fermentation processes. Waste-water treatment and municipal composting of solid wastes represents the largest fermentation capacity practised throughout the world.

Introduction of sterility to biotechnological processes
In the 1940s complicated engineering techniques were introduced to the mass production of microorganisms to exclude contaminating microorganisms. Examples include the production of antibiotics, amino acids, organic acids, enzymes, steroids, polysaccharides, vaccines and monoclonal antibodies.

Applied genetics and recombinant DNA technology
Traditional strain improvement of important industrial organisms has long been practised; recombinant DNA techniques together with protoplast fusion allow new programming of the biological properties of organisms.

breeding approaches. Some of the most exciting advances will be in new pharmaceutical drugs and therapies to improve the treatment of many diseases, and in the production of healthier foods, selective pesticides and innovative environmental technologies.

There is also a considerable danger that biotechnology will be viewed as a coherent, unified body of scientific and engineering knowledge and thinking to be applied in a coherent and logical manner. This is not so; the range of biological, chemical and engineering disciplines that are involved are having varying degrees of application to the industrial scene.

Traditional biotechnology has established a huge and expanding world market, and in monetary terms represents a major part of *all* biotechnology financial profits. 'New' aspects of biotechnology founded in recent advances in molecular biology, genetic engineering and fermentation process technology are now increasingly finding wide industrial application. A breadth of relevant biological and engineering knowledge and expertise is ready to be put to productive use; but the rate at which it will be applied will depend less on scientific or technical considerations and more on such factors as adequate investment by the relevant industries, improved systems of biological patenting, marketing skills, the economics of the new methods in relation to currently employed technologies and, possibly of most importance, public perception and acceptance.

Since the 1980s biotechnology has been recognised and accepted as a strategic technology by most industrialised nations. The economic returns from investing in strategic technologies accrue not just to the companies conducting research and development (R&D) but more importantly returns to society overall are estimated to be even higher!

The present industrial activities to be affected most will include human and animal food production, provision of chemical feedstocks to replace petrochemical sources, alternative energy sources, waste recycling, pollution control, agriculture, aquaculture and forestry. From a medical dimension, biotechnology will focus on the development of complex biological compounds rather than chemical compounds. Use will be made of proteins, hormones and related substances that occur in the living system or may even be created in vitro. The new techniques will also revolutionise many aspects of medicine, veterinary science and pharmaceutics. The recent mapping of the human genome must be recognised as one of the most significant breakthroughs in human history.

The use of microorganisms to replace certain existing procedures could make many industries more efficient and environmentally friendly and greatly contribute towards industrial sustainability. Waste will be reduced, energy consumption and greenhouse gas emissions will be lowered, and greater use of renewable raw materials will be made. In the European Union (EU) this has been termed 'white biotechnology', while healthcare and agricultural-related biotechnologies have respectively been termed 'red' and 'green' biotechnologies.

Many biotechnological industries will be based largely on renewable and recyclable materials, and so can be adapted to the needs of a society in which energy is ever-increasingly expensive and scarce. In many ways, biotechnology is a series of embryonic technologies and will require much skilful control of its development, but the potentials are vast and diverse and undoubtedly will play an increasingly important part in many future industrial processes. Can biotechnology contribute to real-world challenges such as climate change, bioenergy, healthier ageing and agricultural sustainability? This question will be answered in later chapters.

1.3 | Biotechnology: an interdisciplinary pursuit

Biotechnology is a priori an interdisciplinary pursuit. In recent decades a characteristic feature of the development of science and technology has been the increasing resort to multidisciplinary strategies for the solution of various problems. This has led to the emergence of new interdisciplinary areas of study, with the eventual crystallisation of new disciplines with identifiable characteristic concepts and methodologies.

Chemical engineering and biochemistry are two well recognised examples of disciplines that have done much to clarify our understanding of chemical processes and the biochemical bases of biological systems.

The term *multidisciplinary* describes a quantitative extension of approaches to problems that commonly occur within a given area. It involves the marshalling of concepts and methodologies from a number of separate disciplines and applying them to a specific problem in another area. In contrast, interdisciplinary application occurs when the blending of ideas that occur during multidisciplinary cooperation leads to the crystallisation of a new disciplinary area with its own concepts and methodologies. In

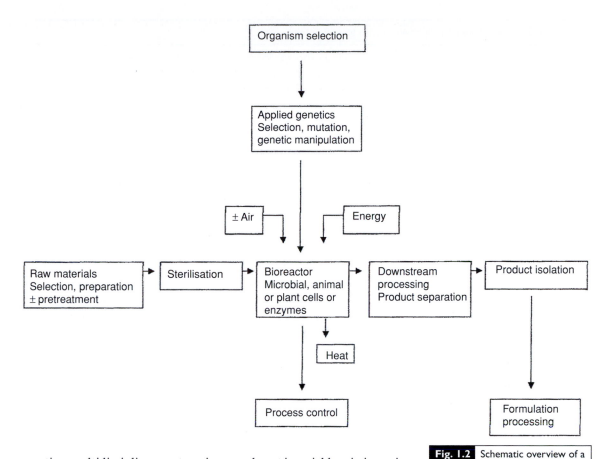

Fig. 1.2 Schematic overview of a biotechnological process.

practice, multidisciplinary enterprises are almost invariably mission orientated. However, when true interdisciplinary synthesis occurs the new area will open up a novel spectrum of investigations. Many aspects of biotechnology have arisen through the interaction between various parts of biology and engineering.

A biotechnologist can utilise techniques derived from chemistry, microbiology, biochemistry, chemical engineering and computer science (Fig. 1.1). The main objectives will be the innovation, development and optimal operation of processes in which biochemical catalysis has a fundamental and irreplaceable role. Biotechnologists must also aim to achieve a close working cooperation with experts from other related fields, such as medicine, nutrition, the pharmaceutical and chemical industries, environmental protection and waste process technology. Biotechnology has two clear features: its connections with practical applications and interdisciplinary cooperation.

The industrial application of biotechnology will increasingly rest upon each of the contributing disciplines to understand the technical language of the others and, above all, to understand the potential as well as the limitations of the other areas. For instance, for the fermentation bioindustries the traditional education for chemical engineers and industrial plant designers has not normally included biological processes. The nature of the materials required, the reactor vessels (bioreactors) and the operating conditions are so different that complete retraining is required (Fig. 1.2).

Table 1.3	Types of companies involved with biotechnology
Therapeutics	Pharmaceutical products for the cure or control of human diseases, including antibiotics, vaccines, gene therapy.
Diagnostics	Clinical testing and diagnosis, food, environment, agriculture.
Agriculture/Forestry/Horticulture	Novel crops or animal varieties, pesticides.
Food	Wide range of food products, fertilisers, beverages, ingredients.
Environment	Waste treatment, bioremediation, energy production.
Chemical intermediates	Reagents including enzymes, DNA/RNA, speciality chemicals.
Equipment	Hardware, bioreactors, software and consumables supporting biotechnology.

Biotechnology is a demanding industry that requires a skilled workforce and a supportive public to ensure continued growth. Economies that encourage public understanding and provide a competent labour force should achieve long-term benefits from biotechnology. The main types of companies involved with biotechnology can be placed in seven categories (Table 1.3).

A key factor in the distinction between biology and biotechnology is their scale of operation. The biologist usually works in the range between nanograms and milligrams. The biotechnologist working on the production of vaccines may be satisfied with milligram yields, but in many other projects aims are at kilograms or tonnes. Thus, one of the main aspects of biotechnology consists of scaling-up biological processes.

Many present-day biotechnological processes have their origins in ancient and traditional fermentations, such as the brewing of beer and the manufacture of bread, cheese, yoghurt, wine and vinegar. However, it was the discovery of antibiotics in 1929 and their subsequent large-scale production in the 1940s that created the greatest advances in fermentation technology. Since then we have witnessed a phenomenal development in this technology, not only in the production of antibiotics but in many other useful, simple or complex biochemical products, for example organic acids, polysaccharides, enzymes, vaccines, hormones, etc. (Table 1.4). Inherent in the development of fermentation processes is the growing close relationship between the biochemist, the microbiologist and the chemical engineer. Thus, biotechnology is not a sudden discovery but rather a coming of age of a technology that was initiated several decades ago. Looking to the future, the *Economist*, when reporting on this new technology, stated that it may launch 'an industry as characteristic of the twenty-first century as those based on physics and chemistry have been of the twentieth century'.

If it is accepted that biotechnology has its roots in distant history and has large, successful industrial outlets, why then has there been such increased public awareness of this subject in recent years? Undoubtedly, the main dominating reason must derive from the rapid advances in molecular biology, in particular recombinant DNA technology, which are giving humans dominance over nature. By these new techniques (to be discussed in later chapters) it is possible to manipulate directly the heritable material (DNA)

Table 1.4 World markets for biological products in 1981	
Product	Sales (US$ millions)
Alcoholic beverages	23 000
Cheese	14 000
Antibiotics	4500
Penicillins	500
Tetracyclines	500
Cephalosporins	450
Diagnostic tests	2000
Immunoassay	400
Monoclonal	5
Seeds	1400
High fructose syrups	800
Amino acids	750
Baker's yeast	540
Steroids	500
Vitamins, all	330
Vitamin C	200
Vitamin B_{12}	14
Citric acid	210
Enzymes	200
Vaccines	150
Human serum albumin	125
Insulin	100
Urokinase	50
Human factor VIII protein	40
Human growth hormone	35
Microbial pesticides	12

of cells between different types of organisms in vitro creating new hybrid DNA molecules not previously known to exist in nature. The potential of this series of techniques first developed in academic laboratories is now being rapidly exploited in industry, agriculture and medicine. While the benefits are immense, the inherent dangers of tampering with nature must always be appreciated and respected.

While in theory the technology is available to transfer a particular gene from any organism into any other organism, microorganism, plant or animal, in actual practice there are numerous constraining factors, such as which genes are to be cloned and how they can be selected. The single, most limiting factor in the application of genetic engineering is the dearth of basic scientific knowledge of gene structure and function.

The developments of biotechnology are proceeding at a speed similar to that of microelectronics in the mid-1970s. Although the analogy is tempting, any expectations that biotechnology will develop commercially at the same spectacular rate should be tempered with considerable caution. While the potential of 'new' biotechnology cannot be doubted, a meaningful commercial realisation is now only slowly occurring and will accelerate throughout the twenty-first century. New biotechnology will have a considerable impact across all industrial uses of the life sciences. In each case the relative merits of competing means of production will influence the economics of a biotechnological route. Biotechnology will undoubtedly have great benefits in the long term in all sectors and, above all, will save countless lives.

The growth in awareness of modern biotechnology parallels the serious worldwide changes in the economic climate arising from the escalation of oil prices since 1973. There is a growing realisation that fossil fuels (although at present in a production glut period) and other non-renewable resources will one day be in limited supply. This will result in the requirement for cheaper and more secure energy sources and chemical feedstocks, which biotechnology could perhaps fulfil. Countries with climatic conditions suitable for rapid biomass production could well have major economic advantages over less climatically suitable parts of the world. In particular, the tropics must hold high future potential in this respect.

Another contributory factor to the growing interest in biotechnology has been the current recession in the Western world, in particular the depression of the chemical and engineering sections, in part due to the increased energy costs. Biotechnology has been considered as one important means of restimulating the economy, whether on a local, regional, national or even global basis, using new biotechnological methods and new raw materials. In part, the industrial boom of the 1950–1960s was due to cheap oil; while the information technology advances in the 1970s and 1980s resulted from developments in microelectronics. It is quite feasible that the twenty-first century will increasingly be seen as the era of biotechnology. There is undoubtedly a worldwide increase in molecular biological research, the formation of new biotechnological companies, large investments by nations, companies and individuals, and the rapid expansion of databases, information sources and, above all, extensive media coverage.

It is perhaps unfortunate that there has been an over-concentration on the new implications of biotechnology, and less identification of the very large traditional biotechnological industrial bases that already function throughout the world and contribute considerably to most nations' gross national profits. Indeed, many of the innovations in biotechnology will not appear a priori as new products, but rather as improvements to organisms and processes in long-established biotechnological industries, e.g. brewing and antibiotics production.

New applications are likely to be seen earliest in the areas of healthcare and medicine, followed by agriculture and food technology. Exciting new medical treatments and drugs based on biotechnology are appearing with ever-increasing regularity. Prior to 1982, insulin for diabetics was derived from beef and pork pancreases. The gene for human insulin was then isolated and cloned into microorganisms that were then mass-produced by fermentation. This genetically engineered human insulin, identical to the natural human hormone, was the first commercial pharmaceutical product of recombinant DNA technology and now supplies millions of insulin users worldwide with a safe, reliable and unlimited source of this vital hormone. Biotechnology has also made it easier to detect and diagnose human, animal and plant diseases. In clinical diagnosis there are now hundreds of specialised kits available for simple home use or for complex laboratory procedures, such as blood screening.

Over the past decade the generation of biopharmaceutical products has greatly expanded both in numbers and types of products approved by the US Food and Drug Administration (FDA); in 1996 there were 39 products and by 2006 there were well over a hundred on the market. Similarly, there has been a wide adoption of transgenic crops, with world acreage increasing from about 4 million acres in 1996 to over 222 million acres in just over ten years. Biotech revenues in the USA have increased from $15 billion in 1996 to $60 billion by 2004.

Biotechnology will be increasingly required to meet the global population's current and future needs for food products that are safe and nutritious, while also ensuring a continuous improvement in the efficiency of food production. Acceptance of new food products produced using new biotechnology may be greater when consumers can readily see the benefits derived from novel production methods. Biotechnology methods can now improve the nutrition, taste and appearance of plants and various food products, enhance resistance to specific viruses and insect pests, and produce safer herbicides. For food safety, new probes can rapidly detect and accurately identify specific microbial pathogens in food, e.g. *Salmonella*, *Listeria* and fungal toxins such as aflatoxin.

Increasingly, biotechnology will evolve as a powerful and versatile approach that can compete with chemical and physical techniques of reducing energy and material consumption and minimising the generation of waste and emissions. Biotechnology will be a valuable, indeed essential, contribution for achieving industrial sustainability in the future. There is an ever-increasing diversity and scale of raw material consumption and this means that it is becoming urgent to act to minimise the increasing pressures on the environment. Applications in chemical production, fuel and energy production, pollution control and resource recovery will possibly take longer to develop and will depend on changes in the relative economics of currently employed technologies.

The use of biotechnology with respect to the environment could have contrasting effects. On the one hand there would be many positive effects on environmental conservation, e.g. reduced contamination, improved recycling and soil utilisation, while on the other hand, the liberation of genetically modified organisms could generate some potential environmental risks, e.g. natural population displacements, ecological interactions and transfer of undesirable genetic characteristics to other species.

Figure 1.3 shows how the USA is currently applying R&D funding to industrial biotechnology.

Biotechnology-based industries will not be labour intensive, and although they will create valuable new employment the need will be more for brains than muscle. Much of modern biotechnology has been developed and utilised by large companies and corporations. However, many small and medium-sized companies are realising that biotechnology is not a science of the future but provides real benefits to their industry today. In

| Table 1.5 | Some unique features of biotechnology companies |

Technology driven and multidisciplinary: product development can involve molecular biologists, clinical researchers, product sales force.

Must manage regulatory authorities, public perception; issues of health and safety; risk assessment.

Business climate characterised by rapid change and considerable risk – one biotechnology innovation may quickly supersede another.

Biotechnology business growth highly dependent on venture capital – usually needs exceptionally high level of funding before profit sales return.

Fig. 1.3 Distribution of research and development funding in industrial biotechnology in the USA.

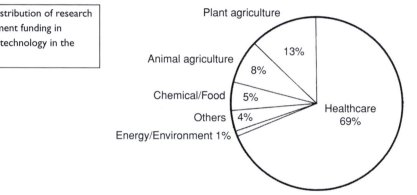

many industries traditional technology can produce compounds causing environmental damage, whereas biotechnology methods can offer a 'green' alternative promoting a positive public image and also avoiding new environmental penalties. Knowledge of biotechnology innovations must be translated through to all sectors of industry.

Many new, high-technology biotech companies have arisen from entrepreneurs from academia who are often dominant, charismatic individuals whose primary aim has been to develop a new technology. New biotechnology companies have certain features not often seen in others (Table 1.5). The position of new biotechnology at the interface between academia and industry creates a unique need for abstracting information from a wide range of sources, and companies spend large sums on information management.

Biotechnology is high-technology par excellence. The most exciting and potentially profitable facets of new biotechnology in the next decade will involve R&D at the very frontiers of current knowledge and techniques. Translating research into application is neither easy nor inevitable and requires a unique investigator and also a unique environment.

In the late 1970s molecular biologists were putting forward vague promises about the wonders of this scientific discipline while the realising technologies were still being developed and were still requiring immense levels of research and product development funding. Biotechnologists now make predictions with more confidence since many of the apparently insurmountable problems have been more easily overcome than had been predicted, and many transitions from laboratory experiments to large-scale industrial processes have been achieved. Truly, new biotechnology has come of age.

For biotechnology to be commercially successful and exploited there is a need both to recruit a specialist workforce and also for the technology to be understood and applied by practitioners in a wide range of other areas including law, patents, medicine, agriculture, engineering, etc. Higher education will supply the range of specialist disciplines encompassing biotechnology, while some courses will endeavour to produce 'biotechnology' graduates who have covered many of the specialist areas at a less rigorous level than the pure degree specialisation. Also many already employed in biotechnology-based industries must regularly have means of updating their knowledge or even retraining. To this end, there are now many books on specific aspects of biotechnology together with software programs. The European-based BIOTOL (Biotechnology by Open Learning) has now produced a wide range of learning programmes. Such programmes are designed not only for the needs of students but also for company training activities and are written in the user-friendly style of good, open-learning materials. The currency of biotechnology throughout the world will be an educated, skilled workforce with ready access to the ever-widening knowledge and resource base. Science has defined the world in which we live and biotechnology, in particular, will become an essential and accepted activity of our culture.

1.4 | Biotechnology: a three-component central core

Many biotechnological processes may be considered as having a three-component central core, in which one part is concerned with obtaining the best biological catalyst for a specific function or process, the second part creates (by construction and technical operation) the best possible environment for the catalyst to perform, and the third part (downstream processing) is concerned with the separation and purification of an essential product or products from a fermentation process.

In the majority of examples developed to date, the most effective, stable and convenient form for the catalyst for a biotechnological process is a whole organism, and it is for this reason that so much of biotechnology revolves around microbial processes. This does not exclude the use of higher organisms; in particular, plant and animal cell culture will play an increasingly important role in biotechnology.

Microorganisms can be viewed both as primary fixers of photosynthetic energy and as systems for bringing about chemical changes in almost all types of natural and synthetic organic molecules. Collectively, they have an immense gene pool, which offers almost unlimited synthetic and degradative potential. Furthermore, microorganisms can possess extremely rapid growth rates far in excess of any of the higher organisms such as plants and animals. Thus immense quantities can be produced under the right environmental conditions in short time periods.

The methodologies that are in general use enable the selection of improved microorganisms from the natural environmental pool, the modification of microorganisms by mutation and, more recently, the mobilisation of a spectacular array of new techniques deriving from molecular biology, which may eventually permit the construction of microorganisms, plants and animals with totally novel biochemical potentials. These new techniques have largely arisen from fundamental achievements in molecular biology over the last two decades.

These manipulated and improved organisms must be maintained in substantially unchanged form and this involves another spectrum of techniques for the preservation of organisms, for retaining essential features during industrial processes and, above all, retaining long-term vigour and viability. In many examples the catalyst is used in a separated and purified form, as enzymes, and a huge amount of information has been built up on the large-scale production, isolation and purification of individual enzymes and on their stabilisation by artificial means.

The second part of the core of biotechnology encompasses all aspects of the containment system or bioreactor within which the catalysts must function (Fig. 1.2). Here the combined specialist knowledge of the bioscientist and bioprocess engineer will interact, providing the design and instrumentation for the maintenance and control of the physico-chemical environment, such as temperature, aeration, pH, etc., thus allowing the optimum expression of the biological properties of the catalyst. Having achieved the required endpoint of the biotechnological process within the bioreactor, e.g. biomass or biochemical product, in most cases it will be necessary to separate the organic products from the predominantly aqueous environment. This third aspect of biotechnology, downstream processing, can be a technically difficult and expensive procedure, and is the least understood area of biotechnology. Downstream processing is primarily concerned with initial separation of the bioreactor broth or medium into a liquid phase and a solids phase, and subsequent concentration and purification of the product. Processing will usually involve more than one stage. Downstream processing costs (as approximate proportions of selling prices) of fermentation products vary considerably, e.g. for yeast biomass, penicillin G and certain enzymes processing costs as percentages of selling price are 20%, 20–30% and 60–70% respectively.

Successful involvement in a biotechnological process must draw heavily upon more than one of the input disciplines. The main areas of application of biotechnology are shown in Table 1.6, while Fig. 1.4 attempts to show how the many disciplines input into the biotechnological processes together with the differing enabling technologies.

Biotechnology will continue to create exciting new opportunities for commercial development and profits in a wide range of industrial sectors including health care and medicine, agriculture and forestry, fine and bulk chemicals production, food technology, fuel and energy production,

Table 1.6	The main areas of application of biotechnology

Bioprocess technology
Historically, the most important area of biotechnology (brewing, antibiotics, mammalian cell culture, etc.), extensive development in progress with new products envisaged (polysaccharides, medically important drugs, solvents, protein-enhanced foods). Novel fermenter designs to optimise productivity.

Enzyme technology
Used for the catalysis of extremely specific chemical reactions; immobilisation of enzymes; to create specific molecular converters (bioreactors). Products formed include L-amino acids, high fructose syrup, semi-synthetic penicillins, starch and cellulose hydrolysis, etc. Enzyme probes for bioassays.

Waste technology
Long historical importance but more emphasis is now being placed on coupling these processes with the conservation and recycling of resources; foods and fertilizers, biological fuels.

Environmental technology
Great scope exists for the application of biotechnological concepts for solving many environmental problems (pollution control, removing toxic wastes); recovery of metals from mining wastes and low-grade ores.

Renewable resources technology
The use of renewable energy sources, in particular lignocellulose, to generate new sources of chemical raw materials and energy – ethanol, methane and hydrogen. Total utilisation of plant and animal material. Clean technology, sustainable technology.

Plant and animal agriculture
Genetically engineered plants to improve nutrition, disease resistance, maintain quality, and improve yields and stress tolerance will become increasingly commercially available. Improved productivity etc. for animal farming. Improved food quality, flavour, taste and microbial safety.

Healthcare
New drugs and better treatment for delivering medicines to diseased parts. Improved disease diagnosis, understanding of the human genome – genomics and proteomics, information technology.

pollution control and resource recovery. Biotechnology offers a great deal of hope for solving many of the problems that the world faces!

1.5 | Product safety

In biotechnology, governmental regulations will represent a critical determinant of the time and total costs in bringing a product to market. Regulatory agencies can act as 'gate-keepers' for the development and availability of new biotechnology products, but can also erect considerable barriers to industrial development. In practice, such barriers come from the costs of testing products to meet regulatory standards, possible delays and uncertainties in regulatory approval, and even outright disapproval of new products on grounds of safety. The very considerable costs that may be required to ensure product safety can often discourage new research or curtail product development if a future new product is not likely to have a high financial

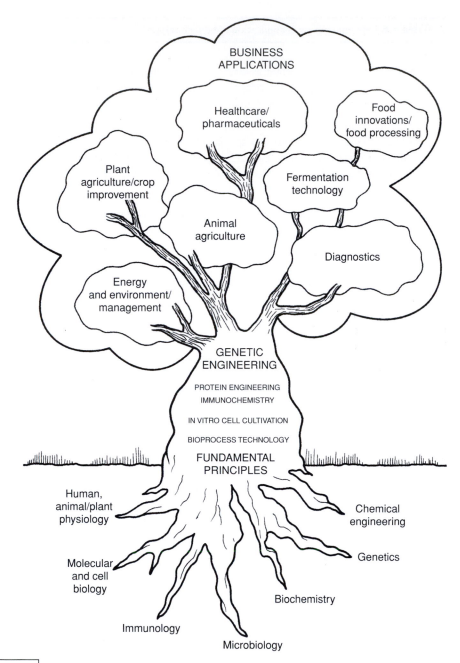

Fig. 1.4 The biotechnology tree.

market return. Concern has been expressed in the USA that over-zealous and perhaps unrealistic regulatory requirements are damaging the future industrial development of some areas of biotechnology and, consequently, they are systematically reassessing their regulatory requirements. The use of recombinant DNA technology has created the greatest areas of possible safety concern. Public attitudes to biotechnology are most often related to matters of perceived or imaginary dangers in the techniques of genetic manipulation.

1.6 | Public perception of biotechnology

While biotechnology presents enormous potential for healthcare and the production, processing and quality of foods through genetic engineering of crops, fertilisers, pesticides, vaccines and various animal and fish species, the implications of these new biotechnological processes go well beyond the technical benefits offered. The implementation of the new techniques will be dependent upon their acceptance by consumers. As stated in the Advisory Committee on Science and Technology (1990) report *Developments in Biotechnology*: 'Public perception of biotechnology will have a major influence on the rate and direction of developments and there is growing concern about genetically modified products. Associated with genetic manipulation are diverse questions of safety, ethics and welfare.'

Public debate is essential for new biotechnology to grow up, and undoubtedly for the foreseeable future biotechnology will be under scrutiny. Public understanding of these new technologies could well hasten public acceptance. However, the low level of scientific literacy (e.g. in the USA where only 7% are scientifically literate) does mean that most of the public will not be able to draw informed conclusions about important biotechnology issues. Consequently, it is conceivable (and indeed the case) that a small number of activists might argue the case against genetic engineering in such emotive and ill-reasoned ways that both the public and the politicians are misled. The biotechnology community needs to sit up and take notice of, and work with, the public. People influence decision-making by governments through the ballot box or through the presence of public opinion.

Until quite recently most biotechnology companies concentrated almost exclusively on raising financial support, research, clinical trials (if relevant), manufacturing problems and regulatory hurdles. Most companies, however, neglected certain essential marketing questions such as, who will be buying the new products and what do these people need to understand? These companies have, by and large, failed to appreciate the general public's inability to understand the basic scientific concepts involved in new biotechnology. They must now seriously invest resources to foster a better understanding of the scientific implications of new biotechnology, especially among the new generation. What biotechnology needs with the public is dialogue! To ignore public understanding will be to the industry's peril!

Ultimately, the benefits of biotechnology will speak for themselves as will be seen in the following chapters.

1.7 | Biotechnology and the developing world

Successful agriculture holds the answer to the poverty gap between the rich and poor nations. In the developed world agricultural sciences are well developed producing an abundance of high-quality products. Agricultural

Table 1.7 Top eight biotechnologies to improve health in developing countries

Molecular diagnostics
Recombinant vaccines
Sequencing pathogen genomes
Female-controlled protection against sexually transmitted diseases
Bioremediation
Bioinformatics
Nutritionally enhanced genetically modified crops
Recombinant therapeutic proteins

Source: after Acharya *et al.* (2003) *Nature Biotechnology*, **21**, 1434–6.

biotechnology will further improve quality, variety and yield. Will these new plant species, improved by genetic engineering, find their way to the developing countries ensuring higher productivity, greater resistance to disease and be more marketable? It is not yet clear what will happen other than that the affluent nations will become increasingly well endowed with an abundance of food. Worldwide there will be enough food for all, but will it always continue to be disproportionately distributed? Biotechnology developments need high inputs in terms of finance and a skilled workforce – both of which are in short supply in most developing nations. Sadly, there is a growing gap between biotechnology in highly industrialised countries and the biotechnology-based needs of developing countries.

While many developing nations have successfully collaborated in the past with Western biotechnology companies, it is salutary to note that between 1986 and 1991 the percentage of arrangements implemented by US biotechnology companies with developing countries dropped from 20% to 3%! The ability of developing nations to avail themselves of the many promises of new biotechnology will to a large extent depend on their capacity to integrate modern developments of biotechnology within their own research and innovation systems, in accordance with their own needs and priorities.

The United Nations Millenium Development Goal for 2015 has targeted poverty alleviation, improved education and health, together with environmental sustainability. The main areas of biotechnology that can contribute to these aims are listed in Table 1.7. In the following chapters some of the most important areas of biotechnology are considered with a view to achieving a broad overall understanding of the existing achievements and future aims of this new area of technology. However, it must be appreciated that biotechnological development will not only depend on scientific and technological advances, but will also be subject to considerable political, economic and, above all, public acceptance. Finally, it has been said that most scientific disciplines pass through golden ages when new approaches open the door to rapid and fundamental expansion. Biotechnology is just now entering this golden period. A spectacular future lies ahead.

Chapter 2

Biomass: a biotechnology substrate?

2.1 | A biomass strategy

It has been estimated that the annual net yield of plant biomass arising from photosynthesis is at least 120 billion tonnes of dry matter on land and around 50 billion tonnes from the world's oceans. Of the land-produced biomass, approximately 50% occurs in the complex form of lignocellulose.

The highest proportion of land-based biomass (44%) is produced as forest (Table 2.1). It is surprising to note that while agricultural crops account for only 6% of the primary photosynthetic productivity, from this amount is derived a major portion of food for humans and animals as well as many essential structural materials, textiles and paper products (Table 2.2). Many traditional agricultural products may well be further exploited with the increasing awareness of biotechnology. In particular, new technological approaches will undoubtedly be able to utilise the large volume of waste material from conventional food processing that presently finds little use.

Biomass agriculture, aquaculture and forestry may hold great economic potential for many national economies particularly in tropical and subtropical regions (Fig. 2.1). Indeed, the development of biotechnological processes in developing areas where plant growth excels could well bring about a change in the balance of economic power.

It should be noted that the non-renewable energy and petrochemical feedstocks on which modern society is so dependent (oil, gas and coal) were derived from ancient types of biomass. Modern industrialised nations have come to rely heavily on fossil reserves for both energy and as feedstocks for a wide range of production processes. In little over a century the industrialised world has drawn heavily on fossil fuels that took millions of years to form beneath the beds of the oceans or in the depths of the earth. Furthermore, it is a very unequal pattern of usage. At present, the USA with 6% and Western Europe with 8% of the world's population use 35% and 25% respectively of the world's oil and gas production.

While coal stocks may last for many hundreds of years this is not true for oil and gas, and at current usage levels the world's known available sources of oil and gas will have been almost fully exploited by the end of

Table 2.1 | Breakdown of world primary productivity

	Net productivity (% of total)
Forests and woodlands	44.3
Grassland	9.7
Cultivated land	5.9
Desert and semi-desert	1.5
Freshwater	3.2
Oceans	35.4

Table 2.2 | Approximate annual world production of some agricultural and forestry products

Sector	Product	Tonnes	Value in US$ billion
Food and feed	Cereals (including milled rice)	1.8 billion	250
	Sugar (cane and beet)	120 million	–
	Fish	85 million	17
	Crude starch	1.0 billion	–
	Refined starch	20 million	–
Materials	Potential wood	13 billion	–
	Harvested wood	1.6 billion	–
	Fuel wood	–	100
	Saw wood	–	60
	Panels	–	35
	Paper	–	110
Chemicals	Oils and fats	70 million	–
	Soybean oil	17 million	8
	Palm oil	10 million	3
	Sunflower oil	8 million	4
	Rape seed oil	8 million	3
	Starch	2 million	–
	Natural pulses	4 million	4
Other	Cut flowers and bulbs	–	10
	Tobacco	4 million	15

Source: OECD (1992), *Biotechnology, Agriculture and Food.*

Fig. 2.1 The distribution of world forestry resources.

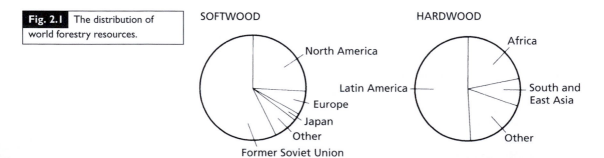

SOFTWOOD — North America, Latin America, Europe, Japan, Other, Former Soviet Union

HARDWOOD — Africa, South and East Asia, Other

Table 2.3	Important products derived from biomass
Fuels	Methane (biogas) especially in the developing world
	Pyrolysis products (gas, charcoal)
	Ethanol (via cane juice and cellulose fermentation)
	Oils (from hydrogenation)
	Direct combustion of waste biomass
Feedstocks	Ethanol (potential feedstock for industry)
	Synthesis gas (from chemical gasification)
Fertilisers	Compost
	Sludge
Feeds	Direct feed supplements
	Single-cell proteins

this century. The answer to these problems must be the use of photosynthetically derived biomass for energy and industrial feedstocks. Currently more than ten times more energy is generated annually by photosynthesis than is consumed by mankind. At present, large-scale exploitation of biomass for fuel and chemical feedstocks is restricted by the cost of fossil alternatives, the heterogeneous nature of biomass sources and their diffuse distribution.

The use of biomass directly as a source of energy has long been practised in the less industrialised nations such as Latin America, China, India and Africa. In developed nations, biomass derived from agriculture and forestry has largely been directed to industrial and food uses (Table 2.3).

At present biomass is used to derive many products of industrial and commercial importance (Table 2.3), and those involving biotechnology will be highlighted and expanded on in subsequent chapters.

2.2 | Natural raw materials

Natural raw materials originate mostly from agriculture and forestry. These are mainly carbohydrates of varying chemical complexity, and include sugar, starch, cellulose, hemicellulose and lignin. The wide range of by-products obtained from raw materials that are of use in biotechnological processes is shown in Table 2.4.

Sugar-bearing raw materials such as sugar beet, sugar cane and sugar millet are the most suitable and available to serve as feedstocks for biotechnological processing. As traditional uses of sugar are replaced by more efficient alternatives, the sugar surplus on the commodity market will give further incentive to develop new uses. Many tropical economies would collapse if the markets for sugar were to be removed. Already cane sugar serves as the substrate for the Brazilian gasohol programme, and many other nations are rapidly seeing the immense potential of these new technologies.

Table 2.4	A range of by-products that could be used as substrates in biotechnology
Agriculture	Forestry	Industry
Straw	Wood waste hydrolysate	Molasses
Bagasse	Sulphite pulp liquor	Distillery wastes
Maize cobs	Bark, sawdust, branches	Whey
Coffee, cocoa and coconut hulls	Paper and cellulose	Industrial waste water from food
Fruit peels and leaves	fibres	industries (olive, palm-oil, potato,
Tea wastes		date, citrus, cassava)
Oilseed cakes		Wash waters (dairy, canning,
Cotton wastes		confectionery, bakery, soft drinks,
Bran		sizing, malting, corn steep)
Pulp (tomato, coffee, banana,		Fishery effluent and wastes
pineapple, citrus, olive)		Meat by-products
Animal wastes		Municipal garbage
		Sewage
		Abattoir wastes

Starch-bearing agricultural products include the various types of grain such as maize, rice and wheat, together with potatoes and other root crops such as sweet potato and cassava. A slight disadvantage of starch is that it must usually be degraded to monosaccharides or oligosaccharides by digestion or hydrolysis before fermentation. However, many biotechnological processes using starch are being developed, including fuel production.

There can be little doubt that cellulose, both from agriculture and forestry sources, must contribute a major source of feedstock for biotechnological processes such as fuels and chemicals. However, cellulose is a very complex chemical and invariably occurs in nature in close association with lignin. The ability of lignocellulose complexes to withstand the biodegradative forces of nature is witnessed by the longevity of trees, which are mainly composed of lignocellulose.

Lignocellulose is the most abundant and renewable natural resource available to man throughout the world. However, massive technological difficulties must be overcome before economic use may be made of this plentiful compound. At present, expensive energy-demanding pre-treatment processes are required to open up this complex structure to wide microbial degradation. Pure cellulose can be degraded by chemical or enzymatic hydrolysis to soluble sugars, which can be fermented to form ethanol, butanol, acetone, single cell protein (SCP), methane and many other products. Exciting advances are being made in laboratories throughout the world, and it is only a matter of time before these difficulties are overcome. It has been realistically calculated that approximately 3.3×10^{14} kg of CO_2 per year are fixed on the surface of the Earth, and that approximately 6% of this, i.e. 22 billion tonnes per year, will be cellulose. On a worldwide basis land plants produce 24 tonnes of cellulose per person per year. Time will surely show that lignocellulose will be the most useful carbon source for biotechnological developments.

2.3 | Availability of by-products

While biotechnological processes will use many agricultural products (such as sugars, starches, oils, etc.) as substrates, the vast array of waste products derived from agriculture, and currently not creatively used, will undoubtedly be subjected to detailed examination and future utilisation. Agricultural and forestry wastes come in many diverse types: cereal straws, corn husks and cobs, soy wastes, coconut shells, rice husks, coffee bean husks, wheat bran, sugar cane bagasse and forestry wastes including trimmings, sawdust, bark, etc. (Table 2.4). Only a modest fraction of these wastes is utilised on a large scale due primarily to economic and logistical factors.

A primary objective of biotechnology is to improve the management and utilisation of the vast volumes of agricultural, industrial and domestic waste organic materials to be found throughout the world. The biotechnological utilisation of these wastes will eliminate a source of pollution, in particular water pollution, and convert some of these wastes into useful by-products.

Not all processes will involve biosystems. In particular, the processes of reverse osmosis and ultrafiltration are finding increasing uses. Reverse osmosis is a method of concentrating liquid solutions in which a porous membrane allows water to pass through but not the salts dissolved in it. Ultrafiltration is a method of separating the high and low molecular weight compounds in a liquid by allowing the liquid and low molecular weight compounds to pass through while holding back the high molecular weight compounds and suspended solids. Some current applications of these technologies include concentration of dilute factory effluents, concentration of dilute food products, sterilisation of water, purification of brackish water and separation of edible solids from dilute effluents.

Waste materials are frequently important for economic and environmental reasons. For example, many by-products of the food industry are of low economic value and are often discharged into waterways, creating serious environmental pollution problems. An attractive feature of carbohydrate waste as a raw material is that, if its low cost can be coupled with suitable low handling costs, an economic process may be obtained. Furthermore, the worldwide trend towards stricter effluent control measures, or the parallel increase in effluent disposal charges, can lead to the concept of waste as a 'negative cost' raw material. However, the composition or dilution of the waste may be so dispersed that transport to a production centre may be prohibitive. On these occasions biotechnology may only serve to reduce a pollution hazard.

Each waste material must be assessed for its suitability for biotechnological processing. Only when a waste is available in large quantities and preferably over a prolonged period of time can a suitable method of utilisation be considered (Table 2.5).

Two widely occurring wastes that already find considerable fermentation uses are molasses and whey. Molasses is a by-product of the sugar industry and has a sugar content of approximately 50%. Molasses is widely used as a fermentation feedstock for the production of antibiotics, organic

Table 2.5	Biotechnological strategies for utilisation of suitable organic waste materials

1. Upgrade the food-waste quality to make it suitable for human consumption.
2. Feed the food waste directly or after processing to poultry, pigs, fish or other single-stomach animals that can utilise it directly.
3. Feed the food waste to cattle, or other ruminants, if unsuitable for single-stomach animals because of high fibre content, toxins or other reasons.
4. Production of biogas (methane) and other fermentation products if unsuitable for feeding without expensive pre-treatments.
5. Selective other purposes such as direct use as fuel, building materials, chemical extraction, etc.

Table 2.6	Pre-treatments required before substrates are suitable for fermentation	

Substrate	Pre-treatment
Sugary materials Sugar cane, beet, molasses, fruit juices, whey	Minimal requirements are dilution and sterilisation
Starchy materials Cereals, rice, vegetables, process-liquid wastes	Some measure of hydrolysis by acid or enzymes. Initial separation of non-starch components may be required
Lignocellulosic materials Corn cobs, oat hulls, straw, bagasse, wood wastes, sulphite liquor, paper wastes	Normally requires complex pre-treatment involving reduction in particle size followed by various chemical or enzymic hydrolyses. Energy intensive and costly

acids and commercial yeasts for baking, and is directly used in animal feeding. Whey, obtained during the production of cheese, could also become a major fermentation feedstock.

More complex wastes such as straw and bagasse are widely available and will be increasingly used as improved processes for lignocellulose breakdown become available (Table 2.6). Wood wastes will include low-grade wood, bark and sawdust, as well as waste liquors such as sulphite waste liquor from pulp production, which already finds considerable biotechnological processing in Europe and former Communist bloc countries.

The largest proportion of the total volume of waste matter is from animal rearing (faeces, urine), followed by agricultural wastes, wastes from the food industries and finally domestic wastes. The disposal of many waste materials, particularly animal wastes, is no problem in traditional agriculture and is particularly well exemplified in China where recycling by composting has long been practised. However, where intensive animal rearing is undertaken, serious pollution problems do arise.

Future biotechnological processes will increasingly make use of organic materials that are renewable in nature or occur as low-value wastes that may presently cause environmental pollution. Table 2.7 summarises the many technical considerations that must be made when approaching the

Table 2.7	Technical considerations for the utilisation of waste materials
Biological availability	low (cellulosics)
	moderate (starch, lactose)
	high (molasses, pulping sugars)
Concentration	solid (milling residues, garbage)
	concentrated (molasses)
	weak (lactose, pulping sugars)
	very dilute (process and plant-wash liquors)
Quality	clean (molasses, lactose)
	moderate (straw)
	dirty (garbage, feedlot waste)
Location	collected (large installation, small centres)
	collected specialised (olive, palm-oil, date, rubber, fruit, vegetable)
	dispersed (straw, forestry)
Seasonally	prolonged (palm-oil, lactose)
	very short (vegetable-cannery waste)
Alternative uses	some (straw)
	none (garbage)
	negative (costly effluents)
Local technology potential	high (USA)
	middle (Brazil)
	low (Malaysia)

utilisation of waste materials. Some processes may also more economically utilise specific fractions of fossil fuels as feedstocks for biotechnological processes.

In the 1960s there was a worldwide glut of chemical and petrochemical feedstocks and alternative uses were being actively pursued. At this time also there was concern that there would be a worldwide shortage of protein. The energy companies producing these excess feedstocks were then drawn into the concept of using them as fermentation substrates to produce bacterial protein – single-cell protein or SCP. The main commercial interest was concerned with n-paraffins, methanol and ethanol, which were available in large quantities in many parts of the world. While massive fermentation programmes were initiated and operated in the developed nations (e.g. Europe, USA and Russia) full commercialisation was never achieved, due in part to the change in oil prices in the 1970s and to the lack of appearance of a worldwide protein shortage.

2.4 | Raw materials and the future of biotechnology

It is now clear that the future development of large-scale biotechnological processes is inseparable from the supply and cost of raw materials. During the early and middle parts of the last century the availability of cheap oil

Table 2.8 Prices of available raw materials for biotechnological processes

Substrate	Mid-1984 US price (US$ per tonne)	Carbon content (mol C per mol substrate)	Carbon content relative to glucose (%)	Corrected price relative to glucose (US$ per tonne)[a]
Corn starch	70–100[b]	0.44	100	64–91
Glucose	290[c]	0.4	100	290
Sucrose (raw)	140[d]	0.42	105	133
Sucrose (refined)	660[e]	0.42	105	140
Molasses	79	0.2[f]	50	140
Acetic acid	550	0.4	100	550
Ethanol	560	0.52	130	430
Methane	n.a.	0.75	188	–
Corn oil (crude)	330	0.8	200	165
Palm-oil	600	0.8	200	300
n-alkanes (n-hexadecane)	n.a.	0.87	218	–

n.a. Not available

[a] Assumes equivalent conversion efficiencies can be obtained.
[b] Approximate guessed price in a wet-milling operation.
[c] Glucose syrups on a dry-weight basis.
[d] Daily spot price.
[e] US price fixed by government tariffs.
[f] On the basis of molasses being 48% by weight fermentable sugars.
Source: Hacking (1986)

led to an explosive development of the petrochemical industry, and many products formerly derived from the fermentation ability of microorganisms were superseded by the cheaper and more efficient chemical methods. However, escalating oil prices in the 1970s created profound reappraisals of these processes, and as the price of crude oil approached that of some major cereal products there was a reawakening of interest in many fermentation processes for the production of ethanol and related products. However, the decrease in oil prices in 1986 again widened the gap and left uncertainty in the minds of industrial planners. However, once again, oil prices have escalated and it is doubtful if they will ever again decrease. Oil has a finite longevity.

The most important criteria that will determine the selection of a raw material for a biotechnological process will include price, availability, composition, form and oxidation state of the carbon source. Table 2.8 gives interesting details on the mid-1984 prices of existing and potential raw materials of biotechnological interest. At present the most widely used and of commercial value are corn starch, molasses and raw sugar.

There is little doubt that cereal crops, particularly maize, rice and wheat, will be the main short- and medium-term raw materials for biotechnological processes. It is hoped that this can be achieved without seriously disturbing human and animal food supplies. Throughout the world there is an uneven distribution of cereal production capacity and demand. Overproduction of cereals occurs mostly where extensive biotechnological processes are in practice. Areas of poor cereal production will undoubtedly benefit from the developments in agricultural biotechnology now at an early, but highly optimistic, stage.

Although much attention has been given to the uses of wastes in biotechnology there are many major obstacles to be overcome. For instance, availability of agricultural wastes is seasonal and geographical availability problematic; they are also often dilute and may contain toxic wastes. However, their build-up in the environment can present serious pollution problems and therefore their utilisation in biotechnological processes, albeit at little economic gain, can have overall community value.

Although in the long term biotechnology must seek to utilise the components of cellulose and lignocelluloses as fuels or feedstocks, the technological difficulties are still considerable. The chemical complexities of these molecules is legend and it is proving more difficult than had been expected to economically break them down to usable primary molecules.

Biotechnology will have profound effects on agriculture and forestry by enabling production costs to be decreased, quality and consistency of products to be increased, and novel products generated.

Wood is extensively harvested to provide fuel, materials for construction and to supply pulp for paper manufacture. Supplies throughout the world are rapidly decreasing resulting in extensive examples of deforestation: deforestation can often then be followed by desertification and soil erosion. Selective breeding programmes are now producing 'elite' fast-growing hardwood trees, such as eucalyptus and acacia, derived from genetic manipulation programmes coupled with new methods of macro- and micropropagation. Such fast-growing trees could even be used for electricity generation, giving less net overall carbon dioxide production than the use of fossil fuels and so minimising any potential 'greenhouse' effect.

There may also be an increased non-food use of many agriculturally derived substances such as sugars, starches, oils and fats. Biotechnology will significantly aid their overall production by improved plant growth; influence biosynthetic pathways to change production; change the chemical structure of molecules; and improve processing by enzyme technology. The ability of biotechnology to improve disease resistance, quality composition and in some cases to grow crops in marginal lands could surely lead to higher yields of products, and in developing economies this could have profound beneficial effects. Supplies in excess of food needs could allow new industries to develop and reduce poverty.

Cotton is a major agricultural crop in many developing nations and is a major natural textile fibre, with world production exceeding that of synthetic textile fibres. It is not well recognised that cotton accounts for about 10% of the world's annual use of agrochemicals, mainly insecticides. Development of disease-resistant cotton plants by new molecular methods could have major economical and environmental impact. Major yield increases would have considerable benefits to the producing nations.

How successful will biomass be as a crucial raw material for biotechnology? An Organisation for Economic Co-operation and Development (OECD) report (1992) set out the factors that will determine the competitiveness of natural (biomass) and synthetic (fossil biomass) derived products:

(1) the relative price of the basic raw materials
(2) quality, variability, regularity of supply and safety of the raw materials
(3) relative costs of chemical base material conversion compared to conversion of agricultural products
(4) premium accorded by the market to 'natural' as compared to synthetic products and increasing requirement for products to be biodegradable.

Chapter 3

Genetics and biotechnology

3.1 | Introduction

In essence, all properties of organisms depend on the sum of their genes. There are two broad categories of genes – structural and regulatory. Structural genes encode for amino acid sequences of proteins, which, as enzymes, determine the biochemical capabilities of the organism by catalysing particular synthetic or catabolic reactions or, alternatively, play more static roles as components of cellular structures. In contrast, the regulatory genes control the expression of the structural genes by determining the rate of production of their protein products in response to intra- or extracellular signals. The derivation of these principles has been achieved using well known genetic techniques, which will not be considered further here.

The seminal studies of Watson and Crick and others in the early 1950s led to the construction of the double-helix model depicting the molecular structure of DNA, and subsequent hypotheses on its implications for the understanding of gene replication. Since then there has been a spectacular unravelling of the complex interactions required to express the coded chemical information of the DNA molecule into cellular and organismal expression. Changes in the DNA molecule making up the genetic complement of an organism are the means by which organisms evolve and adapt themselves to new environments. The precise role of DNA is to act as a reservoir of genetic information. In nature, changes in the DNA of an organism can occur in two ways:

(1) by *mutation*, which is a chemical deletion or addition of one or more of the chemical parts of the DNA molecule

(2) by the interchange of genetic information or DNA between like organisms normally by *sexual reproduction*, and by *horizontal transfer* in bacteria. In eukaryotes, sexual reproduction is achieved by a process of conjugation in which there is a donor, called male, and a recipient, called female. Often these are determined physiologically and not morphologically. Bacterial conjugation involves the transfer of DNA from a donor to a recipient cell. The transferred DNA (normally plasmid DNA) is always in a single-stranded form and the complementary strand is synthesised in the recipient. *Transduction* is the transfer of DNA mediated by a bacterial virus (*bacteriophage* or *phage*) and cells that have received transducing DNA are referred to as *transductants*. *Transformation* involves the uptake of isolated DNA or DNA present in the organism's environment into a recipient cell, which is then referred to as a *transformant*. Genetic transfer by this way in bacteria is a natural characteristic of a wide variety of bacterial genera such a *Campylobacter, Neisseria* and *Streptomyces*. Strains of bacteria not naturally transformable can be induced to take up isolated DNA by chemical treatment or by *electroporation*.

Classical genetics was, until recently, the only way in which heredity could be studied and manipulated. However, in recent years, new techniques have permitted unprecedented alterations in the genetic make-up of organisms even allowing exchange in the laboratory of DNA between unlike organisms.

The manipulation of the genetic material in organisms can now be achieved in three clearly definable ways – organismal, cellular and molecular.

Organismal manipulation

Genetic manipulation of whole organisms has been happening naturally by sexual reproduction since the beginning of time. The evolutionary progress of almost all living creatures has involved active interaction between their genomes and the environment. Active control of sexual reproduction has been practised in agriculture for decades – even centuries. In more recent times it has been used with several industrial microorganisms, e.g. brewing yeasts. It involves selection, mutation, sexual crosses, hybridisation, etc. However, it is a very random process and can take a long time to achieve desired results – if at all in some cases. In agriculture, the benefits have been immense with much improved plants and animals, while in the biotechnological industries there have been greatly improved productivities, e.g. antibiotics and enzymes.

Cellular manipulation

Cellular manipulations of DNA have been used for over two decades, and involve either cell fusion or the culture of cells and the regeneration of whole plants from these cells. This is a semi-random or directed process in contrast to organismal manipulations, and the changes can be more readily identified. Successful biotechnological examples of these methods include monoclonal antibodies (see later) and the cloning of many important plant species.

Molecular manipulation

Molecular manipulations of DNA and RNA first occurred over two decades ago and heralded a new era of genetic manipulations enabling – for the first time in biological history – a directed control of the changes. This is the much publicised area of *genetic engineering* or *recombinant DNA technology*, which is now bringing dramatic changes to biotechnology. In these techniques the experimenter is able to know much more about the genetic changes being made. It is now possible to add or delete parts of the DNA molecule with a high degree of precision, and the products can be easily identified. Current industrial ventures are concerned with the production of new types of organism, and of numerous compounds ranging from pharmaceuticals to commodity chemicals; these are discussed in more detail in later chapters.

3.2 | Industrial genetics

Biotechnology has so far been considered as an interplay between two components, one of which is the selection of the best biocatalyst for a particular process, while the other is the construction and operation of the best environment for the catalyst to achieve optimum operation.

The most effective, stable and convenient form for the biocatalyst is a whole organism; in most cases it is some type of microbe, for example a bacterium, yeast or mould, although mammalian cell cultures and (to a lesser extent) plant cell cultures are finding ever-increasing uses in biotechnology.

Most microorganisms used in current biotechnological processes were originally isolated from the natural environment, and have subsequently been modified by the industrial geneticist into superior organisms for specific productivity. The success of strain selection and improvement programmes practised by all biologically based industries (e.g. brewing, antibiotics, etc.) is a direct result of the close cooperation between the technologist and the geneticist. In the future, this relationship will be even more necessary in formulating the specific physiological and biochemical characteristics that are sought in new organisms in order to give the fullest range of biological activities to biotechnology.

In biotechnological processes, the aim is primarily to optimise the particular characteristics sought in an organism, for example specific enzyme production or by-product formation. Genetic modification to improve productivity has been widely practised. The task of improving yields of some primary metabolites and macromolecules (e.g. enzymes) is simpler than trying to improve the yields of complex products such as antibiotics. Advances have been achieved in this area by using *screening* and *selection* techniques to obtain better organisms. In a selection system all rare or novel strains grow while the rest do not; in a screening system all strains grow, but certain strains or cultures are chosen because they show the desired qualities required by the industry in question.

In most industrial genetics the basis for changing the organism's genome has been by mutation using X-rays and mutagenic chemicals. However, such methods normally lead only to the loss of undesired characteristics or increased production due to loss of control functions. It has rarely led to the appearance of a new function or property. Thus, an organism with a desired feature will be selected from the natural environment, propagated and subjected to a mutational programme, then screened to select the best progeny.

Unfortunately, many of the microorganisms that have gained industrial importance do not have a clearly defined sexual cycle. In particular, this has been the case in antibiotic-producing microorganisms; this has meant that the only way to change the genome with a view to enhancing productivity has been to indulge in massive mutational programmes followed by screening and selection to detect the new variants that might arise.

Once a high-producing strain has been found, great care is required in maintaining the strain. Undesired spontaneous mutations can sometimes occur at a high rate, giving rise to degeneration of the strain's industrial importance. Strain or culture instability is a constant problem in industrial utilisation of microorganisms and mammalian cells. Industry has always placed great emphasis on strain viability and productivity potential of the preserved biological material. Most industrially important microorganisms can be stored for long periods, for example in liquid nitrogen, by lyophilisation (freeze-drying) or under oil, and still retain their desired biological properties.

However, despite elaborate preservation and propagation methods, a strain has generally to be grown in a large production bioreactor in which the chances of genetic changes through spontaneous mutation and selection are very high. The chance of a high rate of spontaneous mutation is probably greater when the industrial strains in use have resulted from many years of mutagen treatment. Great secrecy surrounds the use of industrial microorganisms and immense care is taken to ensure that they do not unwittingly pass to outside agencies.

There is now a growing movement away from the extreme empiricism that characterised the early days of the fermentation industries. Fundamental studies of the genetics of microorganisms now provide a background of knowledge for the experimental solution of industrial problems, and increasingly contribute to progress in industrial strain selection.

In recent years, industrial genetics has come to depend increasingly on two new ways of manipulating DNA – protoplast and cell fusion, and recombinant DNA technology. These are now important additions to the technical repertoire of the geneticists involved with biotechnological industries. A brief examination of these techniques will attempt to show their increasingly indispensable relevance to modern biotechnology.

3.3 | Protoplast and cell fusion technologies

Plants and most microbial cells are characterised by a distinct outer wall or exoskeleton, which gives the shape characteristic to the cell or organism. Immediately within the cell wall is the living membrane, or plasma membrane, retaining all the cellular components such as nuclei, mitochondria, vesicles, etc. For some years now it has been possible, using special techniques (in particular, hydrolytic enzymes), to remove the cell wall, releasing spherical membrane-bound structures known as *protoplasts*. These protoplasts are extremely fragile but can be maintained in isolation for variable periods of time. Isolated protoplasts cannot propagate themselves as such, requiring first to regenerate a cell wall before regaining reproductive capacity.

In practice, it is the cell wall that largely hinders the sexual conjugation of unlike organisms. Only with completely sexually compatible strains does the wall degenerate allowing protoplasmic interchange. Thus natural sexual-mating barriers in microorganisms may, in part, be due to cell wall limitations, and by removing this cell wall, the likelihood of cellular fusions may increase.

Protoplasts can be obtained routinely from many plant species, bacteria, yeasts and filamentous fungi. Protoplasts from different strains can sometimes be persuaded to fuse and so overcome the natural sexual-mating barriers. However, the range of protoplast fusions is severely limited by the need for DNA compatibility between the strains concerned. Fusion of protoplasts can be enhanced by treatment with the chemical polyethylene glycol, which, under optimum conditions, can lead to extremely high frequencies of recombinant formation that can be increased still further by ultraviolet irradiation of the parental protoplast preparations. Protoplast fusion can also occur with human or animal cell types.

Protoplast fusion has obvious empirical applications in yield improvement of antibiotics by combining yield-enhancing mutations from different strains or even species. Protoplasts will also be an important part of genetic engineering, in facilitating recombinant DNA transfer. Fusion may provide a method of re-assorting whole groups of genes between different strains of macro- and microorganisms.

One of the most exciting and commercially rewarding areas of biotechnology involves a form of mammalian cell fusion leading to the formation of monoclonal antibodies. It has long been recognised that certain cells (B-lymphocytes) within the bodies of vertebrates have the ability to secrete antibodies that can inactivate contaminating or foreign molecules (the antigen) within the animal system. The antibody has a Y-shaped molecular structure and uses one part of this structure to bind the invading antigen and the other part to trigger the body's response to eliminate the antigen/antibody complex. It has been calculated that a mammalian species can generate up to 100 million different antibodies thereby ensuring that most invading foreign antigens will be bound by some antibody. Antibodies have high binding affinities and specificity against the chosen antigen. For the mammalian system they are the major defence against disease-causing organisms and other toxic molecules.

Attempts to cultivate the antibody-producing cells in artificial media have generally proved unsuccessful, with the cells either dying or ceasing to produce the antibodies. It is now known that individual B-lymphocyte cells produce single antibody types. However, in 1975 George Kohler and Cesar Milstein successfully demonstrated the production of pure or *monoclonal antibodies* from the fusion product (*hybridoma*) of B-lymphocytes (antibody-producing cells) and myeloma tumour cells. In 1984 they were awarded the Nobel prize for this outstanding scientific achievement. The commercial importance of their scientific findings can be judged from the estimate that the value of therapeutic antibodies alone in the late 1990s was US$6 billion and steadily increasing.

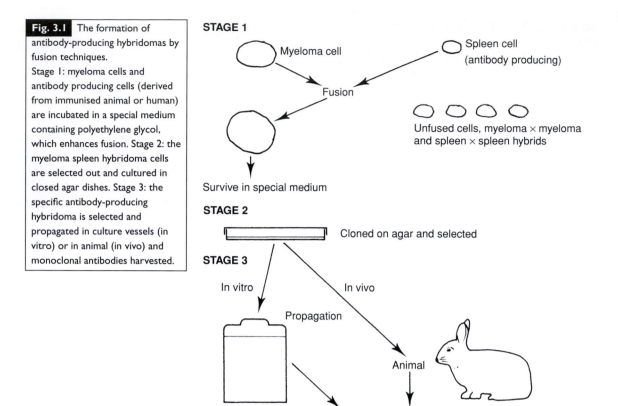

Fig. 3.1 The formation of antibody-producing hybridomas by fusion techniques.
Stage 1: myeloma cells and antibody producing cells (derived from immunised animal or human) are incubated in a special medium containing polyethylene glycol, which enhances fusion. Stage 2: the myeloma spleen hybridoma cells are selected out and cultured in closed agar dishes. Stage 3: the specific antibody-producing hybridoma is selected and propagated in culture vessels (in vitro) or in animal (in vivo) and monoclonal antibodies harvested.

The monoclonal antibody technique changes antibody-secreting cells (with limited life span) into cells capable of continuous growth (immortalisation) while maintaining their specific antibody secreting potential. This immortalisation is achieved by a fusion technique, whereby B-lymphocyte cells are fused to 'immortal' cancer or myeloma cells in a one-to-one ratio, forming hybrids or hybridomas capable of continuous growth and antibody secretion in culture. Single hybrid cells can then be selected and grown as clones or pure cultures of the hybridomas. Such cells continue to secrete antibody, and the antibody is of one particular specificity as opposed to the mixture of antibodies that occurs in an animal's bloodstream after conventional methods of immunisation.

Monoclonal antibody formation is performed by injecting a mouse or rabbit with the antigen, later removing the spleen and then allowing fusion of individual spleen cells with individual myeloma cells. Approximately 1% of the spleen cells are antibody-secreting cells and 10% of the final hybridomas consist of antibody-secreting cells (Fig. 3.1). Techniques are available to identify the right antibody-secreting hybridoma cell, cloning or propagating that cell into large populations with subsequent large formation of the desired antibody. These cells may be frozen and later re-used.

Monoclonal antibodies have now gained wide application in many diagnostic techniques that require a high degree of specificity (this is discussed later). The specificity of monoclonal antibodies can be used for the direct determination of the antigen, even in complex mixtures. By means of suitable standards and controls the detection system can quantify the selected antigen in the system by selectively labelling the antibody with a marker that can be quantitatively determined. Figure 3.2 demonstrates the mechanism of a simple two-site enzyme-linked immunosorbent assay (ELISA) procedure. The antibody is first immobilised onto a surface and then used to capture the antigen in the bathing test solution. Next, an enzyme-labelled antibody specific to a second site on the antigen is added and the excess labelled antibody washed off. A substrate specific to the enzyme is then added and its conversion determined over a specific time interval. Normally a coloured product is produced, which can be monitored using a spectrophotometer. Specific monoclonal antibodies have been combined into test kits for diagnostic purposes, in healthcare, plant and animal agriculture, and in the food industry. Monoclonal antibodies may also be used in the future as antibody therapy to carry cytotoxic drugs to the site of cancer cells. In the fermentation industry they are already widely used as affinity ligands to bind and purify expensive products.

Since the development of the first monoclonal antibody the methodology has developed from a purely scientific tool into one of the fastest expanding fields of biotechnology, which has revolutionised, expanded and diversified the diagnostic industry. The monoclonal antibody market is expected to continue to grow at a very high rate and in healthcare alone the anticipated annual world market could be several billion US dollars within the next few years. It is undoubtedly one of the most commercially successful and useful areas of modern biotechnology and will be expanded on later in several chapters.

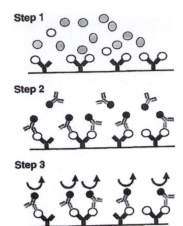

Fig. 3.2 A simple two-site ELISA procedure. In the first step, antibody, which is immobilised onto a surface, is used to capture the antigen from solution. The excess and, therefore, unbound antigen is then washed away. In a second step, an enzyme-labelled antibody specific to a second site on the antigen is added. Again the excess labelled antibody, which does not bind to the antigen, is then washed away. Finally, a substrate is added and the conversion of this by the enzyme is determined over a given time period. Usually a colour change resulting from formation of a coloured product is monitored using a spectrophotometer. (*Source*: from Clark, 2006, with permission.)

3.4 | Genetic engineering

Genes are the fundamental basis of all life, determine the properties of all living forms of life, and are defined segments of DNA. Because DNA structure and composition in all living forms is essentially the same, any technology that can isolate, change or reproduce a gene is likely to have an impact on almost every aspect of society.

Genetic recombination, as occurs during normal sexual reproduction, consists of the breakage and rejoining of the DNA molecules of the chromosomes, and is of fundamental importance to living organisms for the reassortment of genetic material. Genetic manipulation has been performed for centuries by selective breeding of plants and animals superimposed on natural variation. The potential for genetic variation has, thus, been limited to close taxonomic relatives.

In contrast, recombinant DNA techniques, popularly termed gene cloning or genetic engineering, offer potentially unlimited opportunities for creating new combinations of genes that at the moment do not exist under natural conditions.

Genetic engineering has been defined as the formation of new combinations of heritable material by the insertion of nucleic acid molecules, produced by whatever means outside the cell, into any virus, bacterial

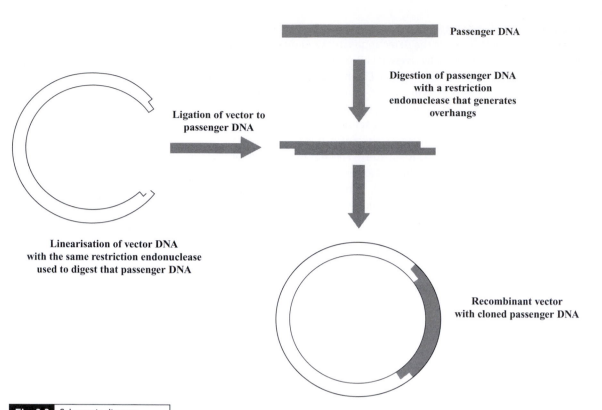

Passenger DNA

Digestion of passenger DNA
with a restriction
endonuclease that generates
overhangs

Ligation of vector to
passenger DNA

Linearisation of vector DNA
with the same restriction endonuclease
used to digest that passenger DNA

Recombinant vector
with cloned passenger DNA

Fig. 3.3 Schematic diagram illustrating the basic concept of genetic engineering using vector and passenger DNA. (*Source:* Harwood and Wipat, 2006.)

plasmid or other vector system so as to allow their incorporation into a host organism in which they do not naturally occur, but in which they are capable of continued propagation. In essence, gene technology is the modification of the genetic properties of an organism by the use of recombinant DNA technology. Genes may be viewed as the biological software and are the programs that drive the growth, development and functioning of an organism. By changing the software in a precise and controlled manner, it becomes possible to produce desired changes in the characteristics of the organism.

These techniques allow the splicing of DNA molecules of quite diverse origin, and, when combined with techniques of genetic transformation etc., facilitate the introduction of foreign DNA into other organisms. The foreign DNA or gene construct is introduced into the genome of the recipient organism host in such a way that the total genome of the host is unchanged except for the manipulated gene(s).

Thus DNA can be isolated from cells of plants, animals or microorganisms (the donors) and can be fragmented into groups of one or more genes. Such passenger DNA fragments can then be coupled to another piece of DNA (the *vector*) and then passed into the host or recipient cell, becoming part of the genetic complement of the new host (Fig. 3.3). The host cell can then be propagated in mass to form novel genetic properties and chemical abilities that were unattainable by conventional ways of selective breeding or mutation. While traditional plant and animal genetic breeding techniques also change the genetic code it is achieved in a less direct and controlled manner. Genetic engineering will now enable the breeder to select the particular gene required for a desired characteristic and modify only that gene.

Although much work to date has involved bacteria, the techniques are evolving at an astonishing rate and ways have been developed for introducing DNA into other organisms such as yeasts and plant and animal cell cultures. Provided that the genetic material transferred in this manner can replicate and be expressed in the new cell type, there are virtually no limits to the range of organisms with new properties that could be produced by genetic engineering. Life forms containing 'foreign' DNA are termed *transgenic* and will be discussed in more detail in later chapters.

These methods potentially allow totally new functions to be added to the capabilities of organisms, and open up vistas for the genetic engineering of industrial microorganisms and agricultural plants and animals that are quite breathtaking in their scope. This is undoubtedly the most significant new technology in modern bioscience and biotechnology. In industrial microbiology it will permit the production in microorganisms of a wide range of hitherto unachievable products such as human and animal proteins and enzymes such as insulin and chymosin (rennet); in medicine, better vaccines, hormones and improved therapy of diseases; in agriculture, improved plants and animals for productivity, quality of products, disease resistance, etc; in food production, improved quality, flavour, taste and safety; and in environmental aspects, a wide range of benefits such as pollution control can be expected. It should be noted that genetic engineering is a way of doing things rather than an end in itself. Genetic engineering will add to, rather than displace, traditional ways of developing products. However, there are many who view genetic engineering as a transgression of normal life processes that goes well beyond normal evolution. These concerns will be discussed in later chapters.

Genetic engineering holds the potential to extend the range and power of almost every aspect of biotechnology. In microbial technology these techniques will be widely used to improve existing microbial processes by improving stability of existing cultures and eliminating unwanted side-products. It is confidently anticipated that within this decade recombinant DNA techniques will form the basis of new strains of microorganisms with new and unusual metabolic properties. In this way fermentations based on these technical advances could become competitive with petrochemicals for producing a whole range of chemical compounds, for example ethylene glycol (used in the plastics industry) as well as improved biofuel production. In the food industry, improved strains of bacteria and fungi are now influencing such traditional processes as baking and cheese-making and bringing greater control and reproducibility of flavour and texture.

A full understanding of the working concepts of recombinant DNA technology requires a good knowledge of molecular biology. A brief explanation will be attempted here, but readers are advised to consult some of the many excellent texts that are available in this field.

The basic molecular techniques for the in vitro transfer and expression of foreign DNA in a host cell (*gene transfer technology*), including isolating, cutting and joining molecules of DNA, and inserting into a vector (carrying)

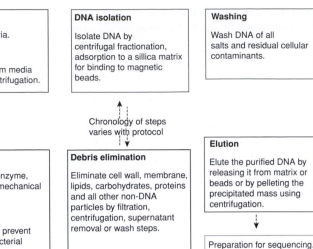

Fig. 3.4 Diagram of a typical series of sample preparation steps required for DNA purification from bacterial cells. (*Source*: Wells and Herron, 2002.)

Culture

Culture the bacteria.

Cell separation

Separate cells from media by filtration or centrifugation.

DNA isolation

Isolate DNA by centrifugal fractionation, adsorption to a sillica matrix for binding to magnetic beads.

Washing

Wash DNA of all salts and residual cellular contaminants.

Chronology of steps varies with protocol

Cell lysis

Lyse cells using enzyme, detergent, pH or mechanical disruption.

Neutralisation

Neutralise lysis to prevent dissociation of bacterial genomic DNA.

Debris elimination

Eliminate cell wall, membrane, lipids, carbohydrates, proteins and all other non-DNA particles by filtration, centrifugation, supernatant removal or wash steps.

Elution

Elute the purified DNA by releasing it from matrix or beads or by pelleting the precipitated mass using centrifugation.

Preparation for sequencing.

molecule that can be stably retained in the host cell, were first developed in the early 1970s. These techniques may be defined thus:

Isolation and purification of nucleic acids. A prerequisite for in vitro gene technology is to prepare large quantities of relatively pure nucleic acids from the desired organism. After disruption of the cells the nucleic acids must be separated from other cellular components using a variety of techniques including centrifugation, electrophoresis, adsorption and various forms of precipitation (Fig. 3.4).

Cutting DNA molecules. DNA can be cut using mechanical or enzymatic methods. The non-specific mechanical shearing will generate random DNA fragments, which are most often used to create genomic libraries. This crude method does not permit the isolation of a specific fragment containing a known gene or operon. In contrast, when specific restriction endonuclease enzymes are used it is possible to recognise and cleave specific target base sequences in double-stranded (ds) DNA. Restriction endonucleases are able to sever the phosphodiester backbone of both strands of the DNA to generate 3′OH and 5′PO$_4$ termini (Fig. 3.5). Large numbers of different restriction endonucleases have been extracted and classified from a wide variety of microbial species. Restriction endonucleases are named according to the species from which they were first isolated, e.g. enzymes isolated from *Haemophilus influenzae* strain Rd are designated *Hind* and when several different restriction enzymes are isolated from the same organism they are designated *HindI*, *HindII* etc. Restriction endonucleases can distinguish between DNA from their own cells and foreign DNA by recognising a certain sequence of nucleotides. This allows the breaking open of a length of DNA into shorter fragments that contain a number of genes determined by the enzyme used. Such DNA fragments can then be separated from each other on the basis of different molecular weight.

Splicing DNA. DNA fragments with either blunt ends or with cohesive overlapping ends can be joined together in vitro by the action of specific DNA ligases. The DNA ligase that is widely used was encoded by phage T4. Such enzymes ensure the formation of phosphodiester bonds between

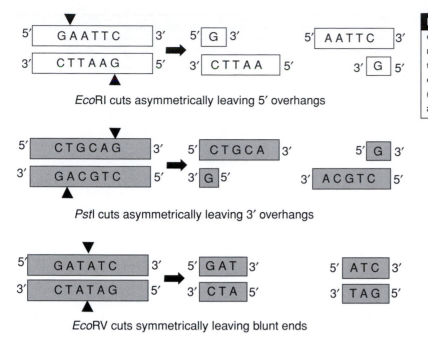

Fig. 3.5 Restriction endonuclease cleavage of molecules of DNA at specific target sites to generate 3′ or 5′ overhangs (overlaps) or blunt ends. (*Source*: adapted from Harwood and Wipat, 2006, with permission.)

EcoRI cuts asymmetrically leaving 5′ overhangs

PstI cuts asymmetrically leaving 3′ overhangs

EcoRV cuts symmetrically leaving blunt ends

3′OH groups at the terminus of one strand with the 5′PO$_4$ terminus of another strand provided that the ends are complementary. The sources of 'passenger' can be quite different, giving an opportunity to replicate the DNA biologically by inserting it into other cells.

The composite molecules in which DNA has been inserted have also been termed 'DNA chimaeras' because of the analogy with the Chimaera of mythology, a creature with the head of a lion, the body of a goat and the tail of a serpent.

The vector or carrier system. Two broad categories of expression vector molecules have been developed as vehicles for gene transfer, *plasmids* (small units of DNA distinct from chromosomes) and *bacteriophages* (or bacterial viruses). Vector molecules will normally exist within a cell in an independent or extrachromosomal form not becoming part of the chromosomal system of the organism. Vector molecules should be capable of entering the host cell and replicating within it. Ideally, the vector should be small, easily prepared and must contain at least one site where integration of foreign DNA will not destroy an essential function. Plasmids will undoubtedly offer the greatest potential in biotechnology and have been found in an increasingly wide range of organisms, for example, bacteria, yeasts and mould fungi; they have been mostly studied in Gram-negative bacteria. Expression vectors can often add an affinity tag to the protein to facilitate its purification by affinity chromatography. The tag can later be removed.

Introduction of vector DNA recombinants. The new recombinant DNA can now be introduced into the host cell by transformations (the direct uptake of DNA by a cell from its environment) or transductions (DNA transferred from one organism to another by way of a carrier or vector system) and if acceptable the new DNA will be cloned with the propagation of the host cell.

Table 3.1	Strategies involved in genetic engineering
Formation of DNA fragments	Extracted DNA can be cut into small sequences by specific enzymes, restriction endonucleases, found in many species of bacteria.
Splicing of DNA into vectors	The small sequences of DNA can be joined or spliced into the vector DNA molecules by an enzyme DNA ligase creating an artificial DNA molecule.
Introduction of vectors into host cells	The vectors are either viruses or plasmids, and are replicons and can exist in an extrachromosomal state; transfer normally by transduction or transformation.
Selection of newly acquired DNA	Selection and ultimate characterisation of the recombinant clone.

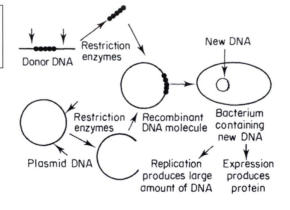

Fig. 3.6 Recombinant DNA: the technique of recombining genes from one species with those of another.

Novel methods of ensuring DNA uptake into cells include *electroporation* and *mechanical particle delivery* or *biolistics*. Electroporation is a process of creating transient pores in the cell membrane by application of a pulsed electric field. Creation of such pores in a membrane allows introduction of foreign molecules, such as DNA, RNA, antibodies, drugs, etc., into the cell cytoplasm. Development of this technology has arisen from synergy of biophysics, bioengineering and cell and molecular biology. While the technique is now widely used to create transgenic microorganisms, plants and animals, it is also being increasingly used for application of therapeutics and gene therapy. The mechanical particle delivery or 'gene gun' methods deliver DNA on microscopic particles into target tissue or cells. This process is increasingly used to introduce new genes into a range of bacterial, fungal, plant and mammalian species and has become a main method of choice for genetic engineering of many plant species including rice, corn, wheat, cotton and soybean.

The strategies involved in genetic engineering are summarised in Table 3.1 and Fig. 3.6.

Although the theory underlying the exchange of genetic information between unrelated organisms and their propagation is becoming better understood, difficulties still persist at the level of some applications. Further research is required before such exchanges become commonplace and the host organisms propagated in large quantities.

Early studies on genetic engineering were mainly carried out with the bacterium *Escherichia coli* but increasingly other bacteria, yeast and filamentous fungi have been used. Mammalian systems have been increasingly developed using the Simian virus (SV40) and oncogenes (genes that cause cancer), while several successful methods are available for plant cells, in particular the *Agrobacterium* system. Thus, in the last four decades, molecular biology has formulated evidence for the unity of genetic systems together with the basic mechanisms that regulate cell functions. Genetic engineering has confirmed the unity of the living world, demonstrating that all living creatures are built of molecules that are more or less identical. Thus, the diversity of life forms on this planet derives from small changes in the regulatory systems that control the expression of genes.

3.5 | The polymerase chain reaction and DNA sequencing

Two molecular biology techniques in recent years have revolutionised the availability of DNA data, the polymerase chain reaction (PCR) and the development of automated DNA sequencing. The polymerase chain reaction is basically a technique that allows the selective amplification of any fragment of DNA (of about 0.2 and 40 kbp (kilo base pairs) in size) provided that the DNA sequences flanking the fragment are known – described as a technique that finds a needle in a haystack and then produces a haystack of needles by specific amplification! The inventor of PCR, Kary Mullis, shared the Nobel prize in Chemistry in 1993.

The polymerase chain reaction process relies on the sequence of 'base-pairs' along the length of the two strands that make the complete DNA molecule. In DNA there are four deoxynucleotides derived from the four bases, adenosine (A), thymidine (T), guanine (G) and cytidine (C). The strands or polymers that comprise the DNA molecule are held to each other by hydrogen bonds between the base pairs. In this arrangement A only binds to T while G only binds to C, and this unique system folds the entire molecule into the now well recognised double-helix structure.

The polymerase chain reaction involves three processing steps – *denaturation, annealing* and then *extension* by DNA polymerase (Fig. 3.7a,b). In Step 1, the double-stranded DNA is heated (95−98 °C) and separates into two complementary single strands. In Step 2 (60 °C) the synthetic oligonucleotide primers (chemically synthesised short-chain nucleotides), short sequences of nucleotides (usually about 20 nucleotide base pairs long), are added and bind to the single strands in places where the strand's DNA complements their own. In Step 3 (37 °C) the primers are extended by DNA polymerase in the presence of all four deoxynucleoside triphosphates resulting in the

Fig. 3.7 (a) The polymerase chain reaction. The double-stranded DNA is heated and separates into two single strands. The synthetic oligonucleotide primers then bind to their complementary sequence and are extended in the direction of the arrows giving a new strand of DNA identical to the template's original partner; (b) PCR temperature cycling profile. (See Graham, 1994.)

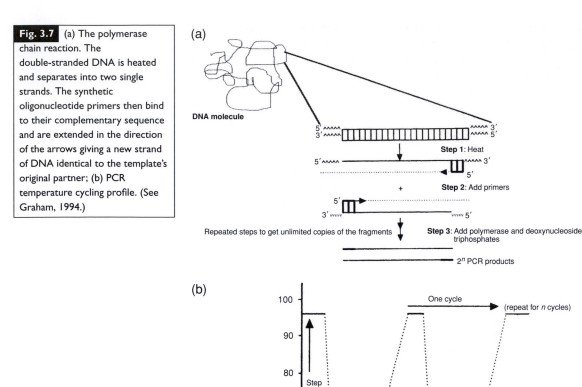

(a)

DNA molecule

Step 1: Heat

Step 2: Add primers

Repeated steps to get unlimited copies of the fragments

Step 3: Add polymerase and deoxynucleoside triphosphates

2^n PCR products

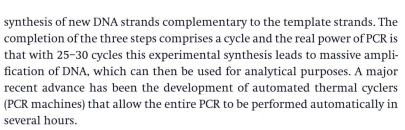

(b)

synthesis of new DNA strands complementary to the template strands. The completion of the three steps comprises a cycle and the real power of PCR is that with 25–30 cycles this experimental synthesis leads to massive amplification of DNA, which can then be used for analytical purposes. A major recent advance has been the development of automated thermal cyclers (PCR machines) that allow the entire PCR to be performed automatically in several hours.

The polymerase chain reaction was first patented in 1987 and then commercialised by the American Cetus Corporation in 1988. However, in 1991 Hoffman La Roche and Perkin Elmer purchased the full operating rights of PCR for $300 million. The applications of PCR increase almost daily and include molecular biology/genetic engineering; infectious and parasitic disease diagnosis; human genetic disease diagnosis; forensic validation; plant and animal breeding; and environmental monitoring. The polymerase chain reaction has been extensively used in the well known procedure of genetic or DNA fingerprinting, the fallibility of which is now being challenged in courts of law (Fig. 3.7).

While the polymerase chain reaction is finding considerable and unique use in archaeology, it is doubtful whether we will ever be able to resurrect woolly mammoths and dinosaurs from ancient animal remains as recently epitomised in Michael Crichton's *Jurassic Park*.

Genomes of all organisms consist of millions of repetitions of the four nucleotides, C, G, A and T. In humans, there are over 3000 million nucleotides. Analysing the sequence of the nucleotides (*DNA sequencing*) has become a critically useful technique for the identification, analysis and directed manipulation of genomic DNA. Originally, methods of separation and identification relied upon gel electrophoresis and autoradiography. However, recent developments in sequencing technology have allowed the process to be automated and greatly speeded up. Fluorescent dye-labelled substrates are used, which allows the use of a laser-induced fluorescent detection system. In many applications automated sequencers can produce over 1000 base pairs of sequence from overnight operations. There are now publicly available databases, such as GenBank, which provide numerous online services for identifying, aligning and comparing sequences. Individual chromosomes contain many thousands of sequences, some organised into genes while others appear to be merely flanking or spacer regions.

3.6 | Nucleic acid probes

Nucleic acid probes are designed to detect specific target DNA molecules. Nucleic acid hybridisation relies on the ability of single-stranded probe nucleic acid (DNA or RNA) to become attached or annealed (hybridisation) to complementary single-stranded target sequences (DNA or RNA) within a population of non-complementary nucleic acid molecules. Test samples must be treated so that the cells are lysed, releasing the double-stranded DNA, which is then denatured into single-stranded forms to which the specific probe is added. The objective of the probe is to be readily detected; this is achieved by the incorporation of radionucleotides such as ^{32}P or ^{35}S or fluorescent compounds (Fig. 3.8). Such techniques are extensively used in biotechnology, e.g. organism identification, cloned DNA, disease diagnosis.

Probe-based technical systems are obtained by immobilising probes to inorganic substances, i.e. dipsticks, to permit the user to easily manipulate the probe, and washing off the unhybridised DNA. This is also referred to as solid-phase hybridisation.

DNA chips or micro-arrays are intrinsically miniaturised extensions of conventional tests of nucleic acid hybridisation. Micro-arrays are miniaturised solid supports (typically a glass slide or grid of single-stranded DNA fragments that can represent all, or a subpopulation of, the genes of an organism). The great advantage of these systems is that they can only require small amounts of resources.

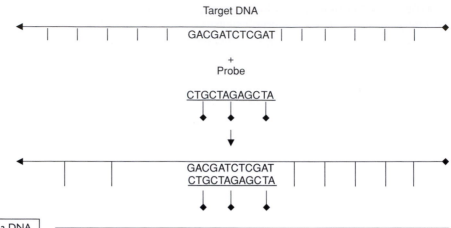

Target DNA

GACGATCTCGAT

+
Probe

CTGCTAGAGCTA

GACGATCTCGAT
CTGCTAGAGCTA

Fig. 3.8 Hybridisation of a DNA probe to a DNA sample.

3.7 | Genomics and proteomics

Chromosomes are the principal receptacles of the genetic information, the site of gene expression and the vehicles of inheritance. The term genome is used in the more abstract sense to refer to the sum total of the genetic information or DNA of an organism. The science of genomics has witnessed intense and dramatic developments over the last 20 years and has become a revolutionary scientific discipline focused on by academics and industrial scientists from many research disciples worldwide. A typical genome project seeks to determine the complete DNA structure for a given organism and to identify and map all of the genes. Arising from the previously described techniques, it was possible in 1995 to determine the first complete genome or DNA sequence of a free-living organism, the bacterium *Haemophilus influenzae*. Since then a considerable number of prokaryotes, the yeast *Saccharomyces cerevisiae*, the fruit-fly *Drosophila melanogaster*, the plant *Arabidopsis thaliani* and many others have been sequenced. However, the major event in molecular genetics was the elucidation of the human genome sequence in 2001. The Human Genome Project cost nearly 3 billion dollars. The scientific benefit is incalculable but translating the potential of the genome into tangible benefits for basic and biomedical research, not to mention personalised medicine, will require vast investments in de novo sequencing in the search for key variables.

While there has been much hype concerning the ethical and commercial implications of these discoveries, this is only the beginning of the understanding of the real functional activity within cells, in tissues and in whole organisms. Throughout this last decade of genomic research there has been insufficient emphasis on other aspects of cellular organisation, and much ill-judged scientific belief that the enigma of cell function in health and disease could be understood solely through knowledge of genes alone.

Biochemical studies over many decades have shown that cellular activity is achieved through a vast array of signalling, regulatory and metabolic pathways, each involving many specific molecules. There still exists a vast gulf between our understanding of individual molecular mechanisms and pathways and how they are integrated into an orderly *homeostatic* system.

Major molecular biology attention has now moved dramatically to the study of the *proteome* – the collective body of proteins made within an organism's cells and tissues. Proteomics aims to describe all the proteins encoded by the genome including their structure, localisation and in humans the clinical profile and also their abundance, interactions and modifications. While the genome supplies the recipes for making the cell's proteins, it is the proteome that represents the bricks and mortar of the cells and carries out the cellular functions. The proteome is infinitely more complex than the genome. While a cell will have only one genome it can have many proteomes. The DNA alphabet is composed of four bases, while proteins in contrast are constructed from approximately 20 amino acids. While the genes through transcription determine the sequence of amino acids in a protein, it is not totally clear what the protein does and how it interacts with other proteins. Unlike genes, which are linear, proteins fold into three-dimensional structures that are difficult to predict. The proteome is extremely dynamic, and minor alterations in the external or internal environment can modify proteome function. Understanding proteomics should give a better holistic view of cellular metabolism.

The dominant biochemical approach to proteomics combines two-dimensional polyacrylamide gel electrophoresis (2D-PAGE), which separates, maps and quantifies proteins, with mass spectrometry (MS)-based sequencing techniques, which identify both the amino acid sequences of proteins and the molecular additions post translation. Proteomics will relate to genomic databases to assist protein identification and consequently indicate which genes within the database are important in specific conditions. The two areas of genomics and proteomics must have a strong synergistic relationship. The potential of proteomics to identify and compare complex protein profiles is now generating highly accurate but sensitive molecular fingerprints of proteins present in human body fluids at a given time. Proteomic data from humans and pathogens are providing major advances in the understanding of all cellular aspects of health and disease, and will surely have a major impact on the diagnosis of diseases and development of suitable specific drugs. Such molecular medicine could well be one of the most remarkable achievements of biotechnology of this century.

The ability to clone DNA or manipulate genes and to obtain successful expression in an organism is nowadays a core technology of quite unparalleled importance in modern bioscience and biotechnology. The expression and acceptance of genetic engineering in the context of biotechnology, where novel gene pools can be created and expressed in large quantities, will offer outstanding opportunities for the well-being of humanity.

3.8 | Antisense and RNA interference

Antisense

It has long been recognised that genes can be silenced by means of antisense technology. An antisense gene can be constructed by reversing the nucleotide sequence of the gene. Transcription of an antisense gene

Table 3.2 Biochemical networks in systems biology
Biochemical networks
Metabolic networks
Regulatory networks
Signalling networks
Mathematical representation of networks
Capabilities of networks

produces an RNA molecule that is complementary to the sense in RNA sequence. The sense and antisense RNA strands are antiparallel and, thus, form a double-stranded RNA molecule similar to double-stranded DNA. The formation of this double-stranded RNA molecule results in decreased translation of the sense RNA. Antisense technology was used in transgenic plants to control ripening – the FlavrSavr tomato. The antisense technology can silence genes using double-stranded complementary synthetic oligonucleotides. This technology has been extensively practised in transgenic organisms and in gene therapy studies.

RNA interference

A central feature of modern molecular biology has been the transcription and translation of the RNA molecule. The molecules were viewed as simple carriers of messages and fetchers of materials (i.e. amino acids) for protein synthesis. In the last decade it has become apparent that the genome produces vast numbers of RNAs with functions other than making proteins.

The discovery in 1993 of a gene expressing small non-protein coding RNAs in a small worm, *Coenorhabditis elegans*, led to the discovery of a previously unknown class of endogenous, single-stranded 19–21 nucleotide molecules called micro RNAs (miRNAs) that can regulate up to 30% of mammalian genes. The discoverer, Craig Mells, was awarded in 2006 the Nobel Prize for Physiology and Medicine. These miRNAs have been shown to inhibit mRNA and prevent translation of large numbers of messages at a time, and have been shown to be deregulated in several diseases. The naturally occurring form of post-translational interference of gene activity within a cell is now being extensively studied worldwide and increasingly being viewed as a possible new therapeutic class. The potential ability to harness the cell's own gene-silencing machinery makes miRNAs most attractive for clinical research. Short interference RNA (siRNA) is double-stranded and exists in the cells of many species and can interact with single genes by cleaving mRNA.

At present, interference RNAs (RNAi) are a most valuable basic research tool while their therapeutic potential is being extensively explored. How can siRNA compounds be delivered to their cellular targets? It can be extremely difficult for oligonucleotides to penetrate cell membranes and to avoid attack by the host immune system. Unless this can be achieved, drug manufacturers will be unable to realise RNAi's therapeutic promise. The means of delivering RNAi-developed drugs to target cells presents difficult challenges and most programmes are still at preclinical stages. Current patent applications with RNAi are almost exclusively related to technical invention, and complex patent applications are now arriving dealing with nucleotide insertion (see later).

Controlling RNA transcription and translation has long been considered as 'the Holy Grail' of molecular biology.

3.9 | Systems biology

Genome sequences now allow us to determine the biological components that make up a cell or an organism. Systems biology is a new discipline, which examines how these components interact and form networks and, furthermore, how such networks generate whole-cell functions and ultimately the organism. Systems biology does not concentrate on individual genes and proteins, one at a time, but encompasses the behaviour and relationships of all components in a particular biological system from a functional perspective. Biological systems are primarily composed of information genes, their encoded products and the regulatory components controlling the expression of these genes.

Systems biology endeavours to interpret complex biological systems by integrating all levels of functional information into a cohesive model. During the twentieth century molecular biologists evolved a 'reductionist approach', acquiring functional information of an organism one gene or one protein at a time. Consequently, this new approach of systems biology represents a paradigm shift from previous molecular biology thinking.

A widely adopted approach to systems biology incorporates bottom-up data collection from all the biological networks (Table 3.2) and top-down computational modelling and simulation by which known functions and behaviour of the biological components are described in mathematical terms and incorporated into complex models that permit the dynamic interaction of large numbers of variables.

Systems analysis has been utilised historically in many areas of biology, including ecology, developmental biology and immunology. However, the genomics and proteomics revolution has catapulted molecular biology into the exciting realms of systems biology. The impact of systems biology on human disease and other biological areas will be highlighted in later chapters.

3.10 | Potential laboratory biohazards of genetic engineering

The early studies on gene manipulation provoked wide discussion and considerable concern at the possible risks that could arise with certain types of experiment. Thus it was believed by some that the construction of recombinant DNA molecules and their insertion into microorganisms could create novel organisms that might inadvertently be released from the laboratory and become a biohazard to humans or the environment. In contrast, others considered that newly synthesised organisms with their additional genetic material would not be able to compete with the normal strains present in nature. The present views of gene manipulation studies are becoming more moderate as experiments have shown that this work can proceed within a strict safety code when required, involving physical and biological containment of the organism.

The standards of containment enforced in the early years of recombinant DNA studies were unnecessarily restrictive, and there has been a steady relaxation of the regulations governing much of the routine genetic engineering activities. However, for many types of study, particularly with pathogenic microorganisms, the standards will remain stringent. Thus, for strict physical containment laboratories involved in this type of study must have highly skilled personnel and correct physical containment equipment, for example negative-pressure laboratories, autoclaves, safety cabinets, etc.

Biological containment can be achieved or enhanced by selecting non-pathogenic organisms as the cloning agents of foreign DNA, or by the deliberate genetic manipulation of a microorganism to reduce the probability of survival and propagation in the environment. *Escherichia coli*, a bacterium that is extremely prevalent in the intestinal tracts of warm-blooded and cold-blooded animals as well as in humans, is the most widely used cloning agent. To offset the risk of this cloning agent becoming a danger in the environment a special strain of *E. coli* has been constructed by genetic manipulation, which incorporates many fail-safe features. This strain can only grow under special laboratory conditions and there is no possibility that it can constitute a biohazard if it escapes out of the laboratory.

The government controlled Health and Safety Executive controls and monitors recombinant DNA work within the UK. This committee seeks advice from the Genetic Manipulation Advisory Group (GMAG) who formulate realistic procedural guidelines, which, in general, have proved widely acceptable to the experimenting scientific community. Most other advanced scientific nations involved in recombinant DNA studies have set up similar advisory committees. The deliberate releasing of genetically manipulated organisms to the environment is discussed in a later chapter.

Chapter 4

Bioprocess/fermentation technology

4.1 | Introduction

Bioprocess or fermentation technology is an important component of most 'old' and 'new' biotechnology processes and will normally involve complete living cells (microbe, mammalian or plant), organelles or enzymes as the biocatalyst, and will aim to bring about specific chemical and/or physical changes in biochemical materials derived from the medium. In order to be viable in any specific industrial context, bioprocessing must possess advantages over competing methods of production such as chemical technology. In practice, many bioprocessing techniques will be used industrially because they are the only practical way in which a specific product can be made (e.g. vaccines, antibiotics). Biochemical engineering covers the design of vessels and apparatus suitable for performing such biochemical reactions or transformations.

The very beginnings of fermentation technology, or as it is now better recognised, bioprocess technology, were derived in part from the use of microorganisms for the production of foods such as cheeses, yoghurts, sauerkraut, fermented pickles and sausages, soya sauce and other Oriental products, and beverages such as beers, wines and derived spirits (Table 4.1). In many cases, the present-day production processes for such products are still remarkably similar. These forms of bioprocessing were long viewed as arts or crafts, but are now increasingly subjected to the full array of modern science and technology. Paralleling these useful product formations was the identification of the roles microorganisms could play in removing obnoxious and unhealthful wastes, which has resulted in the worldwide service industries involved in water purification, effluent treatment and solid waste management.

Bioprocessing in its many forms involves a multitude of complex enzyme-catalysed reactions within specific cellular systems, and these reactions are critically dependent on the physical and chemical conditions that exist in their immediate environment. Successful bioprocessing will only occur when all the essential factors are brought together.

Table 4.1 Fermentation products according to industrial sectors

Sector	Activities
Chemicals	
Organic (bulk)	Ethanol, acetone, butanol
	Organic acids (citric, itaconic)
Organic (fine)	Enzymes
	Perfumeries
	Polymers (mainly polysaccharides)
Inorganic	Metal beneficiation, bioaccumulation and leaching (Cu, U)
Pharmaceuticals	Antibiotics
	Diagnostic agents (enzymes, monoclonal antibodies)
	Enzyme inhibitors
	Steroids
	Vaccines
Energy	Ethanol (gasohol)
	Methane (biogas)
	Biomass
Food	Dairy products (cheeses, yoghurts, fish and meat products)
	Beverages (alcoholic, tea and coffee)
	Baker's yeast
	Food additives (antioxidants, colours, flavours, stabilisers)
	Novel foods (soy sauce, tempeh, miso)
	Mushroom products
	Amino acids, vitamins
	Starch products
	Glucose and high-fructose syrups
	Functional modifications of proteins, pectins
Agriculture	Animal feedstuffs (SCP)
	Veterinary vaccines
	Ensilage and composting processes
	Microbial pesticides
	Rhizobium and other N-fixing bacterial inoculants
	Mycorrhizal inoculants
	Plant cell and tissue culture (vegetative propagation, embryo production, genetic improvement)

Although the traditional forms of bioprocess technology related to foods and beverages still represent the major commercial bioproducts, new products are increasingly being derived from microbial, mammalian and plant cell fermentations, namely the ability:

(1) to overproduce essential primary metabolites such as acetic and lactic acids, glycerol, acetone, butyl alcohol, organic acids, amino acids, vitamins and polysaccharides

Table 4.2 Advantages and disadvantages of producing organic compounds by biological rather than chemical means	
Advantages	Disadvantages
Complex molecules such as proteins and antibodies cannot be produced by chemical means.	Can be easily contaminated with foreign unwanted microorganisms, etc.
Bioconversions give higher yields.	The desired product will usually be present in a complex product mixture requiring separation.
Biological systems operate at lower temperatures, near neutral pH, etc.	Need to provide, handle and dispose of large volumes of water.
Much greater specificity of catalytic reaction.	Bioprocesses are usually extremely slow when compared with conventional chemical processes.
Can achieve exclusive production of an isomeric compound.	

(2) to produce secondary metabolites (metabolites that do not appear to have an obvious role in the metabolism of the producer organism) such as penicillin, streptomycin, cephalosporin, giberellins, etc.

(3) to produce many forms of industrially useful enzymes, e.g. exocellular enzymes such as amylases, pectinases and proteases, and intracellular enzymes such as invertase, asparaginase, restriction endonucleases, etc.

(4) to produce monoclonal antibodies, vaccines and novel recombinant products, e.g. therapeutic proteins.

All of these products now command large industrial markets and are essential to modern society (Table 4.1).

More recently, bioprocess technology is increasingly using cells derived from higher plants and animals to produce many important products. Plant cell culture is largely aimed at secondary product formations such as flavours, perfumes and drugs, while mammalian cell culture has been concerned with vaccine and antibody formation and the recombinant production of protein molecules such as interferons, interleukins and erythropoietins.

The future market growth of these bioproducts is largely assured because, with limited exceptions, most cannot be produced economically by other chemical processes. It will also be possible to make further economies in production by genetically engineering organisms to higher or unique productivities and utilising new technological advances in processing. The advantages of producing organic products by biological as opposed to purely chemical methods are listed in Table 4.2.

The product formation stages in bioprocess technology are essentially very similar no matter what organism is selected, what medium is used or what product formed. In all examples, large numbers of cells are grown under defined controlled conditions. The organisms must be cultivated *and* motivated to form the desired products by means of a physical/technical containment system (*the bioreactor*), and the correct medium composition and environmental growth-regulating parameters such as temperature and aeration. Optimisation of the bioprocess spans both the bio- and the

Table 4.3	Examples of products in different categories in biotechnological industries
Category	Example
Cell mass[a]	Baker's yeast, single-cell protein
Cell components[b]	Intracellular proteins
Biosynthetic products[b]	Antibiotics, vitamins, amino and organic acids
Catabolic products[a]	Ethanol, methane, lactic acid
Bioconversion[a]	High-fructose corn syrup, 6-aminopenicillanic acid
Waste treatment	Activated sludge, anaerobic digestion

[a] Typically conversion of feedstock cost-intensive processes.
[b] Typically recovery cost-intensive process.

Fig. 4.1 The biotechnology process.

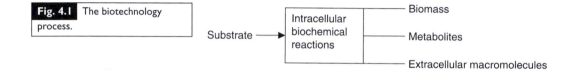

technical systems. The proper exploitation of an organism's potential to form distinct products of defined quality *and* in large amounts will need a detailed knowledge of the biochemical mechanisms of product formation.

Bioprocessing in its many forms is catalysed within each respective cellular system by a large number of intracellular biochemical reactions. Substrates derived from the medium are converted into primary and secondary products, intra- and extracellular macromolecules, and into biomass components such as DNA, RNA, proteins and carbohydrates (Fig. 4.1).

These reactions will be dependent on the physical and chemical parameters that exist in their immediate environments.

The same apparatus with modifications can be used to produce an enzyme, an antibiotic, an amino acid or single-cell protein. In its simplest form, the bioprocess can be seen as just the mixing of microorganisms with a nutrient broth and allowing the components to react, e.g. yeast cells with a sugar solution to give alcohol. More advanced and sophisticated processes operating at large scale need to control the entire system so that the bioprocess can proceed efficiently and be readily and exactly repeated with the same amounts of raw materials and inoculum (the particular organism) to produce precisely the same amount of product.

All biotechnological processes are essentially performed within containment systems or bioreactors. Large numbers of cells are invariably involved in these processes and the bioreactor ensures their close involvement with the correct medium and conditions for growth and product formation. It also should restrict the release of the cells into the environment. A main function of a bioreactor is to minimise the cost of producing a product or service. Examples of the diverse product categories produced industrially in bioreactors are given in Table 4.3.

Table 4.4 Approximate size of cells used in biotechnology processes	
Cell type	Size (μm)
Bacterial cells	1 × 2
Yeast cells	7 × 10
Mammalian cells	40 × 40
Plant cells	100 × 100

4.2 | Principles of microbial growth

The growth of organisms may be seen as the increase of cell material expressed in terms of mass or cell number, and results from a highly complicated and coordinated series of enzymatically catalysed biological steps. Growth will be dependent on the availability and transport of necessary nutrients to the cell and subsequent uptake, and on environmental parameters such as temperature, pH and aeration being optimally maintained.

The quantity of biomass or specific cellular component (X) in a bioreactor can be determined gravimetrically (by dry weight, wet weight, DNA or protein) or numerically for unicellular systems (by number of cells). Doubling time (td) refers to the period of time required for the doubling in the weight of biomass while generation (g) time relates to the period necessary for the doubling of cell numbers. Average doubling times increase with increasing cell size (Table 4.4) and complexity, e.g. bacteria 0.25–1 h; yeast 1–2 h; mould fungi 2–6.5 h; plant cells 20–70 h; and mammalian cells 20–48 h.

It is now possible to develop mathematical equations to describe the essential features of organism growth in bioreactors. The original mathematical equation described by Monod (1942) gives specific growth (μ) as a function of the concentration (S):

$$\mu = \mu_{max} \frac{S}{Ks + S}$$

S is the concentration of a substrate in the medium, which is in limiting concentration when in comparison with other essential nutrients, μ_{max} is the maximum specific growth rate of the organism while Ks represents a saturation constant. Ks is the substrate concentration at which $\mu = \mu_{max}/2$. Exponential growth will occur at specific growth rates having any value between zero and μ_{max} if the substrate concentration can be kept constant at the appropriate value, a factor which will be important for continuous culture. The nutrients essential for growth together with the optimum conditions required for growth have been identified from both batch and continuous bioreactor systems. The rate of increase of concentration of organisms (dx/dt) is the *growth rate* while the *specific growth rate* is the rate of increase/unit of organism concentration (1/x) (dx/dt). A simple relationship exists between growth and utilisation of substrate. In simple systems growth rate is a constant fraction Y of the substrate utilisation rate:

$$\frac{dx}{dt} = -Y\frac{ds}{dt} \tag{1}$$

Y is the *yield constant* and over any finite period of growth:

$$Y = \frac{\text{weight of cells formed}}{\text{weight of substrate used}} \tag{2}$$

Knowing the values of the three growth constants μ_{max}, Ks and Y, equations (1) and (2) can give a complete quantitative description of the growth cycle of a batch culture.

In normal practice an organism will seldom have totally ideal conditions for unlimited growth; rather, growth will be dependent on a limiting factor, for example, an essential nutrient. As the concentration of this factor drops, so also will the growth potential of the organism decrease.

In biotechnological processes there are three main ways of growing microorganisms in the bioreactor: batch, fed-batch or continuous. Within the bioreactor reactions can occur with static or agitated cultures, in the presence or absence of oxygen, and in liquid or low-moisture conditions (e.g. on solid substrates). The microorganisms can be free or can be attached to surfaces by immobilisation or by natural adherence.

In a *batch culture* the microorganisms are inoculated into a fixed volume of medium and as growth takes place nutrients are consumed and products of growth (biomass, metabolites) accumulate. The nutrient environment within the bioreactor is continuously changing and, thus, in turn, enforcing changes to cell metabolism. Eventually, cell multiplication ceases because of exhaustion or limitation of nutrient(s) and accumulation of toxic excreted waste products.

The complex nature of batch growth of microorganisms is shown in Fig. 4.2. The initial *lag phase* is a time of no apparent growth, but actual biochemical analyses show metabolic turnover indicating that the cells are in the process of adapting to the environmental conditions and that new growth will eventually begin. There is then a *transient acceleration* phase as the inoculum begins to grow to be quickly followed by the *exponential phase*. In the exponential phase, microbial growth proceeds at the maximum possible rate for that organism with nutrients in excess, ideal environmental parameters and growth inhibitors absent. However, in batch cultivations exponential growth is of limited duration and as nutrient conditions change growth rate decreases entering the *deceleration phase* to

Fig. 4.2 Growth characteristics in a batch culture of a microorganism. (1) Lag phase; (2) transient acceleration; (3) exponential phase; (4) deceleration phase; (5) stationary phase; (6) death phase.

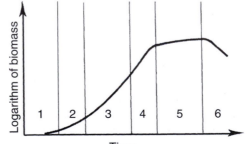

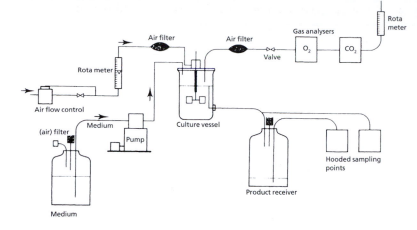

Fig. 4.3 A simple laboratory fermenter operating on a continuous basis.

be followed by the *stationary phase* when overall growth can no longer be obtained due to nutrient exhaustion. The final phase of the cycle is the *death phase* when growth has ceased. Most biotechnological batch processes are stopped before this stage because of decreasing metabolism and cell lysis.

In industrial usage, batch cultivation has been operated to optimise organism or biomass production and then to allow the organism to perform specific biochemical transformations such as end-product formation (e.g. amino acids, enzymes) or decomposition of substances (sewage treatment, bioremediation). Many important products such as antibiotics are optimally formed during the stationary phase of the growth cycle in batch cultivation.

However, there are means of prolonging the life of a batch culture and thus increasing the yield by various substrate feed methods:

(1) by the gradual addition of concentrated components of the nutrient, e.g. carbohydrates, so increasing the volume of the culture (*fed batch*) – used for industrial production of baker's yeast
(2) by addition of medium to the culture (*perfusion*) and withdrawal of an equal volume of used cell-free medium – used in mammalian cell cultivations.

In contrast to batch conditions the practice of *continuous cultivation* gives near balanced growth with little fluctuation of nutrients, metabolites or cell numbers or biomass. This practice depends on fresh medium entering a batch system at the exponential phase of growth with a corresponding withdrawal of medium *plus* cells. Continuous methods of cultivation will permit organisms to grow under steady state (unchanging) conditions, in which growth occurs at a constant rate and in a constant environment. In a completely mixed continuous culture system sterile medium is passed into the bioreactor (Fig. 4.3) at a steady flow rate and culture broth (medium, waste products and organisms) emerges from it at the same rate keeping the volume of the total culture in the bioreactor constant. Factors such as pH and the concentrations of nutrients and metabolic products, which inevitably change during batch cultivation, can be held near constant in continuous cultivations. In industrial practice continuously operated systems are

Table 4.5	Advantages of batch and fed-batch culture techniques in industry

1. Products may be required only in relatively small quantities at any given time.
2. Market needs may be intermittent.
3. Shelf-life of certain products is short.
4. High product concentration is required in broth to optimise downstream processing operations.
5. Some metabolic products are produced only during the stationary phase of the growth cycle.
6. Instability of some production strains requires their regular renewal.
7. Continuous processes can offer many technical difficulties.

Table 4.6	Characteristics of cultivation methods	
Type of culture	Operational characteristics	Application
Solid	Simple, cheap, selection of colonies from single cell possible; process control limited.	Maintenance of strains, genetic studies; production of enzymes; composting.
Film	Various types of bioreactors; trickling filter, rotating disc, packed bed, sponge reactor, rotating tube.	Waste-water treatment, monolayer culture (animal cells); bacterial leaching; vinegar production.
Submerged homogeneous distribution of cells; batch	'Spontaneous' reaction, various types of reactor: continuous stirred tank reactor, air lift, loop, deep shaft, etc.; agitation by stirrers, air, liquid process control for physical parameters possible; less for chemical and biological parameters.	Standard type of cultivation: antibiotics, solvents, acids, etc.
Fed-batch	Simple method for control of regulatory effects, e.g. glucose repression.	Production of baker's yeast.
Continuous one-stage homogeneous	Proper control of reaction; excellent role for kinetic and regulatory studies; higher costs for experiment; problem of aseptic operation, the need for highly trained operators.	Few cases of application in industrial scale; production of single-cell protein; waste-water treatment.

of limited use and include only single-cell protein (SCP) and ethanol productions and some forms of waste-water treatment processes. However, for many reasons (Table 4.5) batch cultivation systems represent the dominant form of industrial usage. The full range of cultivation methods for microorganisms is shown in Table 4.6.

Applied microbial genetics

An essential aspect of microbial biotechnology is concerned with deriving new and improved strains of producer microorganisms. This will involve the selection of microorganisms from natural sources, from culture collections and other organisations, or by further development of 'in-house' company strains. A wide range of techniques is available to modify, delete or add to the genetic complement of an organism. Selection and screening activities remain a major part of biotechnological programmes. Screening is the use of procedures to allow the detection and isolation of only those microorganisms or metabolites of interest among a large population.

Producer microorganisms require to be preserved with minimum degeneration of genetic qualities, and are normally preserved on agar medium, by reduced metabolism, drying, freeze-drying or by ultra-low temperatures. Genomes can be modified by mutagenesis or by various types of hybridisation. Mutational programmes are primarily aimed at strain improvement, and mutagens available include ultraviolet and ionising radiation and a wide range of chemical mutagens. Hybridisation between microorganisms is essentially a procedure that facilitates the recombination of genetic material between microorganisms and can be expressed by sexual and parasexual mechanisms. Protoplast fusion techniques have been used with many microbial cells as well as with plant and animal cells. Fusion rates can be greatly increased by means of the fusogen polyethylene glycol.

Recombinant DNA technologies allow the isolation, purification and selective amplification in specific host cells of discrete DNA fragments or genes from almost any organism. The basic technology is described elsewhere. Recombinant bacteria and fungi are used extensively in certain industrial enzyme productions, while mammalian cell lines are increasingly used for recombinant protein production. Gene manipulations are now widely used to (a) improve yield and quality of existing biomolecules (e.g. metabolites, proteins), (b) improve characteristics of existing products by protein engineering, and (c) alter pathways for synthesis of existing products.

4.3 | The bioreactor

Bioreactors are the containment vehicles of any biotechnology-based production process, be it for brewing, organic or amino acids, antibiotics, enzymes, vaccines or for bioremediation. For each biotechnology process the most suitable containment system must be designed to give the correct environment for optimising the growth and metabolic activity of the biocatalyst. Bioreactors range from simple stirred or non-stirred open containers to complex aseptic integrated systems involving varying levels of advanced computer control (Fig. 4.4).

Bioreactors occur in two distinct types (Fig. 4.4). In the first instance they are primarily non-aseptic systems where it is not absolutely essential to operate with entirely pure cultures, e.g. brewing, effluent disposal systems; while in the second type, aseptic conditions are a prerequisite for successful product formation, e.g. antibiotics, vitamins, polysaccharides and recombinant proteins. This type of process involves considerable challenges on the part of engineering construction and operation.

The physical form of many of the most widely used bioreactors has not altered much over the past forty years; however, in recent years, novel forms

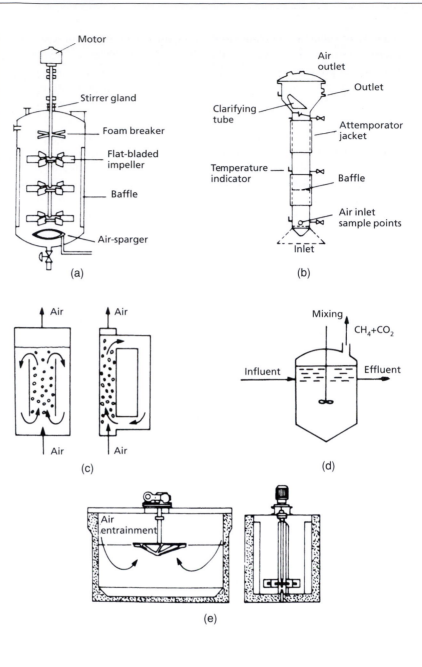

Fig. 4.4 Various forms of bioreactor. (a) Continuous stirred tank reactor. (b) Tower reactor. (c) Loop (recycle) bioreactor. (d) Anaerobic digester or bioreactor. (e) Activated sludge bioreactor. (*Source*: (a) and (b) reproduced by permission from Kristiansen and Chamberlain, 1983.)

of bioreactors have been developed to suit the needs of specific bioprocesses and such innovations are finding increasingly specialised roles in bioprocess technology (Fig. 4.4).

In all forms of fermentation the ultimate aim is to ensure that all parts of the system are subject to the same conditions. Within the bioreactor the microorganisms are suspended in the aqueous nutrient medium containing the necessary substrates for growth of the organism and required product formation. All nutrients, including oxygen, must be provided to diffuse into each cell and waste products such as heat, carbon dioxide and waste metabolites removed.

Table 4.7	Standards of materials used in sophisticated fermenter design

1. All materials coming into contact with the solutions entering the bioreactor or the actual organism culture must be corrosion resistant to prevent trace metal contamination of the process.
2. The materials must be non-toxic so that slight dissolution of the material or components does not inhibit culture growth.
3. The materials of the bioreactor must withstand repeated sterilisation with high-pressure steam.
4. The bioreactor stirrer system, entry ports and end plates must be easily machinable and sufficiently rigid not to be deformed or broken under mechanical stress.
5. Visual inspection of the medium and culture is advantageous, transparent materials should be used wherever possible.

The concentration of the nutrients in the vicinity of the organism must be held within a definite range since low values will limit the rate of organism metabolism while excessive concentrations can be toxic. Biological reactions run most efficiently within optimum ranges of environmental parameters, and in biotechnological processes these conditions must be provided on a micro-scale so that each cell is equally provided for. When the large scale of many bioreactor systems is considered it will be realised how difficult it is to achieve these conditions in a whole population. It is here that the skills of the process or biochemical engineer and the microbiologist must come together.

Fermentation reactions are multiphase, involving a gas phase (containing N_2, O_2 and CO_2), one or more liquid phases (aqueous medium and liquid substrate) and solid microphase (the microorganisms and possibly solid substrates). All phases must be kept in close contact to achieve rapid mass and heat transfer. In a perfectly mixed bioreactor all reactants entering the system must be immediately mixed and uniformly distributed to ensure homogeneity inside the reactor.

To achieve optimisation of the bioreactor system, the following operating guidelines must be closely adhered to:

(1) the bioreactor should be designed to exclude entrance of contaminating organisms as well as containing the desired organisms
(2) the culture volume should remain constant, i.e. no leakage or evaporation
(3) the dissolved oxygen level must be maintained above critical levels of aeration and culture agitation for aerobic organisms
(4) environmental parameters such as temperature, pH, etc., must be controlled and the culture volume must be well mixed.

The standard of materials used in the construction of sophisticated fermenters is important (Table 4.7).

Fermentation technologists seek to achieve a maximisation of culture potential by accurate control of the bioreactor environment. But still there is a great lack of true understanding of just what environmental conditions will produce an optimal yield of organism or product. Organisms with large cell size, such as animal cells compared to bacteria, have a complex demand for nutrients and lower growth rate. On the other hand their ability to produce complicated proteins is increased.

Successful bioprocessing will only occur when all the specific growth-related parameters are brought together, and the information used to improve and optimise the process. For successful commercial operation of these bioprocesses quantitative description of the cellular processes is an essential prerequisite: the two most relevant aspects, *yield* and *productivity,* are quantitative measures that will indicate how the cells convert the substrate into the product. The yield represents the amount of product obtained from the substrate while the productivity specifies the rate of product formation.

To understand and control a fermentation process it is necessary to know the state of the process over a small time increment and, further, to know how the organism responds to a set of measurable environmental conditions. Process optimisation requires accurate and rapid feedback control. In the future, the computer will be an integral part of most bioreactor systems. However, there is a lack of good sensor probes that will allow on-line analysis to be made on the chemical components of the fermentation process.

A large worldwide market exists for the development of new rapid methods monitoring the many reactions within a bioreactor. In particular, the greatest need is for innovatory microelectronic designs.

When endeavouring to improve existing process operations or design it is often advisable to set up mathematical models of the overall system. A model is a set of relationships between the variables in the system being studied. Such relationships are usually expressed in the form of mathematical equations but can also be specified as cause/effect relationships, which can be used in the operation of the specific processes. The actual variables involved can be extensive but will include any parameter that is of importance for the process and can include: pH, temperature, substrate concentration, agitation, feed rate, etc.

Bioreactor configurations have changed considerably over the last few decades. The original fermentation system was a shallow tank agitated or stirred by manpower. From this has developed the basic aeration tower system, which now dominates industrial usage. As fermentation systems were further developed, two design solutions to the problems of aeration and agitation have been implemented. The first approach uses mechanical aeration and agitation devices, with relatively high power requirements; the standard example is the centrally stirred tank reactor (CSTR), which is widely used throughout conventional laboratory and industrial fermentations. Such bioreactors ensure good gas/liquid mass transfer, have reasonable heat transfer, and ensure good mixing of the bioreactor contents.

The vertical shaft of the CSTR will carry one or more impellers depending on size of the bioreactor (Fig. 4.4a). A broad range of impellers have been investigated for stirring and creating homogeneous conditions within the bioreactor. The impellers are usually spaced at intervals equivalent to one tank diameter along the shaft to avoid a swirling type of liquid movement. The six flat-bladed (Rushton) turbine impellers are used in the majority of bioreactors and normally three to five are mounted to achieve good mixing and dispersion throughout the system. The function of the impellers is to create agitation or mixing within the bioreactor and to facilitate aeration. The primary function of agitation is to suspend the cells and nutrient evenly throughout the medium, to ensure that the nutrients, including oxygen, are available to the cells and to allow heat transfer. Most industrial organisms are aerobic and, in most fermentations, the organisms will exhibit a high oxygen demand. Since oxygen is sparingly soluble in aqueous solutions (solubility of CO_2 in water is about 30 times higher than that of O_2) aerobic fermentations can only be supported by vigorous and constant aeration of the medium.

The second main approach to aerobic bioreactor design uses air distribution (with low power consumption) to create forced and controlled liquid flow in a recycle or loop bioreactor. In this way the contents are subjected to a controlled recycle flow, either within the bioreactor or involving an external recycle loop. Thus stirring has been replaced by pumping, which may be mechanical or pneumatic, as in the case of the airlift bioreactor.

The centrally stirred tank reactor consists of a cylindrical vessel with a motor-driven central shaft that supports one or several agitators with the shaft entering either through the top or the bottom of the vessels. The aspect ratio (i.e. height-to-diameter ratio) of the vessel is three to five for microbial systems while for mammalian cell culture the aspect ratios do not normally exceed two. Sterile air is sparged into the bioreactor liquid below the bottom impeller by way of a perforated ring sparger. The speed of the impellors will be related to the degree of fragility of the cells. Mammalian cells are extremely fragile when compared to most microorganisms. In a great many of the high-value processes the bioreactors will be operated in a batch manner under aseptic monoculture. The bioreactors can range from c. 20 l to in excess of 250 m^3 for particular processes. The initial culture expansion of the microorganisms will commence in the smallest bioreactor, and when growth is optimised it will then be transferred to a larger bioreactor, and so forth, until the final operation bioreactor. Throughout such operations it is imperative to maintain aseptic conditions to ensure the success of the process. Bioreactors are normally sterilised prior to inoculation and contamination must be avoided during all subsequent operations. If contamination occurs during the cultivation this will invariably lead to process failure since more often than not the contaminant can outgrow the participating monoculture.

The number of distinct types of bioreactor is quite limited when measured against the wide range of production processes and the varied biological systems involved. In industrial practice, and less as a result of special advantage than as a need for flexibility in production equipment, the CSTR now occupies a dominant position and is virtually the only bioreactor design used in full-scale bioprocessing.

Large amounts of organic waste waters from domestic and industrial sources are routinely treated in aerobic and anaerobic systems. Activated sludge processes are widely used for the oxidative treatment of sewage and other liquid wastes (Fig. 4.4d). Such processes use batch or continuous agitated bioreactor systems to increase the entrainment of air to optimise oxidative breakdown of the organic material. These bioreactors are large and for optimum functioning will have several or many agitator units to facilitate mixing and oxygen uptake. They are widely used in most municipal sewage treatment plants.

Anaerobic bioreactors or digestors have long been used to treat sewage matter. In the absence of free oxygen certain microbial consortia are able to convert biodegradable organic material to methane, carbon dioxide and new microbial biomass. Most common anaerobic digesters work on a continuous or semi-continuous manner.

An outstanding example of methane generation is the Chinese biogas programme where millions of family-size anaerobic bioreactors are in operation. Such bioreactors are used for treatment of manure, human excreta, etc., producing biogas for cooking and lighting and the sanitisation of the waste, which then becomes an excellent fertiliser.

In almost all fermentation processes performed in a bioreactor there is generally a need to measure specific growth-related and environmental parameters, record them and then use the information to improve and optimise the process. Bioreactor control measurements are made in either an on-line or an off-line manner. With an on-line measurement the sensor is placed directly within the process stream whereas for off-line measurement a sample is removed aseptically from the process stream and analysed. Bioreactor processing is still severely limited by a shortage of reliable instruments capable of on-line measurement of important variables such as DNA, RNA, enzymes and biomass. Off-line analysis is still essential for these compounds and since the results of these analyses are usually not available until several hours after sampling, they cannot be used for immediate control purposes. However, on-line measurement is readily available for temperature, pH, dissolved oxygen and carbon dioxide analyses.

The continued discovery of new products such as therapeutic drugs from microorganisms and mammalian cells will continue to depend on the development of innovative exploratory culture systems, which encourage the biosynthesis of novel compounds. New miniaturised, computer-controlled incubator systems with automated analysis units are now available as single units that can perform hundreds of experiments simultaneously, thus producing a wealth of data in a short time to facilitate optimum fermentation conditions for product formation.

A new and quite novel approach involving combinatorial biology generates new products from genetically engineered microorganisms. DNA fragments or genes derived from unusual microorganisms that are not easily cultivated (recalcitrant microorganisms) can be transferred into easily cultivated or surrogate microorganisms and the resulting mixing and matching of genes encoding biosynthetic machinery is now offering the opportunity to discover new or modified molecules or drugs. This could be of great significance in antibiotic discovery.

While most high-value biotechnological compounds such as antibiotics and therapeutic proteins are produced in monoculture under strict conditions of asepsis there are now new avenues of research exploring product formation from mixed culture systems. Such systems may well produce different patterns of metabolites or indeed novel metabolites as a result of interactions that can occur between competing microorganisms. Because of the complexity of these mixed organism processes, they have all but been ignored by the scientific community. Monoculture under aseptic conditions is totally unnatural and rarely, if ever, occurs in nature. The norm is for microorganisms to exist together in the environment and to compete and respond to substrate availability and to the prevailing environmental conditions.

4.4 | Scale-up

Most biotechnological processes will have been identified at laboratory scale, and ultimate commercial success will be dependent on the ability to scale-up the process, first from laboratory to pilot plant level and then to full commercial scale. The achievement of successful process scale-up must fit within a range of physical and economic restraints. The identification of some of the controlling parameters can usually be made with laboratory scale bioreactors (5–10 l) and then moved to pilot scale level. A pilot plant is in reality a large-scale laboratory, which has been designed to give flexibility for equipment accommodation and adaptability for process operation. Pilot plant bioreactors range from 100–10 000 l total volume and the larger pilot bioreactors can, on occasion, be used as production units. Full-scale industrial bioreactors can range between 20 000 l and 400 000 l in volume (Fig. 4.5). The management of scale-up requires high capital investment in mixing and aeration, in monitoring and control devices, and in stringent maintenance of sterility.

4.5 | Media design for fermentation processes

Water is at the centre of all biotechnological processes and in most cases will be the dominant component of the media in which organisms (microorganisms, plant and animal cells) will grow. After liquid fermentation processes have achieved optimum production the removal of water is a major factor in the cost of bioproduct recovery and downstream processing. The quality of water is highly relevant as it affects organism growth and the production of specific bioproducts. In the past, traditional brewing centres were established in localities where natural sources provided water of high quality without having to resort to extensive pre-treatment.

In media production there is usually quality control of the raw materials. It is increasingly being realised that, in respect of volume, water is one of the most important raw materials in many biotechnological processes and that its supply and use must be carefully monitored and controlled.

The basic nutritional requirements of microorganisms are an energy or carbon source, an available nitrogen source, inorganic elements, and for some cell types, specific growth factors. In most biotechnological processes, carbon and nitrogen sources are more often derived from relatively complex mixtures of cheap natural products or by-products (Table 4.8).

Availability and type of nutrient can exert strong physiological control over fermentation reactions and product formation. Raw material input to

Fig. 4.5 A typical industrial stirred tank bioreactor. (1) reactor vessel; (2) jacket; (3) insulation; (4) shroud; (5) inoculum; (6) ports for pH, temperature and dissolved oxygen sensors; (7) agitator; (8) gas sparger; (9) mechanical seals; (10) reducing gearbox; (11) motor; (12) harvest nozzle; (13) jacket connections; (14) sample valve with steam connections; (15) sight glass; (16) connections for acid, alkali and antifoam chemicals; (17) air inlet; (18) removable top; (19) medium or feed nozzle; (20) air exhaust nozzle; (21) instrument parts (several); (22) foam breaker; (23) sight glass with light (not shown) and steam connection; (24) rupture disc nozzle. (*Source*: from Chisti, 2006, with permission.)

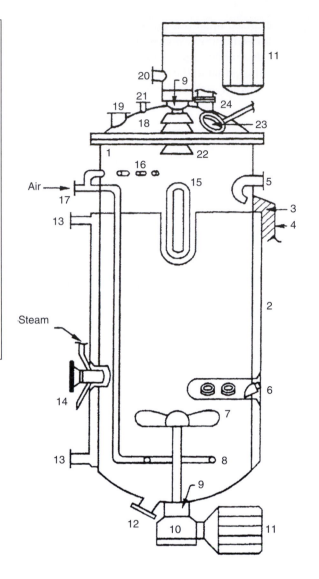

a fermentation will be largely dependent on the cost of the material at a particular time, since commodity market prices do alter with seasonal and other variables.

If biomass or a growth-associated product is the aim of the fermentation then it is required that the medium must allow maximum growth potential throughout the fermentation, whereas for a compound not growth-limited, e.g. organic acids, antibiotics, etc., a medium must be formulated that after an initial growth phase will become deficient in one or more nutrients. Depending on the process, limitation of phosphorus, nitrogen, carbohydrates or trace metals can induce product formation. In some fermentations high levels of glucose can create catabolite repression of, for example, enzyme synthesis; this can be overcome by using other slowly fermentable carbohydrates or by incremental or continuous feeding of the glucose.

Table 4.8 | Sources of carbohydrate and nitrogen for industrial media

Sources of carbohydrate	Sources of nitrogen (% nitrogen by weight)
Glucose: pure glucose monohydrate, hydrolysed starch	Barley (1.5–2.0) Beet molasses (1.5–2.0)
Lactose: pure lactose, whey powder	Corn-steep liquor (4.5)
Starch: barley, groundnut meal, oat flour, rye flour, soybean meal	Groundnut meal (8.0) Oat flour (1.5–2.0) Pharmamedia (8.0)
Sucrose: beet molasses, cane molasses, crude brown sugar, pure white sugar	Rye flour (1.5–2.0) Soybean meal (8.0) Whey powder (4.5)

Sterilisation practices for biotechnological media must achieve maximum destruction of contaminating microorganisms, with minimum temperature damage to medium components. Mostly, batch-wise sterilisation in the bioreactor is still the most widely used method, although continuous methods are gaining increased acceptability.

Media preparation may seem to be a relatively uninteresting part of the overall bioprocess but it is in fact the cornerstone of the whole operation. Poor media design will lead to low efficiency of growth and concomitant poor product formation.

4.6 | Solid substrate fermentation

There are many biotechnological processes that involve the growth of microorganisms on solid substrates in the absence or near absence of free water (Table 4.9). The most regularly used solid substrates are cereal grains, legume seeds, wheat bran, lignocellulose materials such as straws, sawdust or wood shavings, and a wide range of plant and animal materials. Most of these compounds are polymeric molecules, insoluble or sparingly soluble in water, but are mostly cheap, easily obtainable and represent a concentrated source of nutrients for microbial growth.

Many of these fermentations have great antiquity and in many instances there are records dating back hundreds of years. In the Orient there is a wide array of food fermentations, including soy sauce and tempeh, as well as many large industrial enzyme processes. In the West, the fermentation processes have centred on the production of silage, mushroom cultivation, cheese and sauerkraut production, and the composting of plant and animal wastes. Solid substrate fermentations using recyclable raw materials such as straw, wood and other waste materials could well be industries of the future producing ethanol, methane and edible biomass.

Table 4.9 | Some examples of solid-substrate fermentations

Example	Substrate	Microorganism(s) involved
Mushroom production (European and Oriental)	Straw, manure	*Agaricus bisporus* *Lentinus edodes* *Volvariella volvaceae*
Sauerkraut	Cabbage	Lactic acid bacteria
Soy sauce	Soybeans and wheat	*Aspergillus oryzae*
Tempeh	Soybeans	*Rhizopus oligosporus*
Ontjom	Peanut press cake	*Neurospora sitophila*
Cheeses	Milk curd	*Penicillium roquefortii*
Leaching of metals	Low-grade ores	*Thiobacillus* spp.
Organic acids	Cane sugar, molasses	*Aspergillus niger*
Enzymes	Wheat bran etc.	*Aspergillus niger*
Composting	Mixed organic material	Fungi, bacteria, actinomycetes
Sewage treatment	Components of sewage	Bacteria, fungi and protozoa

The microbiological components of solid substrate fermentations can occur as single pure cultures, mixed identifiable cultures or totally mixed indigenous microorganisms.

Solid substrate fermentations using indigenous microorganisms are primarily ensiling and composting. Ensiling is an anaerobic process involving agricultural materials, mostly grasses, in which the bacterium *Lactobacillus bulgaricus* gradually becomes the dominant organism producing lactic acid, which inhibits potential putrefactive bacteria. The end-product – silage – is massively produced in temperate countries as a winter feed for farm animals. Composting is examined in detail in a later chapter.

Solid substrate fermentations involving pure fungal cultures have long been practised in the ancient Oriental Koji process in which grains and soy beans are fermented with the fungus *Aspergillus oryzae* to produce a range of enzymes, e.g. proteases and amylases. In soy sauce production the grain is fermented to produce the above enzymes and then subjected to a mixed bacterial/yeast fermentation. In mushroom production the substrate is derived by a composting process, which then supports the pure culture growth of the specific fungus, e.g. *Agaricus bisporus*. Again, mushroom cultivation by solid substrate fermentation is a huge worldwide industry.

The Japanese Koji bioreactor provides a good environment for fungus growth and product formation, controlled mechanical agitation, reasonable process control and sterile operation conditions. Most are operated in a batch system but can be semi-continuous or continuous.

In many solid substrate fermentations there is a need to pre-treat the substrate raw materials to enhance the availability of the bound nutrients and also to reduce the size of the components, e.g. pulverised straw, shredded vegetable materials, to optimise the physical aspects of the process. However, cost aspects of pre-treatment must be balanced with eventual product value. Bioreactor designs for solid substrate fermentations are inherently simpler than for liquid cultivations. They are classified into

| Table 4.10 | Advantages and disadvantages of solid-substrate compared with liquid fermentation |

Advantages	Disadvantages
Simple media with cheaper natural rather than costly fossil-derived components.	Processes limited mainly to moulds that tolerate low moisture levels.
Low moisture content of materials gives economy of bioreactor space, low liquid effluent treatment, less microbial contamination, often no need to sterilise, easier downstream processing.	Metabolic heat production in large-scale operation creates problems.
	Process monitoring, e.g. moisture levels, biomass, O_2 and CO_2 levels, is difficult to achieve accurately.
Aeration requirements can be met by simple gas diffusion or by aerating intermittently, rather than continuously.	Bioreactor design not well developed.
Yields of products can be high.	Product limitation.
Low energy expenditure compared with stirred tank bioreactors.	Slower growth rate of microorganisms.

fermentations (a) without agitation; (b) with occasional agitation; and (c) with continuous agitation. The relative advantages and disadvantages of solid substrate fermentations when compared with liquid fermentations are represented in Table 4.10.

4.7 | Technology of mammalian and plant cell culture

Mammalian cell culture

The main impetus to achieve mass in vitro cultivation of mammalian cells dates from the early 1950s with the need to produce large quantities of polio vaccine. Polio virus was produced from cultured cells derived from primate neural and kidney tissue, and polio viral vaccines from monkey kidney cells. Shortly afterwards other viral vaccines, mumps, measles and adenovirus, were produced from various cultured animal cells. During the second half of the twentieth century there was a major drive to develop media and cultivation practices to produce viable and actively proliferating cell cultures from a wide range of different organisms including mammals such as humans, rats, mice, hamsters, monkeys, cattle, sheep, horses and, more recently, from fish and insects. Specific cell lines have been obtained from human organs such as the liver, kidney, lungs, lymph nodes, heart and ovaries, together with an extensive range of various cancer cell lines. A cell line can be viewed as a population of genetically identical cells (clones) derived from a single parent cell.

In living systems mammalian cells do not exist in isolation, like a microbial cell, but are organised into functioning organs (e.g. liver, heart) and will obtain the necessary nutrients for metabolism and growth by way of blood circulation. To mimic the complexity of the blood supply has been a continuing area of study, and now many successful media formulations have been achieved that will vary in make-up depending on the cell type. Most media will normally contain a complex mixture of organic compounds, such as amino acids, vitamins, organic acids and others, together with buffering inorganic salts. Some media still contain blood serum (5–20%) for the supply of growth factors, trace elements, lipids and other unknown factors. However, the use of serum creates many problems including variability of nutrient content between batches, irregularity of supply, and now more recently the concern that serum may be contaminated with virions or prion particles.

When mammalian cells are cultured they grow as unicellular organisms, multiplying by division provided suitable nutrient and correct environmental conditions are available. Such cells differ from microbial and plant cells in lacking a rigid outer cell wall, making them vulnerable to shear forces and to changes in osmolarity. Furthermore, they are extremely sensitive to impurities in water, to the cost and quality control of media, and the need to avoid contamination by more rapidly growing microorganisms.

Freshly isolated cultures from mammalian systems are known as *primary cultures* until subcultured. At this stage they are usually heterogeneous but still closely representative of the parent cell types and in the expression of tissue-specific properties. After several subcultures onto fresh media, the cell line will either die out or 'transform' to become a *continuous or immortalised cell line*. Such cell lines show many alterations from the primary cultures including changes in cytomorphology, increased growth rate, increase in chromosome variation and increase in tumorigenicity. In vitro transformation is primarily the acquisition of an infinite lifespan.

Mammalian cells can be grown either in an unattached suspension culture or attached to a solid surface. Cells such as Hela cells (cells derived from a human malignancy) can grow in either state, lymphoblastoid cells can grow in suspension culture, while primary or normal diploid cells will only grow when they are attached to a solid surface. Most future commercial development with mammalian cells will be dominated by the cultivation of anchorage-dependent cell types.

Monolayer cultivation of animal cells is governed by the surface area available for attachment, and design considerations have been directed to methods of increasing surface area. Early designs relied mainly on roller tubes or bottles to ensure exchange of nutrients and gases. A recent sophisticated system supports the growth of cells in coils of gas-permeable Teflon tubing, each tube having a surface area of $10\,000\,cm^2$, and up to 20 such coils can be incorporated into an incubator chamber. A wide range of cells has been successfully cultured under these conditions.

Suspension cultures have been successfully developed to quite large bioreactor volumes thus allowing all the engineering advantages of the stirred tank bioreactor that have accrued from microbial studies to be used to advantage. Such studies have only been on a batch-culture basis.

A combination of attachment culture and suspension culture by the use of porous microcarrier beads has been a major recent innovation in this area. In principle, the anchorage-dependent cells attach to special DEAE-Sephadex beads (having a surface area of $7\,cm^2\,mg^{-1}$), which are able to float in suspension. In this way, the engineering advantages of the stirred bioreactor may be used with anchored cells. Many cell types have been grown in this manner with successful production of viruses and human interferon. The undoubted success of the microcarrier beads may eventually lead to the demise of conventional monolayer systems. New bioreactor designs involving the microcarrier bead concept will surely create a wider commercial development of animal and human cell types.

While such cell lines have allowed extensive studies in mammalian cell biochemistry, the major practical applications have included vaccine production (polio, mumps, rabies, etc.), toxicological and pharmaceutical research with the aim to reduce animal testing, the production of artificial organs and skin, and the extensive use of mammalian cell lines as producers of proteins for diagnostic (monoclonal antibodies) (see later) and for recombinant therapeutic applications (interferons, hormones, insulin, etc.). Monoclonal antibodies are the most important mammalian cell culture glycoprotein products and make up at least one quarter of therapeutic achievements in the biotechnology industry, and were valued at almost US$3 billion in 2001, and increasing. The introduction of foreign genes into mammalian cell lines is now relatively commonplace and will be relevant to improving cell lines in many ways such as extending productivity, the ability to grow on serum-free media and to increase the range of productivity of human therapeutic molecules (see later for details of recombinant proteins).

All biological products used for therapeutic purposes and on the market today are manufactured in either a mammalian or microbial cell line. Mammalian cell lines (e.g. immortalised Chinese hamster ovary cells, mouse myeloma, human embryo kidney and human retinal cells) are now the dominant system for production of recombinant proteins for clinical applications because they can achieve proper protein folding, assembly and post-translational modifications. While most mammalian culture processes involve suspension cultivation there is still considerable diversity in manufacturing methods, in particular, adherent cell culture. Almost all of the high-yielding processes being used are extended batch suspension cultures to which medium components are added in small aliquots or semi-continuously. The productivity of mammalian cells cultivated in bioreactors has achieved gram per litre range in many cases, more than a one hundred-fold yield improvement compared with similar processes in the mid-1980s. Such improvements are mainly due to media composition and process control.

Tissue engineering is a form of regenerative medicine, and the main products such as skin are becoming a clinical success. However, such products are expensive to manufacture and as with experimental drugs, their development costs are high. In essence, most human tissue engineering products are processed in the laboratory by growing cells in culture derived from the actual patient or a donor and then seeding them on to a suitable scaffold and stimulating the cells to proliferate and form specific tissues, e.g. skin. The scaffolds are constructed from natural biomaterials, synthetic or semi-synthetic materials, which offer support for the cells to grow and maintain their differentiated formation. The architecture of the scaffold will determine the shape and pattern of the new tissue. For burns victims the ability to produce new skin from the patient by tissue engineering has been a major success story. In the foreseeable future it is anticipated that tissue-engineered products could offer alternatives to organ donor transplants and many forms of surgical reconstructions. However, much has yet to be done on process design and manufacture to achieve affordable and assured products.

Plant cell culture

The use of plant cell or organ culture techniques for micropropagation of certain plants is discussed later. In such cases, plant cell cultures will progress through organogenesis, plantlet amplification and eventual establishment in soil. However, large-scale production in bioreactors of suspension cell cultures of many plant species has now been achieved and yields of products typical of the whole plant have been impressive, e.g. nicotine, alkaloids and ginseng. It is now envisaged that large-scale fermentation programmes may be able to produce commercially acceptable levels of certain high-value plant products, e.g. digitalis, jasmine, spearmint, codeine, etc. Such processes are considered as plant cell biotechnology.

The fermentation methods used to grow plant cells in liquid agitated culture have been largely derived from microbial techniques. Plant cell culture is much slower than with microorganisms (e.g. doubling times c. 24–72 h), though most of the other characteristics of fermentation are quite similar. The volume of an average cultured plant cell can be up to 200 000 times that of a bacterial cell. A common feature of plant cell culture is that growth and production phases are generally separated, and require two-stage processes in which the conditions for growth and production are separately optimised. Batch and fed-batch operation are the most common bioreactor systems. Although some plant products are now appearing on the market, it is not expected to be commercially attractive for some time.

4.8 | Metabolic engineering

Metabolic engineering (systems biology) is a systems-orientated approach to the analysis and synthesis of entire biological systems with the aim of controlling cellular properties. Outstanding examples are the experimental studies with microbial, plant and mammalian cells under controlled and reproducible conditions in bioreactors accompanied by a broad spectrum of modern bioanalysis. The accurate control of the environment within the bioreactor can promote perturbations of the biological systems leading to improvements of yield, selectivity and productivity when the contained organisms are involved in productive, biotechnological processes. Such systems also allow analysis of flow distribution and mathematical modelling and simulation experiments.

Table 4.11	Downstream processing operations
Separation	Filtration
	Centrifugation
	Flotation
	Disruption
Concentration	Solubilisation
	Extraction
	Thermal processing
	Membrane filtration
	Precipitation
Purification	Crystallisation
	Chromatography
Modification	
Drying	

4.9 | Downstream processing

Downstream processing refers to the isolation and purification of a biotech-nologically formed product to a state suitable for the intended use. In most, but not all, biotechnology processes the desired product(s) will be in dilute aqueous solution and the ultimate level of downstream processing will mir-ror the type of product and required degree of purity. The range of products is considerable and varied in form and can include whole cells, amino acids, vitamins, organic acids, solvents, enzymes, vaccines, therapeutic proteins and monoclonal antibodies. Within these products there will be consider-able variation in molecular size and chemical complexity, and a wide range of separation methods will be required for recovery and purification. While many of the products are relatively stable in structure others can be highly labile and require careful application of the methodology.

The design and efficient operation of downstream processing operations are vital elements in getting the required products into commercial use, and should reflect the need not to lose more of the desired product than is absolutely necessary. An example of the effort expended in downstream processing is provided by the plant Eli Lilly built to produce human insulin (Humulin). Over 90% of the 200 staff were involved in recovery processes. Thus, downstream processing of biotechnological processes represents a major part of the overall costs of most processes, but is also the least heralded aspect of biotechnology. Improvements in downstream processing will benefit the overall efficiency and costs of the processes.

Downstream processing will primarily be concerned with initial sepa-ration of the bioreactor broth into a liquid phase and a solid phase, and subsequent concentration and purification of the product. Downstream processing is a multistage operation (Table 4.11).

Fermentation broths are normally unstable and prone to microbial con-tamination when removed from the bioreactor. Downstream processing will depend largely on the chemical and physical properties of the products.

Initial pre-treatment or conditioning of the broth can involve flocculation of cells or solids, or the breakdown of cells to release intracellular products such as enzymes. Separation of components in the liquid phase of the broth can involve settling, filtration, centrifugation or electrokinetic separation, with the final degree of processing dependent on the final use of the products. When the product has been separated from the liquid phase and the solid phase (e.g. microbial biomass), the broth will be disposed of by standard sewage treatment.

Final product isolation will utilise established chemical and biochemical technologies. Molecular size or centrifugation will determine the extraction processes that will be most suitable, and will be influenced by product quality and overall economics. Final product purity will reflect the type of product and the standard of purity required. A wide range of methods are currently used and include evaporation and distillation, precipitation, membrane filtration, adsorption, affinity, ion-exchange and gel-filtration chromatographies.

Final products of the downstream purification stages should have some degree of stability for commercial distribution. Stability is best achieved for most products by using some form of drying. In practice this is achieved by spray-drying, fluidised-bed drying or by freeze-drying. The method of choice is product and cost dependent. Products sold in the dry form include organic acids, amino acids, antibiotics, polysaccharides, enzymes, single-cell protein and many others. Many products cannot be supplied easily in a dried form and must be sold in liquid preparations. Care must be taken to avoid microbial contamination and deterioration and, when the product is proteinaceous, to avoid denaturation.

The role of downstream processing will continue to be one of the most challenging and demanding parts of many biotechnological processes. Purity and stability are the hallmarks of most high-value biotechnological products.

It can be said that biotechnological processes will, in most part, need to be contained within a defined area or bioreactor and to a large extent the ultimate success of most of the processes will depend on the correct choice and operation of these systems. For most high-value products cultivation of the producer organism will normally be by monoculture requiring complete asepsis to maximise product formation. On the industrial side, the scale of operation will, for economic reasons, mainly be very large, and in almost all cases the final success will require the closest cooperation between the bioscientist, the chemist and the process or biochemical engineer – in this way demonstrating the truly interdisciplinary nature of biotechnological processes.

Chapter 5

Enzyme technology

5.1 | The nature of enzymes

Enzymes are complex globular proteins present in living cells where they act as catalysts that facilitate chemical changes in substances. In 1878 Kühne introduced the term 'enzyme' from the Greek *enzumos*, which refers to the leavening of bread by yeast. With the development of the science of biochemistry has come a fuller understanding of the wide range of enzymes present in living cells and of their modes of action. Without enzymes there can be no life. Although enzymes are only formed in living cells, many can be extracted or separated from the cells and can continue to function in vitro. This unique ability of enzymes to perform their specific chemical transformations in isolation has led to an ever-increasing use of enzymes in industrial and food processes, bioremediation and in medicine, and their production is collectively termed enzyme technology.

The activity of an enzyme is due to its catalytic nature. An enzyme carries out its activity without being consumed in the reaction, while the reaction occurs at a very much higher rate when the enzyme is present. Enzymes are highly specific and function only on designated types of compounds, the substrates. A minute amount of enzyme can react with a large amount of substrate. The catalytic function of the enzyme is due not only to its primary molecular structure but also to the intricate folding configuration of the whole enzyme molecule. It is this configuration that endows the protein with its specific catalytic function; to disturb the configuration by, for example, a change in pH or temperature, may result in the activity being lost. For some enzymes there is an obligatory need for additional factors, termed co-factors, which can be metal ions, nucleotides, etc. Because of their specificity enzymes can differentiate between chemicals with closely related structures and can catalyse reactions over a wide range of temperatures (0–110°C) and in the pH range 2–14. In industrial application this can result in high-quality products, fewer by-products and simpler purification procedures. Furthermore, enzymes are non-toxic and biodegradable (an attractive 'green' issue) and can be produced especially from microorganisms in large amounts without the need for special chemical-resistant equipment.

Table 5.1 Distribution of bulk-produced enzymes by value

Specific area	Percentage
Food	41
Detergents	34
Textiles	11
Leather	3
Pulp/paper	1
Other applications	6

Table 5.2 Approximate annual world production of some industrial enzymes

Enzyme	Tonnes pure enzyme
Bacillus protease	550
Amylo glucosidase	350
Bacillus amylase	350
Glucose isomerase	60
Microbial rennet	25
Fungal amylase	20
Pectinase	20
Fungal protease	15

Enzyme technology embraces production, isolation, purification and use in soluble or immobilised form. Commercially produced enzymes will undoubtedly contribute to the solution of some of the most vital problems with which modern society is confronted, e.g. food production, energy shortage and preservation, improvement of the environment, together with numerous medical applications. This new technology has its origins in biochemistry, but has drawn heavily on microbiology, chemistry and process engineering to achieve the present status of the science. For the future, enzyme technology and genetic engineering will be two very closely related areas of study dealing with the application of genes and of their products. Together these sciences will attempt to creatively exploit the continuous flow of discoveries being made by molecular geneticists and enzymologists.

It is estimated that the world market for enzymes is over US$2 billion and will double over the next decade. Enzyme production and utilisation is one of the most successful areas of modern biotechnology and has increased by *c.* 12% annually over the past ten years. There are now over 400 companies worldwide involved in enzyme production, with European companies dominating (60%) and the USA and Japan with 30%. Bulk enzyme distribution in various industries is shown in Table 5.1, and production of specific bulk enzymes is shown in Table 5.2.

5.2 | The application of enzymes

For thousands of years processes such as brewing, breadmaking and production of cheeses have involved the serendipitous use of enzymes (see Table 5.3). The Greek epic poems *The Odyssey* and *The Iliad*, dating from around 700 BC, both refer to the use of what we now recognise as enzymes in cheese-making. In this way, traditional practices and technologies that relied on enzymic conversions were well established before any coherent body of knowledge on their rational application had been developed.

In the West the industrial understanding of enzymes revolved around yeast and malt where traditional baking and brewing industries were rapidly expanding. Much of the early development of biochemistry was centred around yeast fermentations and processes for conversion of starch to sugar. In the Orient the comparable industries were saké production and many food fermentations, all of which made use of bacteria and filamentous fungi as the sources of enzyme activity. The considered beginnings of modern microbial enzyme technology was the first marketing in the West of takadiastase, a rather crude mixture of hydrolytic enzymes prepared by growing the fungus *Aspergillus oryzae* on wheat bran. A patent was lodged with the US Patent Office in 1884 by a Japanese scientist, Dr Jokichi Takamine. The method of takadiastase production varied little from that practised for thousands of years in Asia, but it did represent an important transfer of technology from East to West.

Leather has always been an important commodity, and originally the process by which hides were softened before tanning, termed 'bating', was most obnoxious, requiring the use of dog faeces and pigeon droppings. However, at the turn of the twentieth century, Otto Rohm, a distinguished German chemist, determined that the active components in dog faeces were proteases – enzymes that degrade proteins. He was able to demonstrate that extracts from animal organs that produced similar enzymes could be used instead of the faeces, and from 1905 pig and cow pancreases were to provide a more socially acceptable and reliable source of these enzymes.

The early local use of enzymes in various processes relied on plant and animal sources. Proteases such as papain from papaya, ficin from figs and bromelain from pineapple are still important commercial sources. From animals there are still considerable viable sources for esterases, proteases and lipases, such as rennets, pepsin, chymosin and lysozyme. While these sources of enzymes continue to have industrial importance they do have limitations including lack of consistent quality and availability and in the case of some plant enzymes, disturbance of supply due to weather and political instability at source.

It was not until the mid-1950s that rapid development in enzyme technology occurred, using, in particular, microbial enzyme sources. The reasons for this are varied but depended largely on the following.

(1) There was a major development in submerged cultivation practices with microorganisms primarily associated with the World War II penicillin production processes, and this newly acquired knowledge was readily

Table 5.3 | Industrial applications of enzymes

Application	Enzymes used	Uses	Problems
Biological detergents	Primarily proteinases, produced in an extracellular form from bacteria. Amylase enzymes.	Used for pre-soak conditions and direct liquid applications. Detergents for machine dishwashing to remove resistant starch residues.	Allergic response of process workers; now overcome by encapsulation techniques.
Baking industry	Fungal alpha-amylase enzymes; normally inactivated about 50°C, destroyed during baking process. Proteinase enzymes.	Catalyse breakdown of starch in the flour to sugar, which can be used by the yeast. Used in production of white bread, buns, rolls. Biscuit manufacture to lower the protein level of the flour.	
Brewing industry	Enzymes produced from barley during mashing stage of beer production.	Degrade starch and proteins to produce simple sugars, amino acids and peptides used by the yeasts to enhance alcohol production.	
	Industrially produced enzymes: amylases, glucanases, proteinases; beta glucanase; amyloglucosidase proteinases.	Now widely used in the brewing process: split polysaccharides and proteins in the malt; improve filtration characteristics; low-calorie beer, remove cloudiness during storage of beers.	
Dairy industry	Rennin, derived from the stomachs of young ruminant animals (calves, lambs, kids). Microbially produced enzymes. Lipases. Lactases.	Manufacture of cheese, used to split protein. Now finding increasing use in the dairy industry. Enhance ripening of blue-mould cheeses (Danish Blue, Roquefort). Break down lactose to glucose and galactose.	Older animals cannot be used as with increasing age rennin production decreases and is replaced by another proteinase, pepsin, which is not suitable for cheese production. In recent years the great increase in cheese consumption together with increased beef production has resulted in increasing shortage of rennin and escalating prices.

Table 5.3 | *(cont.)*

Application	Enzymes used	Uses	Problems
Starch industry	Amylases, amyloglucosidases and glucoamylases.	Convert starch into glucose and various syrups.	
	Glucose isomerase.	Converts glucose into fructose (high-fructose syrups derived from starchy materials have enhanced sweetening properties and lower calorific values).	
	Immobilised enzymes.	Production of high-fructose syrups.	Widely used in USA and Japan but EEC restrictive practices to protect sugar-beet farmers prohibits use.
Textile industry	Amylase enzymes.	Now widely used to remove starch, which is used as an adhesive or size on threads of certain fabrics to prevent damage during weaving. (Traditionally, desizing using strong chemicals has prevailed).	
	Bacterial enzymes.	Generally preferred for desizing since they are able to withstand working temperatures up to 100–110°C.	
Leather industry	Enzymes found in dog and pigeon dung.	Traditionally used to treat leather to make it pliable by removing certain protein components. (The process is called bating; strong bating required to achieve a soft, pliable leather; slight bating for the soles of shoes).	Offensive preparation.
	Trypsin enzymes from slaughterhouses and from microorganisms.	Now largely replacing the enzymes mentioned above for bating. Also used for removing the hair from hides and skins.	
Medical and pharmaceutical uses	Trypsin.	Debridement of wounds, dissolving blood clots.	
	Pancreatic trypsin.	Digestive aid formulations, treatment of inflammations, etc.	
		Many enzymes used in clinical chemistry as diagnostic tools.	

applied to the large-scale cultivation of other microorganisms and subsequently for microbial enzyme production.

(2) Basic knowledge of enzyme properties was rapidly expanding and this led to the realisation of the potential for using enzymes as industrial catalysts.

(3) Most enzymes of potential industrial importance could be produced from some microorganism.

The more recent expansion of the enzyme industry came with the advent of genetic engineering. Recombinant microorganisms are now the largest source of enzymes for a wide variety of applications.

The further development of enzymes as additives was largely to provide enhancement of traditional processes rather than to open up new possibilities. Even now, most bulk production of crude enzymes is concerned largely with enzymes that hydrolyse the glucosidic links of carbohydrates such as starch and pectins, and with the proteases that hydrolyse the peptide links of proteins.

Approximately 90% of bulk enzyme production is derived from microorganisms such as filamentous fungi, bacteria and yeasts, and the remainder from animals (6%) and plants (4%).

Cell-free enzymes have many advantages over chemical processes where a number of sequential reactions are involved. In fermentation processes the use of microbial cells as catalysts can have some limitations.

(1) A high proportion of the substrate will normally be converted to biomass.

(2) Wasteful side reactions may occur.

(3) The conditions for growth of the microorganisms may not be the same for product formation.

(4) The isolation and purification of the desired product from the fermentation liquor may be difficult.

Many, if not all, of these limitations may be alleviated by the use of purified enzymes and possibly by the further use of enzymes in an immobilised form. In the future, many traditional fermentations may be replaced by multienzyme reactors that would create highly efficient rates of substrate utilisation, higher yields and higher product uniformity.

There is now a rapid proliferation of uses and potential uses for more highly purified enzyme preparations in industrial processing, clinical medicine and laboratory practice. The range of pure enzymes now available commercially is rapidly increasing. Enzymes that are sold at over 10 000 tonnes annually cost US$5–30 per kilogram, speciality enzymes less than 1 tonne, US$50 000 per kilogram, while therapeutic enzymes can cost over US$5 000 per kilogram.

In many operations, such as clarifying wines and juices, chill proofing of beer and improving bread doughs, the use of crude enzymes is likely to add very little to the cost of the product. Most of the enzymes used on an industrial scale are extracellular enzymes, i.e. enzymes that are normally excreted by the microorganism to act upon their substrate in an external environment, and are analogous to the digestive enzymes of humans and animals. Thus, when microorganisms produce enzymes to split large external molecules into an assimilable form, the enzymes are usually excreted into the fermentation media. In this way the fermentation broth from the cultivation of certain microorganisms, for example, bacteria, yeasts or filamentous fungi, then becomes a major source of proteases, amylases and (to a lesser extent) cellulases, lipases, etc. Most industrial enzymes are hydrolases and are capable of acting without complex co-factors; they are readily separated from microorganisms without rupturing the cell walls and are water soluble.

Some intracellular enzymes are now being produced industrially and include glucose oxidase for food preservation, asparaginase for cancer therapy and penicillin acylase for antibiotic conversion. Since most cellular enzymes are by nature intracellular, more advances can be expected in this area.

The sales of industrial enzymes were relatively small up until about 1965 when enzymes in detergents came into general use. There was a massive increase in the use of enzymes in detergents between 1966 and 1969 but this was to collapse between the years 1969 and 1970, when apparent allergic symptoms were discovered in workers handling enzymes at the factory level. There was much press hysteria and enzymes were mostly taken out of detergents. However, with proper precautions in the factories and by encapsulating the enzymes before reaching the customer, the postulated risks were eliminated; careful studies found neither any adverse environmental effects from the use of enzymes nor any effects on domestic users. Once again the application of enzymes in detergents has achieved good levels and there is a steady growth in the use of enzymes in that part of the detergent industry where enzymes can improve washing results. Indeed, the widest application of enzymes is now with their detergent use, in household laundry, dishwashing and in industrial and institutional operations.

In Western Europe hot-water washes (c. 65–70°C) have been considered essential for most clothes-cleaning operations, whereas in the USA and Canada most machines operate at 55°C. In complete contrast, in Japan clothes are usually washed for longer periods with cold water. Thus, universally there is increased interest in the use of detergent enzymes that function well at relatively low temperatures, i.e. 20–30°C. While proteases have dominated the detergent market there is increasing use of amylases and lipases, for the removal of starches and fats. Cellulase has recently entered the detergent market and unlike the other enzymes, which degrade particular stains, the cellulases act directly on the fabric. When new, cotton consists of smooth fibres, but with prolonged use and washing microfibrils or broken strands of fibre create a 'fuzz' or roughness on the fabric surface. The cellulases remove this and so improve the appearance and feel or smoothness of the fabric. Cellulases are also used to restore colour of cotton that has been washed several times and to give jeans the so-called 'stone-wash' look.

In the starch processing industry corn starch is the most widely used raw material followed by wheat, tapioca and potatoes. A wide range of sweeteners can be derived from the enzymatic processing of starch (Fig. 5.1).

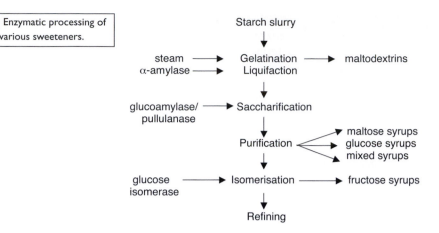

Fig. 5.1 Enzymatic processing of starch to various sweeteners.

Heat-stable α-amylases were discovered in the early 1970s and have revolutionised industrial starch saccharification, replacing acid hydrolysis.

Starch from renewable raw materials such as corn, wheat, rice and cassava is now being hydrolysed to glucose, which is, in turn, converted to ethanol by yeast fermentations and used for the production of biofuel or bioethanol (see later).

However, a vast proportion of the chemical and energy reserves in renewable plant material is locked up in the form of cell-wall material comprising cellulose, complex polysaccharides and phenolic polymers such as lignin. While starch will always be a major substrate for bioethanol production the ultimate raw material will be renewable lignocellulose. Novel hydrolysis and enzymatic methods are now being considered to achieve a commercially feasible disruption of this complex structure. There is a strong requirement for better and more diverse catalysts (biological and chemical) to break down these complex biopolymers into the vast array of chemical compounds that are currently derived from fossil fuels (see later).

The relevance of enzymes in the beverage and food industries will be examined in later chapters.

Enzyme prices have fallen in real terms over the past decades. For example, the bulk quantities of enzymes for most food applications are now at least in relative terms 20–35% cheaper than in the mid-1970s. More specialised enzymes, used in smaller concentrations and in higher purities, have increased in use because of improved production methods. Further large-scale uses of enzymes as catalysts will be achieved only if their costs continue to fall. Current sales of industrial enzymes worldwide are between US$650 and US$750 million according to the US Department of Commerce. In financial terms, 80% of industrial enzyme sales goes to three principal markets – starch conversion (40%), detergents (30%) and dairy applications particularly rennets (10%). Animal rennet sales for cheese manufacturing are approaching US$100 million and are being strongly augmented by microbial and genetically engineered rennets. However, the growth of enzyme sales has been and continues to be heavily influenced by the starch and detergent industries. Innovations such as recombinant DNA technologies and improved fermentation methods and downstream processing will

Table 5.4 Production of industrial enzymes by tonnage in the Western world

Nation	Tonnes	%
USA	6360	12
Japan	4240	8
Denmark	24910	47
France	1590	3
Germany (former West)	3180	6
Netherlands	10070	19
UK	1060	2
Switzerland	1060	2
Others	530	1
Total	53000	100

increasingly reduce production costs, particularly of high-cost enzymes, making them more competitive with other chemical processes.

Although many specific enzymes are being increasingly used in clinical or diagnostic applications, the amount of enzymes actually needed is quite small. This arises from the development of automated procedures that use immobilised enzymes and seek to miniaturise the system, with the enzyme becoming analogous to the microchip in a computer. Thus, although the enzyme is essential, the market need is quite small.

When enzymes are used as bulk additives, only one or two kilograms will normally be required to react with 1000 kilograms of substrate. In this way the cost of the enzyme will be between US$3 and US$25 per kilogram, or 10–14% of the value of the end-product. Such enzymes are usually sold in liquid formulations and are rarely purified. In contrast, diagnostic enzymes will generally be used in milligram or microgram quantities and can cost up to US$100 000 per kilogram. Such enzymes will be required in a high state of purity.

The further growth of world enzyme markets will revolve around (a) high-volume, industrial-grade enzyme products, and (b) low-volume, high-purity enzyme products for analytical, diagnostic or therapeutic applications. In the world production of industrial enzymes it is of interest that two small European countries (the Netherlands and Denmark) dominate the markets (Table 5.4).

5.3 | Selection and development of producer strains for enzyme production

The basic strategy of culture collection (screening) and strain improvement for enzyme production is the same as that carried out for other microbial activities. Clearly devising satisfactory tests to select the desired cultures, whether new isolates or improved strains, is paramount. Enzyme companies maintain large collections of microorganisms derived from a vast range

Table 5.5 | Production organisms for selected enzyme products

Enzyme activity	Application/industry	Host organism	Donor organism
Amylase (fungal)	Baking, brewing, starch	*Aspergillus oryzae*	*Aspergillus* spp.
Amylase (bacterial)	Starch	*A. niger* *Bacillus amylolique faciens*	*Bacillus* spp.
Cellulase	Baking, brewing, detergents, textiles	*B. subtilis* *Trichoderma tsesei*	*Trichoderma, Aspergillus*
Pectate lyase	Fruits and vegetables, textiles	*Bacillus licheniformis*	*Bacillus* spp.
Protease (alkaline)	Detergents	*Bacillus subtilis*	*Bacillus* spp.
Protease (acidic)	Dairy (milk clotting)	*Aspergillus oryzae, A. niger*	Calf stomach *Mucor, Rhizamucor*
Xylanase (hemicellulase)	Pulp and paper textiles	*Aspergillus niger, Bacillus subtilis*	*Actinomedira, Trichoderma* spp.

Source: adapted from Berka and Cherry (2006)

of natural sources and can employ a wide array of enrichment techniques to select out required characteristics in a microorganism. Most companies retain gene libraries that can result in molecular screening and genome sequencing, which can lead to the discovery of novel enzymes.

Most industrial enzyme production involves a selected enzyme activity transferred into a production microorganism recognised for the ability to yield high enzyme activity. In general, fungal enzymes are produced in fungal hosts, e.g. *Aspergillus* and *Trichoderma* species, while bacterial enzymes utilise bacterial hosts, usually *Bacillus* species (Table 5.5).

Genetic engineering or recombinant DNA technology has allowed the transfer of useful enzyme-genes from one organism to another. Thus, when a good candidate enzyme for industrial use has been identified, the relevant gene can be cloned into a more suitable production host microorganism (Fig. 5.2) and an industrial fermentation carried out. In this way it becomes possible to produce industrial enzymes of very high quantity and purity.

Recombinant microorganisms are now becoming a dominant source of a wide variety of types of enzymes. This trend will increase in the future due to the ease of genetic engineering and the almost unlimited variety of enzymes available from microorganisms in diverse and extreme environments, from fastidious microorganisms and from others that are potential pathogens. Enzymes from extremophyles such as microorganisms able to grow at high temperatures (90–100 °C) can now be grown in mesophilic microorganisms producing enzymes that have high temperature resistance and can be used in industrial processes.

A recent example of this technology is the detergent enzyme Lipolase produced by Novo Nordisk A/S, which has improved removal of fat stains in fabrics. The enzyme was first identified in the fungus *Humicola lanuginosa* at levels inappropriate for commercial production. The gene DNA fragment for the enzyme was cloned into the production fungus *Aspergillus oryzae* and

Table 5.6 | Objectives for the preparation of modified enzymes

1. To enhance the activity of the enzyme.
2. To improve the stability.
3. To permit the enzyme to function in a changed environment.
4. To change pH or temperature optima.
5. To change the specificity of an enzyme so that it catalyses the conversion of a different substrate.
6. To change the reaction catalysed.
7. To enhance the efficiency of a process.

Source: adapted from Gray (1990)

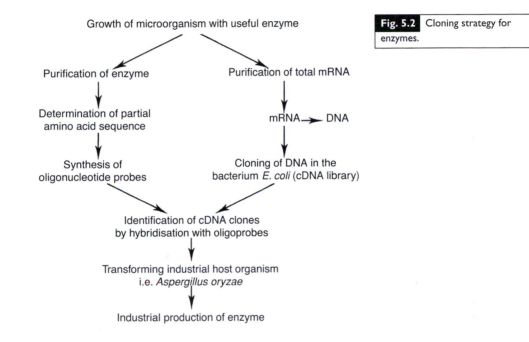

Fig. 5.2 Cloning strategy for enzymes.

commercial levels of enzyme achieved. The enzyme has proved efficient under many wash conditions. The enzyme is also very stable at a variety of temperatures and pH conditions relevant to washing. Furthermore, Lipolase is remarkably resistant to proteolytic activity of the commonly used detergent proteases.

The modification of enzymes to improve/alter their catalytic properties has been carried out for several decades. In the past, this was achieved by random mutational programmes but in recent years advanced technology has brought about major changes in the field. Table 5.6 gives some of the main objectives to which this research has been directed.

Protein engineering or 'molecular surgery' has been used to alter the performance of enzyme molecules. Protein engineering involves the selective replacement of specific amino acids within a protein to deliberately alter specific biochemical characteristics. Protein engineering of enzymes involves the creation of a three-dimensional graphical model of the purified enzyme obtained from X-ray crystallographic data. Changes to the enzyme structure can then be considered that might result in increased stability to, for example, pH and temperature, and the requisite molecular changes made in the gene coding for the enzyme, e.g. amylases with enhanced oxidation stability.

Two main avenues of research have been pursued in order to alter the performance of enzymes. In one approach, mutagenesis of the cloned-gene product, amino acid residues at defined positions in the structure of the enzyme can be replaced by other suitably coded amino acid residues. The altered gene is then transformed into a suitable host organism and the mutant enzyme subsequently produced with the requisite changes in position. This process is known as site-directed mutagenesis. The second method used involves the isolation of the natural enzyme and modifications to its structure carried out by chemical or enzymatic means – sometimes referred to as 'chemical' mutation. A recent successful example of protein engineering is that of the enzyme phospholipase A2, which was modified structurally to resist higher concentrations of acid. This enzyme is widely used as a food emulsifier.

Clearly, genetic engineering and protein engineering will have dramatic impacts on the enzyme industry in its many forms. Genetic engineering will ensure better product economy, production of enzymes from rare microorganisms, faster development programmes, etc. Also extensive tests of the enzymes now used have shown no harmful effects on the environment.

5.4 | The technology of enzyme production

Although many useful enzymes have been derived from plant and animal sources it is clear that most future developments in enzyme technology will rely on enzymes of microbial origin. Even in the malting process of brewing, where the amylases of germinated barley that hydrolyse the starch are relatively inexpensive and around which existing brewing technology has developed, there are now some competitive processes involving microbial enzymes.

The use of microorganisms as a source material for enzyme production has developed for several important reasons.

(1) There is normally a high specific activity per unit dry weight of product.
(2) Seasonal fluctuations of raw materials and possible shortages due to climatic change or political upheavals do not occur.
(3) In microbes a wide spectrum of enzyme characteristics, such as pH range and high-temperature resistance, is available for selection.
(4) Industrial genetics has greatly increased the possibilities for optimising enzyme yield and type through strain selection, mutation, induction and selection of growth conditions and, more recently, by using the innovative powers of gene transfer technology and protein engineering.

Novel enzymes from unusual sources can now be produced by cloning the relevant gene into a well characterised and easily grown microorganism such as *Aspergillus oryzae*.

The rationale for selection between different microorganisms is complex and involves many ill-defined factors such as economics of cultivation, whether the enzyme is secreted into the culture broth or retained in the cell, and the presence of harmful enzymes. Depending on source material, enzymes differ greatly in their stability to temperature and to extremes of pH. Thus *Bacillus subtilis* proteases are relatively heat stable and active under alkaline conditions and have been most suitable as soap-powder additives. In contrast, fungal amylases, because of their greater sensitivity to heat, have been more useful in the baking industry.

When selecting for enzyme production the industrial geneticist must seek to optimise desired properties (high enzyme yield, stability, independence of inducers, good recovery, etc.) while also attempting to remove or suppress undesired properties (harmful accompanying metabolites, odour, colour, etc.). In the past, genetic techniques were not widely practised, most manufacturers relying mainly on mutagenesis combined with good selection methods. A common feature of most early industrial producer organisms was that their genetics was little understood. However, gene transfer technology together with protein engineering is rapidly altering this and presents new horizons to enzyme technology.

The raw materials for industrial enzyme fermentations have normally been limited to substances that are readily available in large quantities at low cost, and are nutritionally safe. Some of the most commonly used substrates are starch hydrolysate, molasses, corn steep liquor, whey and many cereals.

Industrial enzyme production from microorganisms relies predominantly on either submerged liquid conditions or solid substrate fermentation as described in Chapter 4.

Solid substrate methods of producing fungal enzymes have long historical applications, particularly in Japan and other Far East countries. In practice, this method uses moist wheat or rice bran with added nutrient salts as substrates. The growing environment usually consists of rectangular or circular trays held in constant-temperature rooms. Commercial enzymes of importance produced in this way include fungal amylases, proteases, pectinases and cellulases.

Since microbial enzymes are mostly low-volume, medium-cost products, the production methods using submerged liquid systems have generally relied on bioreactors similar in design and function to those used in antibiotic production processes (Fig. 5.3). The choice of fermentation medium is important since it supplies the energy needs as well as carbon and nitrogen sources. Raw material costs will be related closely to the value of the final product.

Enzyme synthesis in microorganisms is often repressed, i.e. the enzyme will only be produced in the presence of an inducer molecule, most often the substrate. The inducer functions by interfering with the controlling repressor as exemplified by starch for amylase production and sucrose for invertase production. Feedback repression can occur in the biosynthesis of small molecules in which usually the first enzyme in the chain of

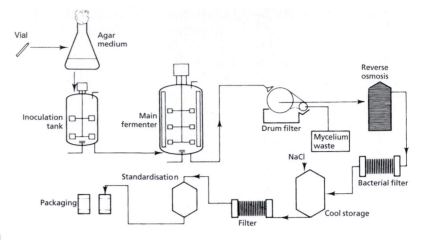

Fig. 5.3 The stages in the production of a liquid enzyme preparation.

production is inhibited by the final product. In some cases excess of specific nutrients such as carbon, nitrogen, etc., can shut down or repress the production of enzymes involved in related or unrelated compounds – catabolic repression.

The use of inducers for industrial enzyme production can often be difficult and the most common solution is to produce regulatory mutants in which inducer dependence has been eliminated by creating constituent mutants. For catabolic repression mutants resistant to this phenomenon have been developed, while it is also possible to control the effect of these substrates by feeding them into the bioreactor by a fed-batch regime.

A typical enzyme-producing bioreactor is constructed from stainless steel and has a capacity of 10–50 m³ (Fig. 5.4). In most cases enzymes are produced in batch fermentations lasting from 30 to 150 hours; continuous cultivation processes have found little application in industrial enzyme production. Sterility of the bioreactor system is essential throughout production.

At the completion of the fermentation the enzyme may be present within the microorganism or excreted into the liquid or solid medium. Commercial enzyme preparations for sale will be either in a solid or a liquid form, crude or highly purified. The concentration and purification of an enzyme is shown in Fig. 5.5. Enzyme recovery and purification are as relevant to the economics of production as the fermentation stage. Enzyme purification will be carried out only if the extra cost is justified by the intended application of the enzyme. The scale of the purification or downstream processing will dictate the choice of separation techniques, as some are difficult to operate on a large scale.

All microbial enzyme products that will be used in foods or medically related applications are required to meet strict specifications with regard to toxicity (Table 5.7). At present only a small number of microorganisms are used for enzyme production. Responsibility for the safety of an enzyme product remains with the manufacturer. In practice, a safe enzyme product should have low allergenic potential, and be free of toxic materials and harmful microorganisms. Enzymes from animal and plant sources do not require toxicological studies to be performed. When enzymes are derived

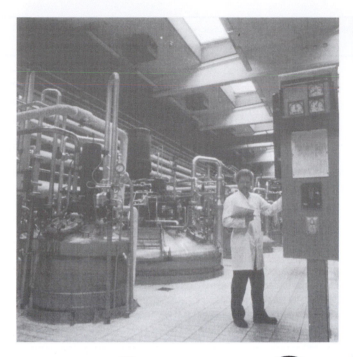

Fig. 5.4 Fermentation plant at Novo, Denmark, used for the production of enzymes.

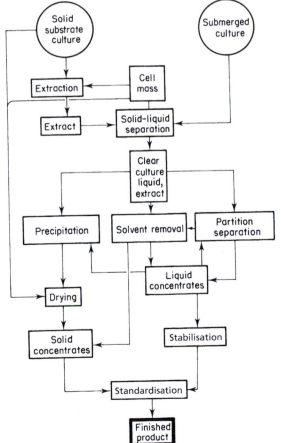

Fig. 5.5 The extraction and preparation of an enzyme.

Table 5.7 Safety testing of food enzymes based on the Association of Microbial Food Enzyme Producers classification

Group tests (× = to be performed)	(a) Microorganisms that have traditionally been used in food, or in food processing	(b) Microorganisms that are accepted as harmless contaminants present in food	(c) Microorganisms that are not included in either (a) or (b)
Pathogenicity	In general no testing required		×
Acute oral toxicity, mouse and rat; sub-acute oral toxicity		×	×
Three-month oral toxicity, rat		×	×
in vitro mutagenicity		×	×
Teratogenicity, rat; in vivo mutagenicity, mouse and hamster			$(×)^a$ $(×)^a$
Toxicity studies on the final food			$(×)^a$
Carcinogenicity, rat; fertility and reproduction			$(×)^a$ $(×)^a$

[a] Only to be performed under exceptional conditions
Source: Godfrey and Reichelt (1983)

from microorganisms traditionally used in food or food processing no testing is required (Table 5.7). Enzymes from other microorganisms may require extensive testing and also analysis for toxic metabolites such as exo- and endotoxins and mycotoxins. All bulk enzymes are supplied with a detailed Material Safety Data Sheet, which covers potential dangers, and also handling procedures for using the enzyme. The Association of Manufacturers and Formulators of Enzyme Products (AMFEP) is an industry organisation that sets the guidelines for environmental health and safety topics related to enzyme manufacturing.

5.5 | Immobilised enzymes

Almost 95% of all commercial enzymes are purchased in a soluble form with the majority being used directly on a single-use basis in the areas listed in Table 5.1. The use of enzymes in a soluble or free form must be considered as very wasteful because the enzyme generally cannot be recovered at the end of the reaction. A new and valuable area of enzyme technology is that concerned with the immobilisation of enzymes on insoluble polymers, such as membranes and particles, which act as supports or carriers for the enzyme activity. The enzymes are physically confined during a continuous catalytic process and may be recovered from the reaction mixture and reused over and over again, thus improving the economy of the process; this is merely a return to the natural immobilised state of most enzymes in

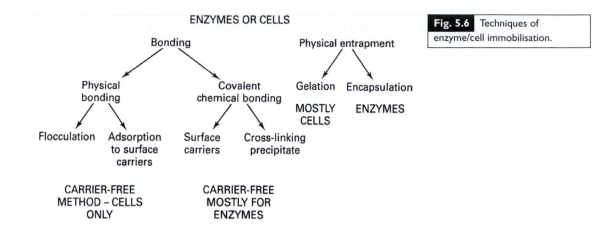

Fig. 5.6 Techniques of enzyme/cell immobilisation.

living systems. Some enzymes that are rapidly inactivated by heat when in cell-free form can be stabilised by attachment to inert polymeric supports, while in other examples such insolubilised enzymes can be used in non-aqueous environments. Whole microbial cells can also be immobilised inside polyacrylamide beads and used for a wide range of catalytic functions. The variety of new enzymes and whole organism systems that are likely to become cheaply available presents exciting possibilities for the future, especially in the pharmaceutical and diagnostic fields.

Present applications of immobilised catalysts are mainly confined to industrial processes, for example, production of L-amino acids, organic acids and fructose syrup. The future potential for immobilised biocatalysts lies in novel applications and the development of new products rather than as an alternative to existing processes using non-immobilised biocatalysts.

Immobilised enzymes are normally more stable than their soluble counterparts and are able to be re-used in the purified, semi-purified or whole-cell form. Catalytic properties of immobilised enzymes can often be altered favourably to allow operation under broader or more rigorous reaction conditions; for example immobilised glucose isomerase can be used continuously for over 1000 h at temperatures between 60 and 65°C.

How are enzymes immobilised? In practice both physical and chemical methods are routinely used for enzyme immobilisation. Physically, enzymes may be absorbed onto an insoluble matrix, entrapped within a gel or encapsulated within a microcapsule or behind a semi-permeable membrane (Fig. 5.6). Chemically, enzymes may be covalently attached to solid supports or cross-linked.

A large number of chemical reactions have been used for the covalent binding of enzymes by way of their non-essential functional groups to inorganic carriers such as ceramics, glass, iron, zirconium and titanium, to natural polymers such as sepharose and cellulose, and to synthetic polymers such as nylon, polyacrylamide and other vinyl polymers and copolymers possessing reactive chemical groups. In many of these procedures the covalent binding of enzymes to the carriers is non-specific, i.e. the binding of the enzyme to the carrier by way of the enzyme's chemically active groups

Table 5.8 | Limitations of immobilised enzyme techniques

Method	Advantages	Disadvantages
Covalent attachment	Not affected by pH, ionic strength of the medium or substrate concentration.	Active site may be modified; costly process.
Covalent cross-linking	Enzyme strongly bound, thus unlikely to be lost.	Loss of enzyme activity during preparation; not effective for macromolecular substrates; regeneration of carrier not possible.
Adsorption	Simple with no modification of enzyme; regeneration of carrier possible; cheap technique.	Changes in ionic strength may cause desorption; enzyme subject to microbial or proteolytic enzyme attack.
Entrapment	No chemical modification of enzyme.	Diffusion of substrate to and product from the active site; preparation difficult and often results in enzyme inactivation; continuous loss of enzyme due to distribution of pore size; not effective for macromolecular substrates; enzyme not subject to microbial or proteolytic action.

distributed at random. More recent studies have attempted to develop techniques of enzyme immobilisation in which the enzyme binds to a carrier with high activity without affecting its catalytic activity. The limitations of immobilised enzyme techniques are shown in Table 5.8.

The entrapment of enzymes in gel matrices is achieved by carrying out the polymerisation or precipitation/coagulation reactions in the presence of the enzyme. Polyacrylamides, collagen, silica gel, etc. have all proved to be suitable matrices, but the entrapment process is relatively difficult and results in low enzyme activity.

Immobilised whole microbial cells are becoming increasingly utilised and tend to eliminate the tedious, time-consuming and expensive enzyme purification steps. Immobilisation of whole cells is normally achieved by the same methods as for cell-free enzymes. The greatest potential for immobilised cell systems lies in replacing complex fermentations, such as secondary product formation (i.e. semi-synthetic antibiotics) in the continuous monitoring of chemical processes (via enzyme electrodes), water analysis and waste treatment, continuous malting processes, nitrogen fixation, synthesis of steroids and other valuable medical products. The advantages of using immobilised biocatalysts are summarised in Table 5.9.

As a consequence of successful immobilisation techniques in the form of enzyme capsules, enzyme beads, enzyme columns and enzyme membranes many types of bioreactors have been developed at a laboratory scale and to a lesser extent at industrial scale. These include *batch-stirred tank* bioreactors, continuous *packed-bed* bioreactors and continuous *fluidised-bed* bioreactors (Fig. 5.7). In industrial practice the catalytic properties of isolated enzymes, immobilised enzymes or immobilised whole cells are generally utilised

Table 5.9 | The advantages of immobilised biocatalysts

1. Permit the re-use of the component enzyme(s).
2. Ideal for continuous operation.
3. Product is enzyme free.
4. Permit more accurate control of catalytic processes.
5. Improve stability of enzymes.
6. Allow development of a multienzyme reaction system.
7. Offer considerable potential in industrial and medical use.
8. Reduce effluent disposal problems.

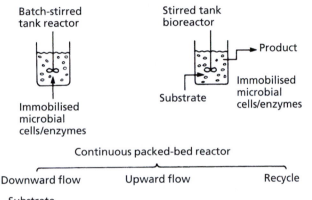

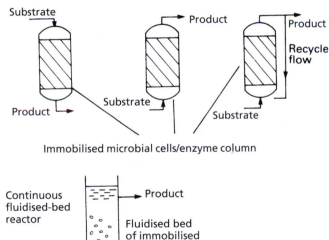

Fig. 5.7 Immobilised cell/enzyme bioreactors.

within the confines of bioreactor vessels. Bioreactor systems can have many forms, depending on the type of reactions and stability of the enzyme.

In Europe, immobilised penicillin acylase is used to prepare 6-amino-penicillanic acid (6-APA) from naturally produced penicillin G or V (Fig. 5.8). This compound is an important intermediate in the synthesis of semi-synthetic penicillins so essential in our fight against bacterial diseases. Two types of penicillins are produced by industrial fermentation: penicillin

Table 5.10 Some industrial applications of immobilised enzymes

Industry	Enzyme	Method of immobilisation	Process
Food	Glucose isomerase	AE-cellulose cell homogenates cross-linked with glutaraldehyde.	Conversion of glucose to fructose.
	Aminoacylase	DEAE-Sephadex	Resolution of DL-amino acids to L-form.
Dairy	Lactase	Cellulose acetate fibres	Hydrolysis of lactose to glucose and galactose.
Pharmaceutical	Penicillin G/V acylases	Br CN-activated Sephadex cellulose triacetate fibres; polyacrylamide	Production of 6-APA from penicillin G.
Chemical	Nitrilase	Polyacrylamide	Production of acrylamide from acrylonitrile.

Fig. 5.8 Formation of 6-APA by hydrolysis of penicillin.

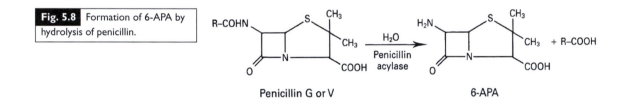

Penicillin G or V → 6-APA

G (phenyl acetyl-6-APA) and penicillin V (phenoxy acetyl-6-APA) each containing a nucleus of 6-APA and a side-chain. The antibiotic activity of the penicillin molecule is governed by the side-chain, which when removed and replaced with another can profoundly alter the antibiotic spectrum and other properties. Many pharmaceutical companies now operate immobilised enzyme processes for the production of 6-APA on an industrial scale. At least 3500 tonnes of 6-APA are produced each year requiring the production of about 30 tonnes of the enzyme (Table 5.10).

Immobilised glucose isomerase is used in the USA, Japan and Europe for the industrial production of high-fructose syrups by partial isomerisation of glucose derived from starch. Thousands of tonnes of high-fructose syrup are produced annually by this enzyme process, which is undoubtedly the most widely used of all the immobilised enzymes. The industrial and commercial success of this process is due to the following facts: glucose derived from starch is relatively cheap; fructose is sweeter than glucose; the high-fructose syrup contains approximately equivalent amounts of glucose and fructose, and from a nutritional aspect is similar to sucrose. The overall production of fructose from starch is shown in Fig. 5.9.

Another important use of immobilised enzymes is aminoacylase production of amino acids. Aminoacylase columns are used in Japan to produce thousands of kilograms of L-methionine, L-phenylalanine, L-tryptophan and L-valine.

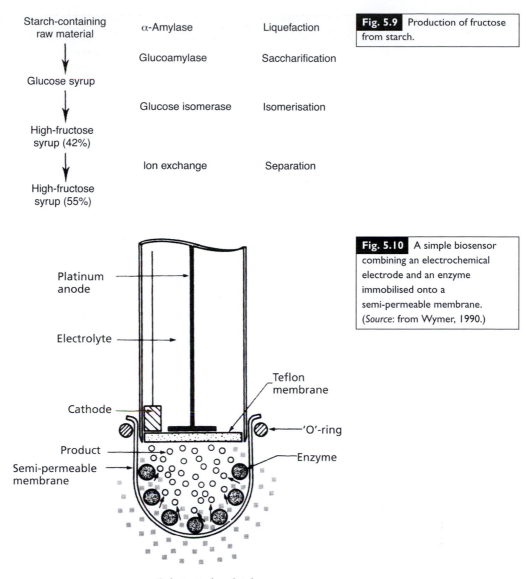

Starch-containing
raw material

α-Amylase   Liquefaction

Glucoamylase   Saccharification

Glucose syrup

Glucose isomerase   Isomerisation

High-fructose
syrup (42%)

Ion exchange   Separation

High-fructose
syrup (55%)

Fig. 5.9 Production of fructose from starch.

Platinum
anode

Electrolyte

Teflon
membrane

Cathode

'O'-ring

Product

Enzyme

Semi-permeable
membrane

Substrate (analyte)

Fig. 5.10 A simple biosensor combining an electrochemical electrode and an enzyme immobilised onto a semi-permeable membrane. (*Source:* from Wymer, 1990.)

Enzyme-polymer conjugates are now being used extensively in analytical and clinical chemistry. Immobilised enzyme columns or tubes can be used repeatedly as specific catalysts in assays of substrates.

Enzymes have long been utilised in a wide range of diagnostics from the widely used end-point assays to complex biosensors. The compound to be analysed (the analyte) becomes the substrate in an enzyme-catalysed reaction that generates a detectable signal such as absorbance change, which can then be recorded and suitable calculations derived. The specificity of the assay system will relate to the substrate specificity of the enzyme employed. Immobilised enzymes are regularly used for analytical purposes. Enzymes can be non-covalently bound to special paper and become test strips for assays in biological samples, e.g. blood, urine, etc. When used in complex biosensors the enzyme is normally an oxidoreductase, which can act as the 'specific' mediating analyte recognition. The resulting enzymatic interaction is then transferred through a 'transducer' component into an electrical signal, then amplified and processed electronically.

Enzyme electrodes are a new type of detector or biosensor designed for the potentiometric or amperometric assay of substrates such as urea, amino acids, glucose, alcohol and lactic acid. In design, the electrode is composed of a given electrochemical sensor in close contact with a thin permeable enzyme membrane capable of reacting specifically with the given substrates. The embedded enzymes in the membrane produce oxygen, hydrogen ions, ammonium ions, carbon dioxide or other small molecules depending on the enzymatic reactions occurring, which are readily detected by the specific sensor; the magnitude of the response determines the concentration of the substrate (Fig. 5.10). While the biological component in a biosensor may more often be an enzyme or multienzyme system, it can also be an antibody, an organelle, a microbial cell or whole slices of tissue.

The application of enzyme technology to existing processes, for example brewing, food processing, medicine, pharmaceuticals, chemical industry, waste treatment, etc., has enormous potential and is examined in later chapters.

Looking to the future, it seems reasonable to expect that the production and application of enzymes will continue to expand. The growing world concern about the environment and natural resources, the rising prices of oil and other raw materials, and fears of global warming are promoting new avenues of research and there is little doubt that enzymes will play a major role in solving some of these problems.

Chapter 6

Biological fuel generation

6.1 | Global warming and the significance of fossil fuels

Energy for industrial, commercial and residential purposes, electricity generation and transportation is primarily supplied by fossil fuels (coal, gas and oil) and nuclear power. It is now widely believed that climate change is strongly linked to the increased level of greenhouse gases in the atmosphere, and that human activity especially through the combustion of fossil fuels is a major contributing factor.

One of the main greenhouse gases, accounting for 65% of global warming, is carbon dioxide. Fossil fuels are the stored energy or 'ancient sunlight' of aeons and millennia ago that mankind has been burning extensively over a few centuries and more prolifically in recent decades. When such fossil fuels are burned for energy, carbon dioxide that has been locked away for all those years is released into the atmosphere greatly adding to global greenhouse gases. In contrast, when present-day plant material is burned the carbon locked into the biomass for a relatively short period of time is released back into the atmosphere thus recycling the carbon dioxide. Consequently, the system is relatively carbon neutral unlike the burning of fossil fuels.

Global emissions of carbon dioxide from fossil fuels over the first five years of this third millennium were four times greater than for the preceding ten years, despite the decisions of the Kyoto Agreement to reduce carbon dioxide emissions. Levels of carbon dioxide in the world atmosphere are 380 ppm, about 100 ppm higher than before the Industrial Revolution 200 years ago. It is believed that should carbon dioxide levels increase to about 450–500 ppm there could be irreversible climate change.

Energy issues have now become a subject of global concern and there has been a noticeable escalation of public and political interest. Everyone has an interest in the future of our planet! Energy demand is expected to double between 2000 and 2050 as a result of the increase in global populations and the consequent growth in gross domestic product. As a result, the future demand for, and supply of, energy is an increasingly important issue for nations worldwide.

Fossil fuel energy sources have been the lifeblood of all industrial civilisations, and have greatly contributed to the current concern over greenhouse gases. While most industrialised nations are now attempting to curtail their carbon emissions it is now required of them to help developing economies who seek to improve living standards by assisting them to bypass their current use of ineffectual and dirty energy technologies that fuelled the industrial development of the former, but mortgaged the environment in the process.

6.2 | Photosynthesis: the ultimate energy source

Throughout the world plants and algae perform a chemical reaction that cannot be repeated by laboratory chemistry – they use energy from sunlight to split water into hydrogen and oxygen. The enzyme responsible for the water-splitting reaction is a photo-oxidase reductase. Within the photosynthetic cell hydrogen will combine with carbon dioxide from the atmosphere to produce a myriad of organic carbon-containing compounds including sugars, starches, proteins, etc., on which life throughout the world depends. The oxygen released into the atmosphere is essential for most forms of life on the planet while it also helps to maintain the ozone layer that protects the planet from damaging ultraviolet radiation.

Photosynthetic organisms, both terrestrial and marine, can be considered as continuous solar energy converters and are constantly renewable. Plant photosynthesis alone fixes about 2×10^{11} tonnes of carbon with an energy content of 2×10^{21} joules, which represents about 10 times the world's annual energy use and 200 times our food energy consumption. The magnitude and role of photosynthesis has gone largely unappreciated because we use such a small proportion of the fixed carbon. Let it not be forgotten that photosynthesis in the past provided all the present fossil carbon sources, namely coal, oil and natural gas. Thus, photosynthetically derived biomass that exists in many available forms in the environment could well be transformed into storage fuels and chemical feedstocks, such as bioethanol, biodiesel and methane gas. The actual efficiency of solar energy capture by green plants can be as much as 3–4%, the more effective photosynthetic plants – such as maize, sorghum and especially sugar cane – being the most productive.

When crops are grown for biofuel production they can be seen as an important part of a renewable and sustainable society – renewable since the crops can be harvested and re-sown, and sustainable because the carbon emissions generated during burning are reabsorbed by new plant growth. As such the cycle can continue indefinitely!

Fossil fuel reserves have a finite nature. The term 'peak oil' has been coined to identify the point in the future when, for example, oil production will peak and start to decline. Taken in association with the current dramatic increase in industrialisation in, for example, China and India, this is generating growing economic and trade pressures for alternative and

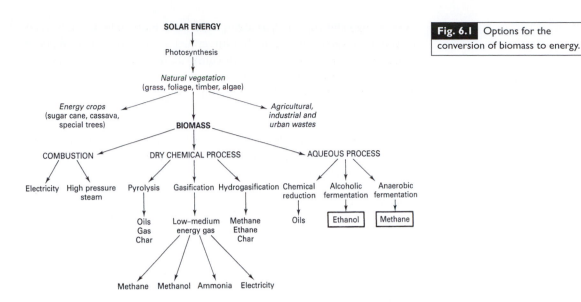

Fig. 6.1 Options for the conversion of biomass to energy.

reliable supplies of energy. This is over and above the continuing world concern about global warming.

Biomass can be considered as a renewable energy source, and can be converted into either direct energy or energy-carrier compounds by direct combustion, anaerobic digestion systems, destructive distillation, gasification, chemical hydrolysis and biochemical hydrolysis (Fig. 6.1).

6.3 | Biofuels from biomass

Bioenergy (biofuel) is basically the production of combustible/usable energy from biological sources. This can be liquid fuels, e.g. bioethanol, biodiesel; gaseous fuels, e.g. methane; or direct solid heat energy, e.g. wood.

What are the main biological energy sources or crops? (Smith, 2006.)

Sugar crops	Sugar cane, sugar beet: sugars extracted and fermented to bioethanol.
Starch crops	Maize (corn), barley, wheat, oats, cassava: starch enzymatically hydrolysed to sugars and fermented to bioethanol.
Cellulose crops/wastes	Straw, bagasse, woody wastes, cropped trees: the hemicelluloses can be enzymatically hydrolysed to sugars and fermented to bioethanol.
Oil crops	Rapeseed, linseed, sunflower, castor oil, groundnut: oils extracted and transesterified to biodiesel.
Organic wastes/manures	Complex microbial fermentations to methane/methanol.
Solid energy crops	Coppiced trees, sorghum, reeds, grasses, Eucalyptus: direct burning alone or with other conventional sources, e.g. coal.

Many woody crops such as alder, willow and birch, which can be readily coppiced, can be grown to offer direct fuel sources to be used in power stations to generate electricity. Some considerable success has already been achieved in Scandinavia and Canada. In other parts of Europe with considerable redundant farmland resulting from reductions in cereal cultivation, this land could be used for the cultivation of woody perennials or coppiced trees for fuel-energy production.

The recent non-food crop initiative in the UK encourages the cultivation of crops that can be processed into biofuels, construction materials, packaging, speciality chemicals and pharmaceuticals. Similar programmes occur in other EU countries using set-aside land to reduce overproduction of food crops.

The conversion of biomass to usable fuels can be accomplished by biological or chemical means or by a combination of both. The main end-products are methane, ethanol and biodiesel, although other products may arise depending on initial biomass and the processes utilised, e.g. solid fuels, hydrogen, low-energy gases, methanol and longer-chain hydrocarbons.

The concept of cultivating plant biomass specifically for energy supply is based on the fact that much higher yields of fixed carbon are attainable from well planned plantation methods than from harvesting natural vegetation or collecting agricultural or industrial wastes. Programmes of this type are now being extensively planned and practised in many countries throughout the world. Sugar cane and corn are the two principal crops that are being developed (primarily for bioethanol production) in Brazil, Australia, the USA and South Africa, whereas more lignocellulose-based programmes are being developed in Sweden, Canada and the USA. In the latter case, plans are being made to grow forests for conversion into liquid fuels. Cost analysis of all of these processes offers considerable encouragement, in particular with sugar cane conversion.

Energy-crop plantations will undoubtedly supply meaningful amounts of energy in the near future. The problem of water deficiency is very real, however, and rainfall is most often the limiting factor operating in otherwise ideal conditions of solar radiation intensity, annual hours of sunshine, mild winters and an abundance of good-quality land. In certain areas of the world it is possible that such plantations will rapidly become a reality, but for most countries development will centre on the use of organic wastes, namely agricultural, municipal and industrial. Conversion to biofuels could well serve as substitutes for petroleum energy and as a chemical feedstock.

The technical processing of the biomass depends on many factors, including moisture level and chemical complexity. With materials having a high water content, aqueous processing is normal to avoid the need for substrate drying. Alcoholic fermentation to ethanol, anaerobic digestion to methane, as well as chemical reduction to oily hydrocarbons, are all possible. Low moisture level materials such as wood, straw and bagasse can be burnt to give heat or to raise steam for electricity generation; subjected to thermochemical processes such as gasification and pyrolysis to produce energy-rich compounds such as gaseous oil, char and eventually methanol and ammonia; or treated by alkaline or biological hydrolysis to produce chemical feedstocks for use in further biological energy conversions.

6.4 | Bioethanol from biomass

The production of alcohol by fermentation of sugars and starch is an ancient art and is often considered to be one of the first microbial processes used by humans.

$$C_6H_{12}O_6 \rightarrow 2CH_3CH_2OH + 2CO_2$$

Production of industrial alcohol by fermentation draws heavily upon the accumulated knowledge of the brewer and the distiller. At present industrial alcohol production is largely synthetic, i.e. non-microbial, deriving from petrochemical processes. Petrochemical ethanol is made by the hydration of ethene, and the decline of microbial production of alcohol dates from the large-scale production of ethene from the 1940s. Within 20 years of development of large-scale petroleum cracking, industrial production of fermentation alcohol fell below potable alcohol production in most industrialised nations. Thus, in technologically more advanced countries ethanol is produced by chemical means. In many developing countries where cheap raw materials are available, ethanol is still produced for industrial purposes using traditional fermentation techniques.

While the benefits of ethanol as a fuel are considerable, it is energy-efficient, does not produce toxic carbon monoxide during combustion and is, therefore, much less polluting than conventional fuels, it is still cheaper to produce ethanol from oil chemically than by fermentation processes at current oil prices. In this way, ethanol usage, as with other alternative fuels, is economically hindered in industrialised countries until oil prices once again take on an upward rise. It is inevitable that it will happen, but exactly when is hard to predict. However, the world concern of global warming is now dramatically influencing fuel choice.

A dramatic change in the economics of alcohol production resulted from the massive increases in the world prices of crude oil in the 1970s. Whereas oil prices have more than quadrupled since 1975, the price of suitable cheap carbohydrates has risen far less on average.

Oil-importing nations are anxious to reduce their import costs and many now subsidise home-produced alternatives. Since ethanol can be used as a partial or complete substitute for motor fuel and can also be converted readily into ethene and related compounds, its production from indigenous and renewable resources is now an attractive alternative strategy.

Historically, ethanol and, to a lesser extent, methanol were used extensively as motor fuels in Europe prior to World War II and, indeed, Henry Ford's model T car was designed to run on alcohol, petrol or any mixture in between.

Nowhere has this been more actively pursued than in Brazil. Vast biotechnological processes operate throughout the country, converting sugar cane and cassava into bioethanol by yeast fermentation. Brazil's

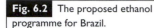

Fig. 6.2 The proposed ethanol programme for Brazil.

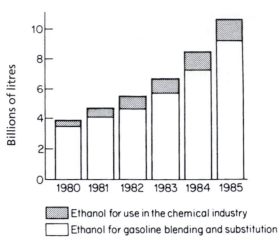

Ethanol for use in the chemical industry
Ethanol for gasoline blending and substitution

National Ethanol Programme (PROALCOOL) was in response to the oil shock of the 1970s and has now succeeded in reducing the country's dependence on fossil fuel. Bioethanol now accounts for 40% of Brazil's driving fuel. A production output of approximately 5 billion litres of ethanol in the early 1980s has now been well surpassed to 15 billion litres in 2005. Brazil's ethanol programme is shown in Fig. 6.2. Brazil's undoubted success in pioneering this production of 'green petrol' has created worldwide interest, particularly among poorer Third World nations with the climate and land to grow their own fuel crops but with limited currency to buy oil. Even developed nations, such as Australia, the USA, Sweden and Canada, have extensive biological ethanol production processes that utilise either large agricultural surpluses or forestry wastes.

Three billion litres of fuel alcohol were fermented in the USA from corn in 1987 and one third of all American gasoline is 10% waste-derived ethanol or gasohol. Brazilian officials now estimate that the country's entire petrol needs could be met from planting 0.3% of the country's vast area with alcohol-producing crops. Over 500 fermentation and distillation plants have been built throughout the country processing the crops produced throughout the year. An additional bonus to the energy generation is the creation of over 700 000 new direct jobs and 300 000 indirect jobs in the rural areas of Brazil.

However, the current economic scenario for Brazil's bioethanol programme is being influenced by current world oil prices. By 1985 ethanol production had increased to 12 billion litres and by 1988, 88% of new cars were powered by ethanol engines. Production of ethanol has remained relatively stable at about 12 billion litres in the 1990s. It is now realistically estimated that the costs of producing bioethanol from sugar cane are at least US$50 per barrel.

There are many indirect advantages to Brazil in using bioethanol instead of gasoline. While there is the obvious reduction in their contribution to global warming, the addition of anhydrous bioethanol to gasoline eliminates the need for octane improvers to raise the octane rating. Studies have further shown that ethanol powered engines produce 57% less carbon

Table 6.1 | Potential raw materials for fuel ethanol production

Starch containing	Cellulosics	Sugar containing	Other

Cereal grains:
  Corn
  Grain sorghum
  Wheat
  Barley.
	Wood
	Sawdust
	Waste paper
	Forest residue
	Agricultural residues
		Sucrose and invert sweet
		  sorghum
		Molasses
		Sugar beet
		Fodder beet
		Sugar cane
			Jerusalem artichoke
			Raisins
			Bananas

Milling products:
  Wheat flour
  Wheat millfeeds
  Corn hominy feed.
	Municipal solid
	  wastes
	Intensive livestock
	  production wastes
		Lactose
		Whey
		Glucose
		Sulphite wastes	

Starchy roots:
  Cassava
  Potatoes.			

monoxide, 64% fewer hydrocarbons and 13% less nitric oxide than gasoline powered vehicles.

Brazil's flex fuel car fleet is the only one in the world that can use 100% of either bioethanol or gasoline. Economic considerations are constantly changing in favour of bioethanol production, with future anticipated fluctuating oil prices and new design concepts for alcohol-based engines. Furthermore, on a global aspect, green petrol production will help to take some of the pressure off oil products for the rest of the world, reducing competitive tensions and perhaps even wars.

Bioethanol for fuel programmes require a considerable capital investment and will be in keeping with large-scale needs and not small on-farm systems (where methane products are more suitable).

To make available the necessary fermentable sugars (Table 6.1), most raw materials require some degree of pre-treatment, depending on their chemical composition. With sugar cane this treatment is minimal and consists mainly of the usual milling operation, whereas corn or cassava, containing starch, require the action of a suitable saccharifying agent – either acid hydrolysis or enzyme hydrolysis. Cellulosic raw materials such as timber and straw require more extensive pre-treatment, and this is reflected in the increased energy inputs required (see Table 6.2). A flow diagram for the production of ethanol from diverse substrates is shown in Fig. 6.3.

The Brazilian programme is almost exclusively based on batch fermentation systems. At present the standards of these fermentations are modest but are steadily improving. Continuous methods of production offer many advantages but are really only studied and operated in developed nations with an interest in ethanol formation. Improvements in continuous fermentations have utilised many approaches, including retention of the yeast cells in the bioreactor by separation and recycling and by continuous evaporation of the fermentation broth.

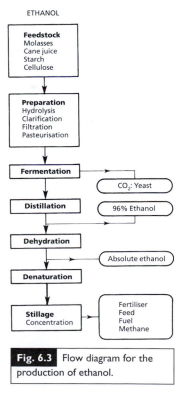

Fig. 6.3 Flow diagram for the production of ethanol.

Table 6.2 | The gross energy requirements of ethanol produced from different substrates by microbial fermentation

Physical inputs	Substrates				
	Sugar cane	Cassava	Timber[a]	Timber[b]	Straw
Substrate	7.27	19.19	12.67	20.00	4.37
Additional chemicals	0.60	0.89	4.74	6.37	4.74
Water	0.30	0.38	0.80	0.30	0.80
Electricity	7.00	10.47	175.70	7.84	166.74
Fuel oil	8.00	29.03	42.13	62.40	42.13
Capital inputs (buildings etc.)	0.46	1.21	3.34	0.64	3.34
Total	24	61	239	98	222

All figures given in MJ kg^{-1} ethanol.
[a] Fermentable sugars formed via enzymic hydrolysis.
[b] Fermentable sugars formed via acid hydrolysis.

So far, innovation in the Brazilian programme has been restricted to some marginal improvements in essentially traditional alcohol fermentation processes. However, biotechnology is having a considerable input with new developments and numerous research programmes in this field, for example, production of more efficient microorganisms by genetic engineering (improved alcohol fermentation, resistance to high temperatures and high alcohol levels, speed of fermentation and higher yields), by improved immobilised enzyme bioreactor technology and by process design improvements. Novel introductions such as fermentation under partial vacuum and recycling of the fermentative yeast cells have increased ethanol productivity to ten or twelve times that of conventional batch fermentation processes, and such increases reduce capital costs and energy requirements for bioreactor operation. Application of these biotechnological improvements to ethanol production is making these processes increasingly economically attractive as a substitute for fossil fuel. This is especially true now in the USA.

In many ways the logistics of distribution are more important than production capacity, e.g. building ports with storage tanks and loading facilities, improving railway and pipeline links between ports and sugar-producing regions. Brazil now exports bioethanol to the USA, India, Nigeria, Venezuela and soon to Japan.

The overall economics of fermentation ethanol from specific crop cultivation in developing countries will achieve support indirectly by the expansion of agriculture, by creating more employment, because oil prices will continue to outstrip agricultural feedstocks, and because new technologies will create further economic uses for the wastes generated in fuel ethanol production.

Vast volumes of wastes or *stillage* result from the Brazilian and other alcohol programmes, and much research is in progress to seek worthwhile end-products. Of particular significance will be:

(1) evaporation to feed or fertilisers
(2) mineralisation to ash
(3) anaerobic fermentation for methanol generation
(4) conversion by microorganisms into SCP.

6.5 | Biodiesel

Conventional diesel, an important transportation fuel, is a by-product of the crude oil distillation process, which also results in the formation of petrol, and has a high aromatic and sulphur content. In contrast, biodiesel is produced from vegetable oils (e.g. rapeseed oil) and is now a viable alternative to conventional diesel fuel.

The most successful method of producing biodiesel is by transesterification of plant oils with methanol (or ethanol) in the presence of a catalyst, sodium hydroxide, at 50°C resulting in the formation of fatty acid methyl esters and glycerol. The glycerol is allowed to settle and the biodiesel purified and used directly, or as a mixture, with diesel as a fuel.

$$\begin{matrix} \text{Rapeseed oil} \\ \text{(1 tonne)} \end{matrix} + \begin{matrix} \text{Methanol} \\ \text{(0.1 tonne)} \end{matrix} \rightarrow \begin{matrix} \text{Biodiesel} \\ \text{(1 tonne)} \end{matrix} + \begin{matrix} \text{Glycerol} \\ \text{(0.1 tonne)} \end{matrix}$$

Biodiesel has chemical characteristics similar to those of conventional diesel fuel in terms of combustion within modern diesel engines. The oils that can be used include rapeseed, soybean, canola and also waste cooking oils; the methanol is readily obtained from natural gas, biogas or coal, while the glycerol is a valuable and easily saleable by-product, which can offset some of the production costs. This basic method is now widely used throughout the world, especially in parts of Europe and the USA.

What are the main advantages of biodiesel over fossil fuel-derived diesel?

• Reduces the dependence on fossil fuel use/imports.
• Has a lower flashpoint and does not ignite.
• Free of toxic aromatic and sulphur compounds.
• Biodegradable – reducing environmental damage due to spillage.
• Biodiesel is renewable.

Conventional diesel engines do not require modification to run on biodiesel used alone or blended with diesel. The fuel economy and power generated are relatively similar. The most important accolade is that unlike diesel there is no net increase in carbon dioxide released into the atmosphere with combustion, i.e. it is carbon neutral.

The EU, particularly France, Italy and Germany, have been the leading proponents of biodiesel – France for agricultural reasons, Italy for environmental reasons and Germany for both. Many urban public transportation systems in these countries burn biodiesel; thus enhancing their 'environmental' image. Italy has given preference to its use as a fuel for heating municipal buildings.

Biodiesel production is still more expensive than conventional diesel fuel but governments are now implementing various forms of tax incentives to stimulate usage, i.e. lower fuel tax derogation compared with fossil fuels. Also the subsidising of rapeseed oil production in EU countries encourages farmers to grow a crop for industrial, economic and ecological importance rather than continuing with conventional (generally over-produced) cash food crops. However, in other parts of the world the substitutability of biodiesel will be determined by the farmland acreage that can be redirected from food production to vegetable oil production to serve as biofuel feedstock. Bioethanol could also be used to replace the methanol of fossil origin used in the esterification reaction. In this way, bioethanol usage would be increased and the biodiesel would be derived from entirely renewable resources.

The USA is the world's largest producer of biodiesel, mainly from soybeans. Current levels of demand of biodiesel are *c.* 150 million gallons per year while newly envisaged government targets have been set for 1 billion gallons per year by 2010.

An exciting new industrial programme in the USA will combine bioethanol production with biodiesel production using corn. In the bioethanol production from corn the oil-rich distillers grain generated through the milling of the corn, which is normally taken for animal feed, is now going to be used for biodiesel production. Creating another renewable fuel from an existing co-product of the bioethanol production process is good environmental business and economic sense. The overall process still produces a more effective feed with higher protein and lower fat content than the previous mix.

It is calculated that for every 100 million gallons of bioethanol, 7–8 million gallons of biodiesel will be produced. It is proposed to use the biodiesel at a 2% blend with fossil fuel-derived diesel. Whereas bioethanol must travel to refineries by rail, the biodiesel will be transported by way of existing oil pipelines. It is expected that this plant will produce 30 million gallons of biodiesel annually, which is five times the production of existing biodiesel facilities.

6.6 | Methane

Methane gas can be used for the generation of mechanical, electrical and heat energy, and is now extensively used as a fuel source for domestic and industrial purposes through national gas pipelines or can be converted to methanol and used as fuel in internal combustion engines. Such natural gas sources were originally derived from biomass in ancient times.

Methane gas also exists in the atmosphere and is mainly derived from microbial action in natural wetlands, rice paddies and enteric fermentation in animals, contributing about 20%, 20% and 15% respectively to the total methane flux. Domestic cattle are the major contributors producing about 75% of all animal emissions whereas humans produce about 0.4%. After carbon dioxide, methane is considered to be the next most important greenhouse gas and is expected to contribute 18% of future warming.

The microbiology of methane production is complex (Fig. 6.4), involving mixtures of anaerobic microorganisms. In principle, anaerobic fermentation of complex organic mixtures is believed to proceed through three

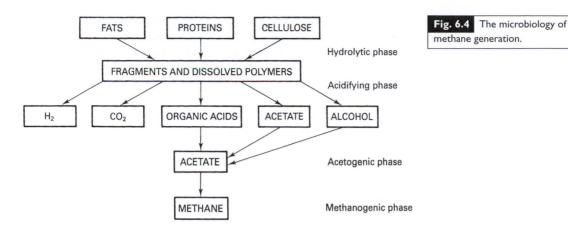

Fig. 6.4 The microbiology of methane generation.

main biochemical phases, each of which requires specific microbiological parameters. The initial stage requires the solubilisation of complex molecules such as cellulose, fats and proteins, which make up most raw organic matter. The resultant soluble, low molecular weight products of this stage are then converted to organic acids; in the final phase of microbial activity, these acids (primarily acetic) are specifically decomposed by the methanogenic bacteria to methane and carbon dioxide.

The most efficient and complex methane-producing system in nature is the rumen. This anaerobic system has never been fully reproduced outside the cow, and is known to be a complex interaction of large numbers of bacteria, protozoa and fungi. All intensively studied bioreactor programmes set up to create methane under controlled conditions have shown that consistent high gas outputs require substantial laboratory monitoring with highly accurate control of environmental variables such as temperature, pH, moisture level, agitation and raw material input and balance. To date, most practical applications of methanogenesis have been at a very low technological level.

There are several possible ways by which methane can be produced in a planned economy: from sewage, from agricultural and urban wastes, and in biogas reactors.

The anaerobic digestion of *sewage* is a long-practised technique and many municipal systems have devised methods of capturing the methane and harnessing the energy for the needs of the sewage plant. The energy returns are modest and large-scale expansion does not seem probable.

In recent years methanogenesis of the abundantly available *agricultural and urban wastes* has appeared as an obvious and profitable way to generate energy. The energetic considerations of methane production from such wastes are complex and subject to many limitations. Using urban wastes it should be possible to convert 30 to 50% of the combustible energy to methane, while with the use of certain other vegetable materials or forages it may be possible to achieve 70% conversion. The overall economics of methane production must recognise the valuable by-products generated by the process, namely the effluent and residue rich in ammonia, phosphates and microbial cells, which may be used as fertiliser, soil conditioner or even as animal feed. Furthermore, the process can convert malodorous and pathogenic wastes into innocuous and useful materials.

However, there are still many inherent problems that must be overcome before there can be any hope of achieving an energy balance. At present, the cost of collection of organic matter only for the purpose of methanogenesis is too expensive; the rate of methane production is inconsistent and low in most processes, and much research needs to be carried out on the balance of nutrients for process optimisation. However, the major problem is the presence of lignin in most agricultural and urban wastes. Lignins are not easily digested by anaerobic processes, and physical and chemical pre-treatment places a considerable energy and cost burden on the overall process.

When methane is produced by the fermentation of animal dung the gaseous products are usually referred to as *biogas* and the installations called biogas plants or bioreactors. Biogas is a flammable mixture of 50–80% methane, 15–45% carbon dioxide, 5% water and some trace gases. Biogas is produced via biomethanation (Fig. 6.4) and is in fact a self-regulating symbiotic microbial process operating under anaerobic conditions, and functions best at temperatures around 30°C. The organisms involved are all found naturally in ruminant manures. In such systems the animal dung is mixed with water and allowed to ferment in near-anaerobic conditions. Production of biogas by such methods goes back into antiquity and is of particular importance in India, China and Pakistan. The Gobar system of biogas production in the Far East ranges from small peasant systems to quite large plants continuously producing large volumes of gas. In energy terms the simple Gobar system is very near to being a net energy producer on a small scale. Small-scale plants of family, farm or village size are in operation throughout the world.

Under ideal conditions, 10 kg dry organic matter can produce $3\,m^3$ of biogas, which will provide 3 h cooking, 3 h lighting or 24 h refrigeration with suitable equipment. Biogas does, in fact, furnish a considerable part of the world's energy source; China is the largest user with over 7 million biogas units providing the equivalent energy of 22 million tons of coal, and with current subsidies a biogas plant in China is cheaper than a bicycle. Larger systems of this type do not achieve a net energy balance.

Biogas combustion has been used to heat steam to drive electricity turbines and in California, USA, one plant provides electricity to 20 000 homes by way of cow-manure biomethanation.

There has also been some consideration of growing crops on a large scale to provide a 'methane economy'. High-yielding crops in terms of megajoules per hectare cultivated on massive land or water areas have been proposed. It has been suggested that 65% of the current gas consumption in the USA could be provided by an energy plantation of area $260\,000\,km^2$ using water hyacinth of energy content 3.8 MJ per kg dry material. Marine algae have also come under special scrutiny.

Methane generated from organic materials by anaerobic fermentation offers a valuable source of energy that could be directly put to many uses. Furthermore, the associated by-products may be useful forms of fertilisers for agriculture. Yet, before the full realisation of these systems can be

| **Table 6.3** | Economic arguments against large-scale methane production by microbial processes |

1. An abundance of methane occurs in nature, particularly in natural gas fields and oil field overlays.
2. Methane production by gasification of coal is commercially more attractive.
3. Microbial production of methane is more expensive than natural gas.
4. Costs of storage, transportation and distribution of gaseous fuels is not yet economically worthwhile.
5. Methane cannot be used in automobiles and is difficult and expensive to convert to the liquid state.

achieved, very considerable biotechnological studies must be undertaken. The biological aspects revolve around complex mixed cultures and it is doubtful that the thermodynamic efficiency of the fermentation can be improved. Thus emphasis must be given to improving process design and to technological improvements of the control systems. New and cheap construction materials for digesters (bioreactors) and gas storage vessels will be required. In time there will be available a complete range of anaerobic technologies to deal with most kinds of biodegradable materials. Although methane will be the principal end-product, fuels such as propanol and butanol as well as fertilisers will undoubtedly add to the cost-effectiveness of the overall process.

Methane as an energy source may well have economic value at local small-scale production levels, but there is considerable doubt about the future of large-scale commercial processes for methane production. Some of the more obvious considerations are shown in Table 6.3.

However, anaerobic digestion of municipal, industrial and agricultural wastes can have positive environmental value, since it can combine waste removal and stabilisation with net fuel (biogas) formation. The solid or liquid residues can further be used as fertiliser, soil conditioner or animal feed.

Biogas production will continue to have high priority in alternative energy research.

6.7 | Hydrogen

Consideration has been given to the use of hydrogen as a fuel or in fuel cells for the production of electricity. Hydrogen production can occur by way of photosynthetic bacteria, biophotolysis of water and by fermentation. In the first two systems, encouraging production of hydrogen has been achieved, but much research is needed to assess the significance of these methods at an applied level. It has been estimated that at least 20 to 30 years of research is needed before any type of functional system is obtained.

Although it is possible to generate hydrogen from glucose by bacterial action, the production rate is too small to make microbial genesis of hydrogen economic.

The efficiency of hydrogen production by anaerobic fermentation is much less than that of methane production by the same method. Since methane also has a higher energy content it would appear that methane production by microbial processes has a much higher practical potential than hydrogen. However, further research may well alter these considerations.

Biohydrogen requires the invention of a practical and economic means of storage, not to mention a large improvement in the efficacy of current fuel-cell technology. Furthermore, most of the world's machines and transport systems were not built for fuels like hydrogen and methane. There is no commercial-scale biohydrogen process yet in use, though some promising processes are under development. Much hope is being attached to a photosynthetic bacterium, *Rhodopseudomonas palustris*, which can produce this without any energy input.

6.8 | The way ahead for biofuels

World energy needs at present are dominated by the continued adaptability of fossil fuels, the same fossil fuels that we now realise are causing continued and permanent damage to world climates. The ability of biofuels to realistically enter the energy market will be determined by several factors: (a) the availability of the existing energy chain to biofuels; (b) the resistance to the adoption of biofuels by the current energy management; (c) the ability to reduce the costs of biofuels; and (d) the retrofitting of the existing energy supply-chain to accommodate biofuels. The entry of biofuels to the current energy supply system will be slow and gradual, but the world must start the slow process of weaning itself from total dependence on fossil fuels.

While there will continue to be entrenched, political, industrial and commercial obfuscating, which may hinder optimal crisis management of the global energy situation, there are also some positive indicators coming from established world renowned energy companies, for example BP. BP plans to establish a dedicated bioscience energy research laboratory to be attached to a major US academic centre and spending US$500 million over the next ten years.

Three aspects of energy bioscience will be explored:

(1) developing new biofuel components and improving the efficiency and flexibility of those currently blended with transport fuels
(2) devising new technologies to enhance and accelerate the conversion of organic matter to biofuel molecules, with the aim of increasing the proportion of a crop that can be used to produce feedstock
(3) using modern plant science to develop species that produce a higher yield of energy molecules and can be grown on land not suitable for food production.

They will also support the need for new biofuels to be blended into traditional fossil-based transport fuels. The biofuel industry will also gain support from the USA automakers since Ford, Chrysler and General Motors have confirmed that half of all the cars they produce by 2010 will be 'flex-fuel'.

A final question must be considered – how eco-friendly are biofuels? Advocates of biofuels consider them as ecological alternatives to fossil fuels,

Table 6.4 | Estimated fossil fuel reserves

Fuel	Reserves (giga tonnes)	Reserves in carbon (giga tonnes)
Oil	175	147
Natural gas	431	323
Coal	984	832

Source: www.glohive.com

since they are primarily manufactured by plants and when utilised as fuel the carbon emitted is recycled back into plants – they are carbon neutral. However, life cycle studies, which examine the overall energy balance for individual biofuels, have identified many aspects of net energy inputs in the making of a biofuel: the type of plants, i.e. sugar-cane, corn, soybean, lignocellulose; level of fertilisers required; collection and transport to the refinery; pre-treatment needs, i.e. maceration, enzymic/acid hydrolysis; bio-fuel recovery; by-product purification and valorisation; waste treatment; and finally biofuel storage and distribution. Furthermore, how much land can be used for biofuels without affecting food production for the world's expanding population?

However, all of these apparent net energy input drawbacks to large-scale bioenergy crops, while real, do not take into consideration future advances in plant and agricultural biotechnology, the potential use of genetically modified plants, enhanced bioprocess technologies, improved carbon-fixation of photosynthesis, improved enzymology and nitrogen-fixation pathways in bioenergy crops.

6.9 | Contrasting views on climate change

Recently, the former Vice-President of America, Al Gore, shared the 2007 Nobel Peace Prize with the Integrated Panel on Climate Change (IPCC), which was established with these predictions of fossil fuel use and climate change. They propose that solar activity has dramatically increased in recent times and consider that the resulting solar winds have reduced cloud cover over the Earth creating an increased warming and release of dissolved carbon dioxide from the world's oceans. The climate system is hugely complex and up to the present time it is believed that no computer modelling is sufficiently accurate for the prediction of future climate to be fully relied upon.

Notwithstanding, there is no doubt that the world's fossil energy sources (Table 6.4) are dwindling and should be used prudently and with proper respect for the environment. Identification of alternative energy sources will continue to be an activity of intense scientific commitment.

Chapter 7

Environmental biotechnology

7.1 | Introduction

As societies throughout the world are increasingly moving to greater levels of urbanisation and industrial development, public concern is mounting over the state of the environment and much attention is now being given to improving the environment for future generations. To achieve this, there has been, particularly in developed nations, major environmental legislation directed towards liquid, solid and hazardous wastes. In most developing countries, the situation is less encouraging where financing is limited, or not available, for the construction of water and waste treatment facilities and there is a shortage of trained personnel to operate the systems. Furthermore, in many developing countries, there is a lack of official regulations and control systems, no administration bodies responsible for waste control and little obligation for existing and emerging industries to dispose of waste properly. Also it is in such countries that there is the greatest movement towards urbanisation and new industrial development with concomitant destruction of the environment.

Waste generation is a side-effect of consumption and production activities and tends to rise with the level of economic advance. Wastes arise from domestic and industrial activity, e.g. sewage, waste waters, agriculture and food wastes from processing, wood wastes and an ever-increasing range of toxic industrial chemical products and by-products. In the final assessment, wastes represent the end of the technical and economic life of products. Costs for properly dealing with wastes are escalating and much attention is presently devoted to efficient and effective waste management, which will include costs of collection, storage, processing and removal of wastes.

Probably the most disturbing aspect of pollution is the increasing presence of toxic chemicals in the natural environment. The large-scale production and application of synthetic chemicals and their subsequent pollution of the environment is now a problem of serious concern in most industrialised countries, and must be viewed as an extreme threat to the self-regulating capacity of the biosphere in which we live. The US

Environmental Protection Agency's list of high awareness pollutants includes most pesticides, halogenated aliphatics, aromatics, polychlorinated biphenyls, polycyclic aromatic hydrocarbons and nitrosamines.

While many of these compounds are used directly by humans in agriculture and public health for obvious and beneficial results, others may be derived from a spectrum of industrial processes used to make a variety of useful products. Some are associated with the petroleum industry and others are solvents. Such toxic and hazardous chemicals are insidiously entering a variety of environments. These synthetic compounds can be found at very high concentrations at the point of discharge, such as factory sites and industrial spillages, where they can exert pronounced deleterious effects, while others occur at low levels in natural environments but because of their inherent toxicity, e.g. the pesticide dioxin, constitute a serious health hazard.

In many parts of the world there is increasing evidence that underground water sources are demonstrating dangerous levels of contamination. In continental Europe a notorious example of such industrially derived pollution is the valley of the River Po in North Italy where there has been permanent abandonment of groundwater sources. Similar examples occur in parts of the Netherlands lying below the level of the notoriously polluted river Rhine. Such chemical pollutants can remain in water-bearing rocks for decades and measures of removal would be lengthy, unbelievably complicated and restrictively costly.

It is now clear that many past and present industrial products and processes can be seen as environmentally unfriendly and are major sources of pollution. Historically, civil engineering or, more specifically, sanitary engineering, dealt mechanistically with such socially important areas as drinking water, catchment and treatment, waste water (domestic and industrial), solid wastes and industrial off-gases. The bio-component of all these processes was largely ignored. While biotechnological processes have always been part of these industrial activities, they are now increasingly being viewed in an overall environmental context. Environmental biotechnology is the application of recognised biotechnology processes for the protection and restoration of the quality of the environment, especially with a long-term perspective.

While industrial biotechnology largely utilises known microorganisms in product formation, environmental biotechnology will mainly rely on microbial consortia of complex and variable composition. New studies are now identifying and characterising the microorganisms that exist and interact in soils, anaerobic systems, and domestic and industrial waste streams. Can such mixed culture systems accept new improved microorganisms and what will be the regulatory constraints on the deliberate introduction of genetically modified microorganisms into the environment? The potential to enhance the degradative potential of microorganisms to degrade recalcitrant pollutants is immense and must be examined cautiously but creatively. Rehabilitation of contaminated land and waters is a major task for present and future generations. Of equal importance is the need to prevent future contamination from ongoing manufacturing processes, by using clean technology.

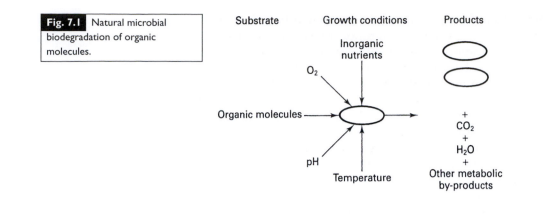

Fig. 7.1 Natural microbial biodegradation of organic molecules.

7.2 | Microbial ecology/environmental biotechnology

The presence and functioning of microbial communities affect our everyday lives in so many ways but none more so than their role in soil, waste and water management. Historically, the need to supply populations with safe drinking water and acceptable sewage disposal has mainly been the concern of sanitary engineers. (Engineering-driven solutions to these basic sanitary problems of communities were evolving long before there was any appreciation of the intrinsic roles of microorganisms.) More recently, the skills and knowledge of the microbiologist are increasingly being employed to develop new systems.

Microbial ecology is the science that studies the interrelationships between microorganisms and their living (biotic) and non-living (abiotic) environments. The increasing scientific and public awareness of microbial ecology since the 1960s derives mainly from the recognition of the central role of microorganisms in maintaining good environmental quality. It is the microbes in their multivarious forms that largely direct the orderly flow of materials and energy (biogeochemical cycles) through the world's ecosystems by way of their immense and varied metabolic abilities to transform inorganic and organic materials. Microbial ecology is an extremely relevant scientific discipline with proven practical applications and must be seen as one of the most critical scientific approaches to environmental problems.

Biodegradation can be defined as the decomposition of substances by microbial activities either by single organisms but most often by microbial consortia. Microorganisms found in soil and water will attempt to utilise any organic substances encountered as sources of energy and carbon by enzymatically breaking them down into simple molecules that can be absorbed. Under suitable environmental conditions all natural organic compounds should be degraded (Fig. 7.1) and for this reason large-scale deposits of naturally formed organic compounds are rarely observed. When such organic deposits do occur, e.g. coal, oil, it has been under conditions hostile to biodegradation.

Environmental biotechnology will include the application of biological systems and processes in waste treatment and management, and for the protection and restoration of the quality of the environment. Many successful biotechnological processes have now been developed for water, gas, soil and solid waste treatments. Modern developments in environmental biotechnology now focus on process optimisation and will no longer accept processes that are inefficient and sometimes merely transform one problem into another, for example, formation of carcinogenic nitrosamine compounds by the reaction of some microorganisms with organic amines and nitrogen dioxide. Environmental safety should not be threatened by environmental processes.

Organic chemicals that cannot easily be degraded by microorganisms or are indeed totally resistant to attack are termed recalcitrant, e.g. lignin. Xenobiotics are man-made synthetic compounds not formed by natural biosynthetic processes and, in many cases, can be recalcitrant. A xenobiotic compound is, therefore, a foreign substance in our ecosystem and may often have toxic effects. All environmental biotechnological processes make use of the metabolic (degradative and anabolic) activities of microorganisms demonstrating, again, the indispensable nature of microbes in our ecosystem.

The term 'biodegradable' is often loosely identified with the term environmentally 'friendly' and numerous advertising campaigns and product packaging have put across the message that because a product is biodegradable, its impact on the environment will be dramatically reduced. This is not always the case and demonstrations of product biodegradability have often only been achieved under highly conducive microbial conditions not easily met in the natural environment. Furthermore, biodegradability itself is a complex multifactorial event whose mechanisms are not completely understood. A range of environmental waste treatment technologies will now be examined.

7.3 | Waste water and sewage treatment

While many ancient civilisations had an appreciation of the need to protect the quality of water to be used for human consumption, it was not until 1855 that it was demonstrated that cholera was transmitted by water contaminated by faeces. A similar route for typhoid fever was shortly to be demonstrated. By the end of the nineteenth century, the microbial ecology of many human diseases had been shown to have an anal–oral route of transmission, which finally confirmed the health hazards associated with water contaminated with faeces. The introduction of sewage systems in developed societies during the nineteenth century allowed, for the first time, the possibility of treatment of municipal and industrial wastes before discharging into natural water systems.

Growth in human populations has generally been matched by a concomitant formation of a wider range of waste products, many of which cause serious environmental pollution if they are allowed to accumulate in the ecosystem. In rural communities recycling of human, animal and

Fig. 7.2 Aerial view of bioreactors at the sewage treatment plant for the city of Glasgow, Scotland.

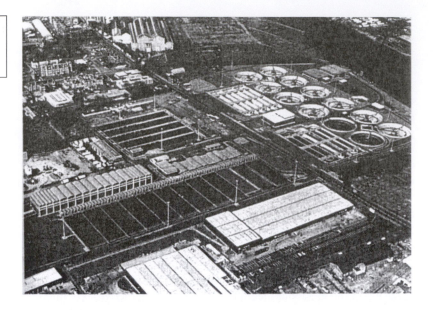

vegetable wastes has been practised for centuries, providing in many cases valuable fertilisers or fuel. However, it was also a source of disease to humans and animals by residual pathogenicity of enteric (intestinal) bacteria. In urban communities, where most of the deleterious wastes accumulate, efficient waste collection and specific treatment processes have been developed since it is impractical to discharge high volumes of waste into natural land and waters. The introduction of these practices in the last century was one of the main reasons for the spectacular improvement in health and well-being in the developed countries.

Mainly by empirical means a variety of biological treatment systems have been developed, ranging from cesspits, septic tanks and sewage farms to gravel beds, percolating filters and activated sludge processes coupled with anaerobic digestion. The primary aims of all of these systems or bioreactors is to alleviate health hazards and to reduce the amount of biologically oxidisable organic compounds, producing a final effluent or outflow that can be discharged into the natural environment without any adverse effects.

Such bioreactor assemblies rely on the metabolic versatility of mixed microbial populations (microbial ecology) for their efficiency. The systems in which they perform their biological functions can be likened to other industrial bioreactors (e.g. antibiotic production); large-scale plants, for example municipal forced aeration tanks (Fig. 7.2), can be extremely complex, requiring the skills of the engineer and the microbiologist for successful operation. The fundamental feature of these bioreactors is that they contain a range of microorganisms with the overall metabolic capacity to degrade most organic compounds entering the system.

The development of these systems was an early example of biotechnology. Indeed, in volumetric terms biological treatment of domestic waste waters and sewerage in the industrialised nations is by far the largest

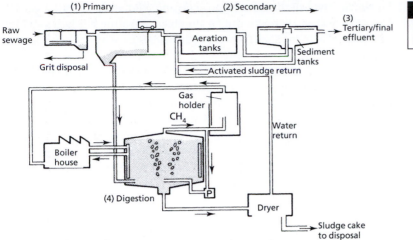

Fig. 7.3 Stages of sewage treatment in a complex incorporating anaerobic digestion.

biotechnological industry, and the least recognised by lay people. Controlled use of microorganisms has led to the virtual elimination of such waterborne diseases as typhoid, cholera and dysentery in these communities. Yet, if water and sewage treatments are seriously interrupted, major epidemics may quickly develop as witnessed in 1968 in Zermatt, Switzerland, where typhoid developed following the breakdown of the water treatment plant.

Thus, biotechnology not only generates a whole new range of useful products, it also plays an indispensable part, through water and sewage treatment processes, in the reduction of infectious diseases of humans and animals.

The biological disposal of organic wastes is achieved in many ways throughout the world. A widely used practice for sewage treatment is shown in Fig. 7.3. This complex but highly successful system involves a series of three stages of primary and secondary processing followed by microbial digestion. An optional tertiary stage involving chemical precipitation may be included. The primary activity is to remove coarse particles and solubles leaving the dissolved organic materials to be degraded or oxidised by microorganisms in a highly aerated, open bioreactor. This secondary process requires considerable energy input to drive the mechanical aerators that actively mix the whole system, ensuring regular contact of the microorganisms with the substrates and air. The microorganisms multiply and form a biomass or sludge, which can either be removed and dumped, or passed to an anaerobic digester (bioreactor) that will reduce the volume of solids, the odour and the number of pathogenic microorganisms. A further useful feature is the generation of methane or biogas, which can be used as a fuel. However, the value of biogas is marginal because of its content of carbon dioxide and hydrogen sulphide.

Another important means of degrading dilute organic liquid wastes is the percolating or trickling filter bioreactor. In this system the liquid flows over a series of surfaces, which may be stones, gravel, plastic sheets, etc., on which attached microbes remove organic matter for essential growth. Excessive microbial growth can be a problem, creating blockages and loss of biological activity. Such techniques are widely used in water purification systems.

Abundant availability of water is vital for modern urban and industrial development. Water makes up more than 70% of the human body and about two litres a day is usually sufficient to keep an adult healthy. Water acts as a transport medium for essential nutrients within the body, helps to remove toxins and waste materials, stabilises body temperature and performs a crucial part in the structure and function of the circulatory system. In essence, water is the elixir of life. In the natural world the ecosystem regenerates and recycles water. Increasingly, human intrusion into nature by industrialisation, extensive farming practices, deforestation, etc., has severely unbalanced this process. It is now accepted that two-thirds of the world's nations are water-stressed – using clean water faster than it is replenished in aquivers or rivers. Biotechnology will play an important role for reclamation and purification of waste waters for re-use. Water must be recycled in the sustainable use of resources. The most important threat mankind faces in the coming decades is not global warming or energy deficiency but an increasing shortage of high-quality water.

What are the future areas of importance? Microbiological effluent treatment will be a major field of biotechnological interest in the future. Integrated systems will be developed for treating complex wastes. The role of the biocatalyst or microbe will be constantly reassessed. Biotechnologists are now designing increasingly specific and efficient bioreactors to contain selected consortia of microorganisms best adapted to a range of different waste streams.

In countries with high annual hours of sunlight there has been considerable development of combined algal/bacterial systems for waste and water treatments. Such processes can lead to the formation of relatively pure water and algal/bacterial biomass, which may be used for animal feeding, biogas formation or, perhaps more ambitiously, for bulk organic chemical formation.

A comparison of several widely used treatment processes for liquid wastes is shown in Table 7.1, while Table 7.2 defines the various operating components.

Water is now being recognised as an increasingly expensive component of many industrial processes. Industries worldwide use vast quantities of quality water in their manufacturing procedures, e.g. steel, textiles, food, etc. For example, for each tonne of steel produced approximately 280 tonnes of water will be used. In the past many of these industries simply discharged the waste water into water courses often resulting in extensive down-river or estuarine pollution. Stringent anti-pollution laws together with greatly increased water charges have prompted such companies to develop new waste-water treatment systems that function in a closed-loop manner.

Almost two-thirds of water consumption worldwide is utilised for agricultural irrigation. In many cases where water is in short supply raw domestic sewage is used, which invariably leads to crop contamination

Table 7.1	Comparison of aerobic biological treatment processes for liquid wastes	
Process	Advantages	Drawbacks
Aerated lagoons	High BOD removal efficiency. Low operating costs. Low operator skills required.	Can foul-up and create smells. Solids carry-over. Considerable land requirements. Sensitive to cold weather.
Activated sludge	High BOD removal efficiency. Moderate ground requirements.	High energy consumption. Requires disposal of excess sludge. Requires skilled operators. Sensitive to sudden high inputs.
Trickling filters	Low operator costs. Moderate space requirements. Resistant to sudden high inputs.	Moderate BOD removal. Disposal of excess sludge necessary.
Rotating biological contactors	High BOD removal efficiency. Compact. Moderate energy input.	Possible odour formation. Requires skilled operators. Disposal of excess sludge required.

BOD: Biological oxygen demand – the amount of dissolved oxygen required by aerobic microorganisms to stabilise organic matter in waste water or sludge.

Sludge: microbial aggregates or flocs that can be separated from the purified effluent via sedimentation.

Table 7.2	Treatment of liquid wastes: definitions
Treatment	Definition
BOD	Biological oxygen demand (after five days of incubation) is a parameter that quantifies the concentration of biodegradable organic matter present in waste water. It is the amount of O_2 used by microorganisms to degrade the organic matter as determined in a standardised laboratory test.
Mixed liquor	The suspension of microbial flocs (tiny aggregates of microorganisms) in the aeration tank of an activated sludge plant.
Sludge	The microbial flocs in an activated sludge plant after these have been separated from the purified effluent via sedimentation in the settling tank.
Nitrification	The biochemical conversion of ammonium to nitrate carried out by autotrophic bacteria.
Denitrification	The biological reduction of nitrate to N_2. It occurs when O_2 is absent (anoxic conditions) and readily oxidisable organic compounds are present.
Anoxic	A liquid wherein O_2 is absent but other oxidised species such as nitrate or ferric iron are present.
Anaerobic	A liquid wherein oxidised species are absent, the redox potential is below zero, and where biochemical reactions such as fermentations, sulphate reduction and methanogenesis take place.

Source: adapted from Vandevivere and Vertstaete (2006)

with human pathogenic viruses. In such places it is important to develop waste treatment processes that will produce pathogen-free waste water without losing the essential nitrogen and phosphorous content required as fertilisers.

7.4 | Landfill technologies

Solid wastes account for an increasing proportion of the waste streams generated by modern urban societies. While part of this material will be made up of glass, plastics, etc., a considerable proportion will be decompostable solid organic material such as paper, food wastes, sewage wastes, wastes from large-scale poultry and pig farms, and, in the USA in particular, cattle feed lot wastes.

There are now many strategies available for solid waste management (a) primary recycling or selecting out from the waste stream materials for direct re-use, e.g. metals; (b) secondary recycling by mechanical (grinding) for re-use, e.g. glass, or chemical breakdown to produce re-usable molecules, e.g. plastics; (c) tertiary recycling – incineration: incineration is only considered recycling if the calorific value of the waste is recovered to generate heat or electricity; and finally (d) landfilling, which is the least desirable for recycling.

In large urbanised communities, the essential disposal of solid wastes is problematic and one well used system is by low-cost anaerobic landfill technology. In this procedure solid wastes are deposited in low-lying, low-value sites and each day's waste deposit is compressed and covered by a layer of soil. The complete filling of such sites can take months or years depending on size of the site and flow of wastes. They can be unsightly, smelly and unhygienic if improperly managed. Also toxic wastes can create severe problems, both to the microbiological process occurring in the site and with toxic run-off.

Improperly prepared and operated landfill sites may result in toxic heavy metals, hazardous pollutants and products of anaerobic decomposition seeping from the site into underground aquifers and subsequently polluting urban water supplies. Properly constructed and sealed landfill sites (Fig. 7.4) can be used to generate methane gas, for commercial use. Much effort is now made to use strong, impermeable liners to avoid leachates damaging surrounding land and water courses.

Current regulations require new landfill sites to be air- and watertight to protect the environment. Regular monitoring is necessary to detect contamination of groundwater, surface water and surrounding air. Landfill owners are now *financially* responsible for the long-term care of the sites *after* final closure. Landfill operations should be viewed as gigantic bioreactors and methane the useable product. Biogas production (which is mostly methane) will usually commence several months or years after proper construction and filling of the site, proceeding through a peak production period and gradually declining after many years.

In the past, landfill sites were seen essentially as 'dumping' sites or storage vessels where the waste was essentially sealed from the surrounding

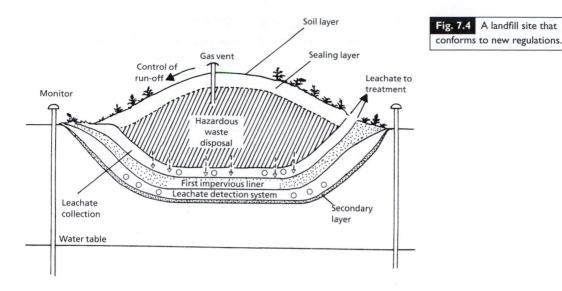

Fig. 7.4 A landfill site that conforms to new regulations.

environment. Nowadays, in sharp contrast, new sites are managed as bioreactor vessels where correct stabilisation enhancement systems are operated during the working life of the landfill site. Current practice in most western nations is to reduce the amount of waste to be landfilled and to increase the safety of the operation. While the practice of landfilling will continue to have a role in the overall management of solid wastes, its weaknesses lie with the inability to recycle re-usable products and poor energy (biogas) recovery. Furthermore, landfill leachates and gas emissions in inefficient sites can pollute the environment.

7.5 | Composting

Composting is an aerobic microbial driven process that converts solid organic wastes into a stable, sanitary, humus-like material that has been considerably reduced in bulk and can be safely returned to the environment. It is, in effect, a low-moisture, solid substrate fermentation process as previously discussed. To be totally effective, it should only use as substrates readily decomposable solid organic waste. In large-scale operations using largely domestic solid organic wastes, the final product is mostly used for soil improvement, but in more specialised operations using specific organic raw substrates (straw, animal manures, etc.), the final product can become the substrate for the worldwide commercial production of the mushroom *Agaricus bisporus*.

Composting has long been recognised not only as a means of safely treating solid organic wastes but particularly as a form of recycling of organic matter. Composting will increasingly play a significant role in future waste management schemes since it offers the means of re-use of organic material derived from domestic, agriculture and food industry wastes. The increased interest in composting derives from the growing awareness of the many environmental problems associated with some of the main ways

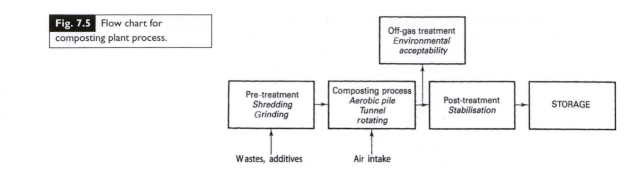

Fig. 7.5 Flow chart for composting plant process.

now practised for treating solid organic wastes, e.g. incineration and land-filling. The overwhelming majority of municipalities and individuals are opposed to having incinerators and landfill sites established within their communities.

Composting has only recently become a serious waste management technology, and both theoretical and practical development of the technology is still in its infancy. The primary aim of a composting operation is to obtain, in a limited time within a limited compost, a final compost with a desired product quality. A composting plant must function under environmentally safe conditions.

Composting is carried out in a packed bed of solid organic particles in which the indigenous microbes will grow and reproduce. Free access to air is an essential requirement. The starting materials are arranged in static piles (windrows), aerated piles or covered tunnels, or in rotating bioreactors (drums or cylinders). Some form of pre-treatment of the waste may be required, such as particle size reduction by shredding or grinding. The basic biological reaction of the composting process is the oxidation of the mixed organic substrates with oxygen to produce carbon dioxide, water and other organic by-products (Fig. 7.5). After the composting process is completed, the final product most often needs to be left for variable time periods to stabilise.

Successful composting requires optimisation of the growth conditions for the microorganisms. It is a mixed culture fermentation and an outstanding example of microbial ecology in action. Because of the large bulk of most operations this acts as insulation and as a result of the biological heat generated by the microbial reactions, there can be rapid internal heat build-up. Overheating can seriously impair microbial activity. Compost processes should be regulated to prevent the temperature rising above 55 °C. Moisture level of the organic substrates should normally be between 45 and 60% – above 60% free moisture will accumulate filling the interparticle spaces and restricting aeration, while below 40% conditions become too dry for successful microbial colonisation.

Solid organic materials are only slowly solubilised by exo-enzyme secretion by the fermenting microbes. This reaction step is generally considered as rate-limiting. Cellulose and lignin are abundantly present in most solid wastes. A high lignin content, for example in straw and wood materials, hampers the overall process of degradation; lignin is especially resistant to degradation and is only slowly degraded and in many instances it can shield other substances that are otherwise more easily degraded. Ready access to air is an essential ingredient for a successful, balanced bioreactor.

For large-scale commercial composting the aerated pile system is carried out in closed buildings to facilitate the control of odour emissions. In these systems forced aeration with regular turning is used to create good composting conditions. There are now several plants in Europe with a capacity of over 60 000 tonnes per year.

Tunnel composting is performed in closed plastic tunnels 30–50 m long and 4–6 m in width and height. Such tunnel systems have been in operation for many years for the composting of sewage sludge and domestic wastes, and for specialised substrate preparation for mushroom production. Some plants can operate at up to 10 000 tonnes per year.

Rotating drum systems in various sizes have been used for composting domestic wastes worldwide. The large Dano process is especially useful for wettish organic waste. Small drum systems have been widely accepted for small quantities of garden waste that can readily be used for recycling.

In some composting processes the waste gas outlets can create odour problems due to the presence of sulphur and nitrogen compounds. Special attention is now being given to reduce or remove these odours by gas scrubbers or filtration, since environmental regulations can lead to the shut down of offending plants. The most widely used form of biofiltration involves a fixed bed or mass of organic material, e.g. mature compost or microbially embedded wood chips. The gases pass through the mixture and the resulting biochemical activity can greatly reduce the offensive chemical smells.

Composting is undoubtedly one of the principal strategies for solid organic waste treatment and recycling back into the environment.

For future expansion of composting and recycling, four criteria will require to be achieved.

(1) A suitable infrastructure must be in place.
(2) Suitable quality and quantity of substrates must be available.
(3) There must be markets for the end-products.
(4) Processes must be environmentally sound and demonstrate economic viability.

In 1992, 7% of all European municipal solid waste was composted and by 2000 this had grown to 18%. In Germany, a renowned 'green' nation, this figure was much higher. During 1992, no fewer than 120 composting plants were being built, enlarged or planned in Germany. This has added a compost production capacity of nearly one million tonnes annually.

A major reason for this expansion has been the separation of domestic waste at source. This is the three-bin approach widely practised in Europe: one bin for recyclables (glass, metals, plastics), one for fully degradables (vegetable wastes, papers – the bio-bin), and finally a third for other materials and hazardous wastes.

In Germany alone it has been calculated that an annual demand for 20 million tonnes of compost can be achieved by: agriculture (10.8 million tonnes); viniculture (1.2 million tonnes); forestry (1 million tonnes);

substrates and soils (3.6 million tonnes); and land reclamation (3.4 million tonnes).

The process of composting has been with us in many forms for centuries, recycling vegetable wastes into useful products. It is simple, natural and invariably costs less than landfill and incineration. But above all, it is safe, free from toxic emissions and needs minimum financial resources.

While aerobic composting is a well practised technology throughout the world, anaerobic composting is a new approach being actively researched by several environmental companies. In dry anaerobic composting the process operates at a thermophilic temperature (55°C), at a high solid concentration and is a single-stage fermentation. While the process bears much similarity to landfill technology, it differs insofar as it is in a closed bioreactor and has a much higher reaction rate due to higher mixing/recirculation inputs. Complete digestion time of the waste organics takes two weeks, as opposed to several years in landfill. Since this process is performed in closed bioreactors anaerobic composting uses less space, produces energy (biogas), produces less odour, and kills pathogens and seeds more efficiently than aerobic composting.

With the growing number of environmental companies now developing and commercialising anaerobic composting facilities, clearly a revolution in composting practices is about to challenge existing concepts.

7.6 | Bioremediation

Large areas of the Earth's surface and the oceans and other waterways have already been contaminated with oil-derived compounds and toxic chemicals. More than 2 million tonnes of oil are estimated to enter the sea each year. Approximately half will be derived from industrial effluents, sewage and river outflows, and the remainder from non-tanker shipping and natural seepage from below the sea floor. It is considered that only about 18% of the total is coming from refineries, offshore operation and tanker activities. Unlike most other pollutants, oil spillages can readily be seen and have become an emotive subject on the TV screen. Most oils do have a relatively low toxicity to the environment in general, but can have catastrophic and immediate effects on bird and animal life associated with water. Some of the major oil spills of recent years are shown in Fig. 7.6. The maintenance of sustainable marine and coastal ecosystems will necessitate the development of effective measures to reduce oil pollution and mitigate the resulting environmental impact.

The contamination of soil normally results from a range of anthropogenic activities. Contaminated land is viewed as land that contains substances that, when present in sufficient quantities or concentrations, can probably cause harm to humans, directly or indirectly, and to the environment in general. Many xenobiotic (industrially derived) compounds can show high levels of recalcitrance and while in many cases only small concentrations get into the environment, they can be subject to biomagnification. Biomagnification in essence implies an increase in the concentration of a chemical substance, e.g. DDT, as the substance is passed through the food chain.

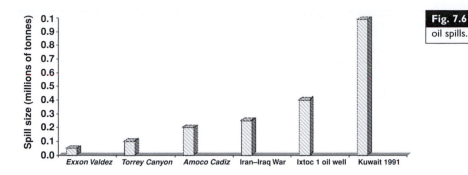

Fig. 7.6 Estimated size of major oil spills.

Hazardous wastes and chemicals have become one of the major problems of modern society worldwide. In the USA in excess of 50 000 contaminated sites and several hundred thousand leaking underground storage tanks have been identified. The estimated cost of treating these polluted sites is US$1.7 × 10^{12} and to date the US Environmental Protection Agency (EPA) has given US$15.2 × 10^9 to clean up hazardous waste sites. Hazardous wastes and toxic chemicals pose complex environmental problems by directly affecting the air, water, soil and sediments, while indirectly and unpredictably affecting living organisms that use these resources. Environmental forensics is a new discipline that has evolved to determine the legal responsibility for remediating the environmental damage caused, for example, by oil spills and chemical leaks etc. Who pays for the damage? Costly and contentious legal cases are now very common.

The commitment of biotechnology for the environmental management of such hazardous wastes or contaminants can be seen as the development of systems that involve biological catalysts to degrade, detoxify or accumulate contaminating chemicals. The application of biological agents, mostly microorganisms, for the treatment of environmental chemicals has mostly been directed towards remedial activities.

There are three main approaches to be assessed in dealing with contaminated sites (a) identification, (b) assessment of the nature and degree of the hazard, and (c) the choice of remedial action.

When dealing with contaminated soil, clean-up operations can involve on-site processing, *in situ* treatment or off-site processing. Up to the present, a considerable degree of remedial activity has centred on physical and chemical methods of separation and/or removal of the pollutants. Such methods will not be further discussed in the present context, but rather attention will be devoted to the increasingly utilised biological methods of remediation variously termed *bioremediation, biorestoration, bioreclamation* or *biotreatment*.

The basic principles of bioremediation are superficially simple: optimise the environmental conditions so that microbial biodegradation can occur rapidly and as completely as possible. Microbes that are naturally present in soils and water environments are potential candidates for the biological transformation of xenobiotic compounds that are introduced into the ecosystem. Microbial populations in natural environments exist in a dynamic equilibrium that can be altered by modifying the environmental conditions, such as nutrient availability.

Table 7.3 | The effect of microbes on chemical pollutants

Category	Chemical change
Degradation	Complex compound transformed into simple products, sometimes mineralisation.
Conjugation	Formation of complex or addition reactions to more complex compounds.
Detoxification	Conversion to non-toxic compound(s).
Activation	Compound converted into more toxic compound.

In almost all cases it will not be individual strains but consortia of microorganisms that will act on pollutant molecules. The metabolic effect of microorganisms on pollutants can take many forms and not always to the environmental advantage of the ecosystems (Table 7.3). While bioremediation treatments around the world rely largely on indigenous microbial ecosystems little is known about the individual microorganisms involved.

The application of bioremediation to environmental clean-up has been applied in two ways.

(1) Promotion of microbial growth *in situ* can be achieved by the addition of nutrients (*biostimulation*). When the indigenous microbial population has been exposed to specific polluting compounds for prolonged periods, subpopulations will have developed a limited metabolic ability to utilise and, thus, degrade the offending pollutant. However, growth of these particular microbes will invariably be nutrient-limited and when essential growth nutrients such as nitrogen and phosphorus are added, growth stimulation will normally occur with a concomitant increase in pollutant breakdown. This method was successfully applied to beaches along Prince William Sound and the Gulf of Alaska in 1989/90 to clean up the oil spillage from the oil tanker *Exxon Valdez*. Fertilisers (nutrients), when applied in various formulations to the beaches, stimulated the indigenous microorganisms to degrade the oil to less harmful products, which subsequently became part of the food chain. Over three million dollars were spent on the bioremediation of the Alaskan beaches and, to date, this has been the largest application of this emerging technology. Soils contaminated with recalcitrant chemicals such as PCBs, previously considered as highly toxic and indestructible industrial pollutants, are now being realistically dechlorinated by this method.

(2) The alternative approach to direct nutrient supplementation and *in situ* microbial growth stimulation has been to remove microbial samples from the polluted site, enrich the useful microbes, scale-up from the mixture by bioreactor cultivation, and re-inoculate large quantities of the 'cocktail' of microbes into the contaminated site (*bioaugmentation*). This has been quite successful in some sites.

Some companies now market microbial inocula that are claimed to significantly increase the rate of biodegradation of oil pollutants. Another approach has been to utilise and market white rot fungi, such as *Phanaerochytae chrysosporium*, a widely used degrader of lignocellulosic materials. Organisms that can degrade complex organic molecules such as lignin have a wide range of enzymic activities capable of degrading many of the most dangerous industrial pollutants, such as polychlorinated biphenols. There are presently some constraints on this approach.

(1) Indigenous degradative microbes are fully adapted to the specific environment to be treated.
(2) Introduced or 'foreign' microbes must be able to survive in the new environment and be able to compete with the established indigenous microbes.
(3) Added inocula must remain in close contact with the pollutant and, in aqueous environments, avoid dilution.

A further possibility of bioaugmentation is to genetically engineer microorganisms to be able to degrade organic pollutant molecules that at present they are unable to. While this has been achieved in some cases there are considerable technical problems including genetic stability and survival of the 'new' microbe in a hostile environment. Furthermore, there are legislative, ethical and perceptional problems concerned with their release into environments such as sewage systems, soils and oceans. To date, no genetically engineered microorganism has left the laboratory and been tested in the field. There is intense research in progress worldwide, particularly in the USA, and it is believed by many informed industrial scientists that within ten years this technology will be widely and safely used for environmental applications.

While microorganisms have dominated bioremediation practices there is a groundswell of interest in using plants to remediate some environmental problems. Plants have evolved an extensive root system that allows efficient acquisition of essential elements from soil. Removing from soil inorganic pollutants such as lead, mercury and cadmium could well be a new, potentially low-cost, environmentally sound remediation strategy.

Decades of military action have led to severe and widespread contamination of land and groundwaters by explosives that are recalcitrant to degradation, e.g. royal demolition explosive RDX (1,3,5-trinitro-1,3,5 triazine) and TNT (2,4,6-trinitrotoluene). RDX is toxic to all classes of organisms tested, including mammals and plants. The US EPA list RDX as a priority pollutant and possible carcinogen. Current treatment for both explosives is by bioaugmentation and detonation, or by excavation and re-burial. For both explosives novel methods of phytoremediation are being successfully explored. For TNT, tobacco plants have been genetically engineered to express a bacterial (*Enterobacter cloacae*) NADPH dependent nitroreductase, which enhances conversion to aminodinitrotoluene within the roots of the engineered plants. Plants expressing the bacterial gene tolerate and degrade TNT, at levels lethal to wild-type plants. Interestingly, the plants also naturally contained an enzyme that could remove the toxic aminodinitrotoluene. In a similar way a gene XplA has been transferred from *Rhodococcus rhodochrous* into the plant *Arabidopsis thaliana* with subsequent decontamination of RDX. However, all of this is still at an early stage of development and must await regulatory acceptance. Sadly, it is the countries that are littered with spent munitions that will continue to suffer,

Table 7.4	Strengths and weaknesses of bioremediation of oils	
Strengths	Weaknesses
Relatively simple techniques	Can be slow when compared with physical clean-up methods
Relatively low cost	Applicable only in certain environments and for compounds suitably biodegradable
Results in mineralisation or easily dispersed by-products	Involves addition of man-made chemicals/nutrients and dispersants – possible source of environmental contamination
Technology can be unobtrusive and non-disruptive	Requires explanation to the public regulators and bodies involved in environmental clean-up because it is a new technology
Accelerated natural biological mechanics avoid associated risks of man-made hazardous wastes	

Source: P. Morgan, Shell International Petroleum Co. Ltd., London.

and *not* the countries (who oppose GM plants) that created and sold the munitions!

Bioremediation is a new technology and will require time for full development and application. Some of the relative strengths and weaknesses of bioremediation for the treatment of oil spillages are shown in Table 7.4.

Advances in environmental biotechnology continue on a global basis and are improving the performances and reliability of microbial-based processes for site reclamation, waste treatments and pollution prevention.

7.7 | Detection and monitoring of pollutants

A wide range of traditional methods have long been used to detect pollutants, including microbial and chemical analyses. More recently improved biological detection methods include biosensors and immunoassays. Such sensors can be designed to be highly selective or sensitive to a wide range of compounds, e.g. pesticides. Microbial biosensors are microorganisms that produce a reaction (such as luminescence) upon contact with the substance to be sensed.

Immunoassays use labelled antibodies and enzymes to measure pollutant levels. Such assays have proved very valuable for sensitive and rapid field use. Another increasingly used technique for microbial detection is direct isolation and amplification of DNA from soil.

7.8 | Microbes and the geological environment

Microbes are increasingly recognised as important catalytic agents in certain geological processes, for example, mineral formation, mineral degradation, sedimentation, weathering and geochemical cycling.

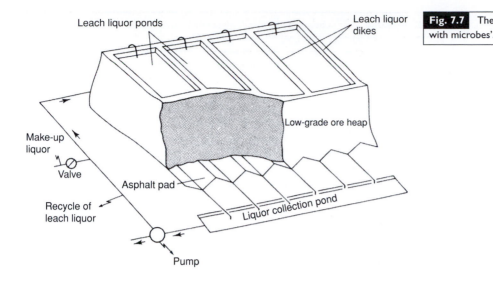

Leach liquor ponds

Leach liquor dikes

Low-grade ore heap

Make-up liquor

Valve

Asphalt pad

Recycle of leach liquor

Liquor collection pond

Pump

Fig. 7.7 The principle of 'mining with microbes'.

One of the most detrimental examples of microbal involvement with minerals occurs in the production of acid mine waters. This occurs from microbial pyrite oxidation when bituminous coal seams are exposed to air and moisture during mining. In many mining communities the huge volumes of sulphuric acid produced in this way have created pollution on an unprecedented scale. Other examples of the detrimental effects of microbes include the microbial weathering of building stone, such as limestone, leading to defacement or structural changes.

In contrast to these harmful effects, microbes are increasingly used beneficially to extract commercially important elements by solubilisation (*bioleaching*). For example, metals such as cobalt, copper, zinc, lead or uranium can be more easily separated from low-grade ores using microbial agents – mining with microbes.

The biological reactions in extractive metal leaching are usually concerned with the oxidation of mineral sulphides. Many bacteria, fungi, yeasts, algae and even protozoa are able to carry out these specific reactions. Many minerals exist in close association with other substances, such as iron sulphide, which must be oxidised to free the valuable metal. A widely used bacterium *Thiobacillus ferrooxidans* can oxidise both sulphur and iron, the sulphur in the ore wastes being converted by the bacteria to sulphuric acid. Simultaneously, the oxidation of iron sulphide to iron sulphate is enhanced.

The commercial process involves the repeated washing of crushed ore, normally in large heaps (Fig. 7.7) with a bioleaching solution containing live microorganisms and some essential nutrients (phosphate/ammonia) to encourage their growth. The leach liquor collected from the heaps contains the essential metal that can easily be separated (downstream processing) from the sulphuric acid into which it has been extracted.

In the USA almost 10% of total copper production is obtained by this method. Countries such as India, Canada, the USA, Chile and Peru are routinely extracting copper at a worldwide annual rate of 300 000 tonnes

Table 7.5 | Chemical reactions associated with microbial bioleaching of low-grade uranium ores

Indirect oxidation of uranium ore with ferric ion catalysed by *Thiobacillus ferrooxidans*

UO_2^{2-} tetravalent uranium, insoluble oxide.
$UO_2SO_4^{2-}$ hexavalent uranium (uranyl ion, UO_2^{2-}), soluble sulphate.
$UO_2 + 2Fe^{3+} + SO_4^{2-} \rightarrow UO_2SO_4 + 2Fe^{2+}$
$(U^{4+} + 2Fe^{3+} \rightarrow U^{6+} + 2Fe^{2+})$

Thiobacilllus ferrooxidans reoxidises the Fe^{2+}

using microbes – with low-grade ores bioleaching costs only half or one-third as much as direct smelting.

Large-scale bioleaching of uranium ores is widely practised in Canada, India, the USA and the former USSR. By means of bacterial leaching it is possible to recover uranium from low-grade ore (0.01–0.5% U_3O_8) which would be uneconomical by any other known process. The USA alone extracts 4000 tonnes of uranium per year in this manner. Uranium is primarily used as a fuel in nuclear power generation and microbial recovery of uranium from otherwise useless low-grade ores can be considered as an important contribution to energy production (Table 7.5). Bioleaching of uranium ores is seen to make an important contribution to the economics of nuclear power stations by providing also a means of recovery of uranium from low-grade nuclear wastes.

Continuous processes have been developed, and the control of the essential bacterial populations is easily achieved because of the acidity and limited substrate availability. Leaching technology will continue to offer more efficient and cheaper ways of extracting the increasingly scarce metals necessary for modern industry. The principal disadvantage of bioleaching is the relative slowness of the process.

Another important potential application for bacterial bioleaching is the removal of the sulphur-containing pyrite from high-sulphur coal. Little use is now made of high-sulphur coal because of the SO_2 pollution that occurs with burning. However, as more and more reserves of coal are brought into use, high-sulphur coals cannot be overlooked. Thus the bacterial removal of pyrite (which contains most of the sulphur) from high-sulphur coal could well have huge economic and environmental significance.

Aliphatic hydrocarbon-utilising bacteria are also being used for prospecting for petroleum deposits. Microbes will soon be commercially used to release petroleum products from oil shelf and tar sands. In all these systems there is rarely any formalised containment vessel or bioreactor. Instead, the natural geological site becomes the bioreactor, allowing water and microorganisms to flow over the ore and to be collected after natural seepage and outflow. Recycling by mechanical pumping can also be used.

When an oil field is opened up, pumping will produce only about one-third of the total petroleum present. Secondary recovery techniques such

Table 7.6	A typical oil well production scenario	
Oil source	Original oil in place (%)
Produced	24.0
Reserves	8.8
Tertiary oil target	13.6
Future technically developed targets	13.6
Unrecoverable	40.0

as gas pressurising, water flooding, miscible flooding and thermal methods can further increase output. Tertiary oil recovery methods involving the use of solvents, surfactants and polymers that are able to dislodge oil from geological formations can further increase or prolong the production life of a well (Table 7.6). Microbially enhanced oil recovery processes involve the use of polymers such as xanthan gum, produced by large-scale fermentation of specific bacteria. Such gums have excellent viscosity and flow characteristics and can pass through small-pore spaces, releasing most trapped oil. Application is usually associated with water-flooding operations. A further possible approach is the use of microorganisms *in situ* for dislodging oil by way of surfactant production, gas formation or even altering the viscosity of the oil by partial microbial degradation. At present, the difficulties outweigh the advantages.

Microorganisms can also be used as metal (bio)accumulators from dilute solutions. The microorganisms, bacteria, yeasts and moulds, can actively uptake the metals by various ways and such processes have a potential use in extracting rare metals from dilute solution, but it is still to be seen whether it will become an important technology.

In a similar way, microorganisms are being used to extract toxic metals from industrial effluents and reduce subsequent environmental poisoning.

Some plants have been shown to accumulate heavy metals such as nickel, cobalt, cadmium and even gold, and studies are now being carried out to assess whether such plants could be used to extract metal from soils or ores that are subeconomical for conventional mining. This area of study is called phytomining and will depend on the use of hyperaccumulating plants. It is envisaged that hyperaccumulating plants would be harvested from soil containing metal, the plant material burnt to give a small volume of plant ash (bio-ore) containing high concentrations of the target metal, and the final bio-ore smelted to yield metal. Such processes are not yet commercially viable. Phytomining could well appeal to conservation movements as an alternative to open cast mining of low-grade ores.

In all these activities, multidisciplinary approaches are necessary, and new biotechnological techniques such as designing an organism for a specific function could yield further benefits. The overall picture of this area of biotechnology is one of rapid and exciting development. There is a growing awareness of the value of an unpolluted environment.

7.9 | Environmental sustainability and clean technology

In the present chapter, attention has been drawn to the various biotechnological technologies that are being used to reduce the impact of societies' wastes on the environment. In a seminal paper 'Sustainable biotechnology development: from high tech to eco-tech', Professor Moser (1994) identified how current utilisation of biotechnology is seen as a 'bolt-on' service for intrinsically unfriendly current environmental processes. While economics is the determining force for most technological changes, efforts towards enhancing environmental biotechnology must surely be seen only as an add-on strategy.

He probingly enunciated how biotechnology with respect to environmental protection has three levels of application.

(1) *Pollution clean-up:* for example, clean-up of oil spills and detoxification of contaminated soil; treatment of domestic and industrial waste water supplies.
(2) *Pollution control:* for example, recovery of heavy toxic metals from mining water; use of enzymes rather than chlorine in pulp and paper manufacture.
(3) *Pollution protection:* for example, closed cycling practice at enzyme production plants where raw materials are renewable, waste material is a biodegradable sludge, which can be used as a local fertiliser.

In past decades there has been extensive investment in the treatment of industrial waste with minimal investment in waste minimisation. The advent of the concepts of clean technology now attempts to shift attention and actions from remediation to prevention of environmental degradation. In this way it is hoped this will lead to the emergence of technologies directed towards waste minimisation or prevention. Ideally, totally environmentally friendly technological processes would have low consumption of energy and non-renewable raw materials (particularly fossil fuel feedstocks) and would reduce or eliminate waste.

It is increasingly becoming evident that human activities within the environment are far exceeding the sustainable capacity of the Earth. In essence, the environmental load equals the size of the world's population × the prosperity or welfare per head of population × the environmental use per unit of prosperity (welfare). It is now apparent that in 50 years' time there will be an unavoidable requirement to reduce the environmental load 20–50 times. As it is doubtful that this can be achieved we must either accept an increasing erosion of environmental values and standards worldwide or set about making processes more efficient by minimising mass and energy flows. Time is running out!

All environmental biotechnology processes and products can have negative implications and such risks must be balanced against ensuring benefits. While such processes must always be put through risk assessment,

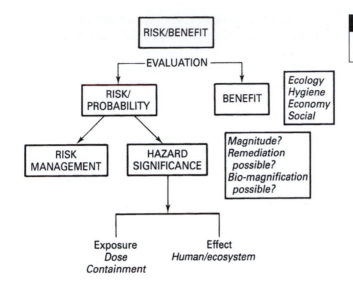

Fig. 7.8 Scheme for environmental biotechnology risk assessment. (*Source:* EFB, 1999.)

it is clear that in the light of legislative awareness and technological realism, a great amount of existing and forthcoming environmental biotechnologies should be capable of achieving maximum environmental safety (Fig. 7.8).

It is now universally accepted that environmental impact is a function of population, affluence or consumption and the technology used to create and support goods and services. If the standard of living currently achieved in the West, especially the USA, was universal, then the environmental impact would already be unsustainable.

The ecosystem must be protected from the adverse environmental effects associated with increased urbanisation and industrialisation. This will involve creative management of effluents and emissions, reducing waste generation and overall producing reliable and clean technologies where possible. Thus, there is now an increased awareness that rather than attempt to remediate after the process the problem should be tackled at source. Biotechnology will increasingly be seen as a means to improve many types of existing biological and chemical engineering processes that presently generate environmentally damaging by-products. There will be increased integrated bioprocess design (Chapter 4), which will develop high-quality bioprocesses that are efficient, controllable and *clean*. Biotechnology will play a central role in 'eco-tech' – a new technology concept embedding technology into the exosphere and human culture by using the whole range of biodiversity in a holistic and low-invasive way in order to achieve benefits for humankind obeying ecological principles.

The principal feature of future clean technologies will be to refocus attention from remediation onto prevention or minimisation of pollution and environmental degradation. Clearly, no single technology is expected to deliver clean products and processes; however, biotechnology will undoubtedly be a major driver of industrial sustainability, competing increasingly with existing chemical and physical systems, reducing material and energy consumption, and waste generation, while being economically competitive.

Sustainable development must ensure the needs of the present without compromising the needs of future generations.

Chapter 8

Plant and forest biotechnology

8.1 | Introduction

Globally, agriculture and food production are committed to produce, in a sustainable way, sufficient, healthful and safe food for the world population. Demographers, who had been until quite recently forecasting a steady exponential rise in world population, have now had to make a major readjustment and now estimate world population peaking at c. 10 billion (ten giga people) by 2050–60. World population growth, in percentage terms, had almost stopped by the 1960s and started to decrease by the 1970s. World population is still growing but adding smaller numbers each year. In many parts of the developing world, child births have decreased by up to 50% by greater awareness of the necessity of using modern methods of birth control. To successfully feed 10 billion people will require 35% more calories than presently produced by world agriculture and, indeed, much more, if any increasing proportion of the 10 billion will want to eat meat more than once a month.

To feed this world population there will need to be substantial increases in the production of the staple food commodities: cereals (40%), meat (63%) (it takes ten calories of wheat to produce one calorie of meat) and roots and tubers (40%). At least 80% of this food will need to be produced in developing countries, yet only about 6% of new virgin soil can be brought into cultivation. Humankind must, somehow, raise yields from areas planted with cereals (two-thirds of all energy in the human diet) to approximately double the present value. Consequently, there can be no alternative other than to plan, with modern scientific inputs, new agricultural systems that are sustainable but yet intensive. Whereas in the last great 'green revolution' in agriculture in the 1960–1970s, the environment was adapted to the plant by increased use of fertilisers, biocides, irrigation, etc., modern sustainable agriculture must increasingly adapt the plant to the environment, breeding high-yielding crops that can grow in places deficient in nitrogen or water, and where plant diseases and pests prevail. Many aspects of modern biotechnology are, and will increasingly be, applied to agriculture.

Agriculture continues to be the world's largest single industry and in advanced societies such as the USA agriculture contributes over 20% of total gross national production. In developed economies agriculture relies heavily on technology to achieve productivity and profitability. Agriculture in many parts of the world is undergoing a major strategic restructuring to achieve vertical integration between production and ultimate utilisation. Whereas the food processor would formerly buy raw agricultural products on the commodity market, they are increasingly establishing breeding programmes to create the desired raw materials with the specific traits required for higher value processing. Genetic engineering is creating a revolution in agricultural practice allowing an ever-increasing range of improved plants and animals. There will be increased stability in the marketplace and much less wastage. Agricultural biotechnology will allow higher quality standards with lower costs of production.

Agriculture is a politically sensitive area with many selective trade barriers and protectionist policies. In many parts of the world, such as Europe and the USA, agriculture is a highly efficient industry and continues to demonstrate annual increases in productivity. In contrast, many countries are still not self-sufficient in food production for many reasons, such as lack of good agricultural practices, hostile or changing climate, or political instability. Many countries are intrinsically poor and lack the ability to take advantage of new agricultural practices and biotechnology. This can only be remedied when the advanced nations make available the training programmes and financial investments required. However, much is already taking place through agencies such as the World Bank and the EEC.

8.2 | Plant biotechnology

By the unique process of photosynthesis, plants are able to fix carbon dioxide into chemical energy using the physical energy of sunlight. This flow of energy from sunlight through plant photosynthesis is at the heart of the importance of plants in world economics. Plants in their myriad forms are the primary producers in almost all ecosystems, and as a result most life on the planet depends for its very existence upon plants. Plants are the basic source of food for the human race (and also a source of energy as described elsewhere) and only by correct management of plant agriculture can the present and future populations of the world survive.

Surprisingly, only a relatively few plant species have been brought into agricultural practice. While there are at least 300 000 known plant species, only a few hundred, but especially wheat, maize and rice, have had any significant impact on agriculture. Manipulating the genetic constitution of plants and then selecting the characteristics that are best suited to human needs has prevailed throughout the history of agriculture. In the highly technology-driven world that we now live in the links between plants and people are easily overlooked (Fig. 8.1).

Since early times humans have sought to improve the quality and productivity of agriculturally important plants. This was done by selection and traditional breeding procedures of natural mutations – a painstakingly

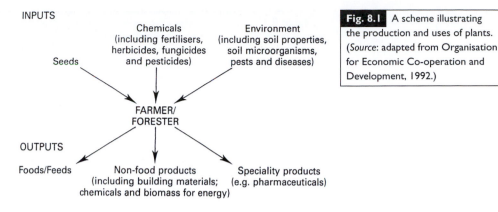

INPUTS

Chemicals
(including fertilisers,
herbicides, fungicides
and pesticides)

Environment
(including soil properties,
soil microorganisms,
pests and diseases)

Seeds

FARMER/
FORESTER

OUTPUTS

Foods/Feeds

Non-food products
(including building materials;
chemicals and biomass for energy)

Speciality products
(e.g. pharmaceuticals)

Fig. 8.1 A scheme illustrating the production and uses of plants. (*Source*: adapted from Organisation for Economic Co-operation and Development, 1992.)

slow and difficult process. But it has been a remarkably successful commitment as witnessed by the high quality of the present food plants such as maize, rice, wheat, potato, etc. – all far removed from their ancestral beginnings. However, from the mid-1950s it became possible to increase the rate of plant mutations by artificial means, in particular, irradiation. Nowadays, plant scientists use thermal neutrons, X-rays or ethyl methane sulphate (a harsh carcinogenic chemical) that can damage DNA – to generate *artificial mutations* in crop plants, especially cereals. It is intriguing to note that this drastic DNA damage has required *no safety tests* and has not generated any protests! The arrival of genetic manipulation in 1983 clearly proved to be a more predictable alternative to an unpredictable mutation breeding system. Thus, instead of a random process, it was now possible to introduce the desired trait that was required. The genetically modified (GM) crop plant had now arrived! The well orchestrated opposition to this safer approach will be discussed elsewhere.

Traditional breeding programmes involving natural or induced mutations and sexual crosses will continue to dominate the approach to improve the agronomic characteristics of food crops, but will be increasingly augmented by new techniques incorporating micropropagation, protoplast fusion and genetic engineering.

The rate of genetic improvement has been historically restricted by the number of suitable genes available and the ability to form and propagate the improved strains. However, by the nature of modern genomics, more useful genes from plants and other sources are now becoming available, together with the development of methods for transforming and then expressing those genes in appropriate crop strains. A major challenge will be to try and understand how to control the way genes act in concert to produce crop traits of value to farmers, processors *and* consumers.

Clonal propagation

As early as 1939 it became possible to isolate small numbers of cells from certain plants and to keep them alive indefinitely in artificial cultivation. The cultivation of these tissues required the presence of a plant hormone, which allowed the cells to propagate in an unorganised manner resulting in an amorphous mass of cells. Advances were soon made in cultivation

Table 8.1 | Potential markets for plant secondary products

Compound	Use	Estimated retail market (US$ million)
Vinblastine/vincristine	Leukaemia	18–20 (USA)
Ajmalicine	Circulatory problems	5–25 (world)
Digitalis	Heart disorders	20–55 (USA)
Quinine	Malaria; flavour	5–10 (USA)
Codeine	Sedative	50 (USA)
Jasmine	Fragrance	0.5 (world)
Pyrethrins	Insecticide	20 (world)
Spearmint	Flavour; fragrance	85–90 (world)

techniques, achieving rapid growth rates in chemically defined media. These individuals or groups of cells were treated like microbial suspensions and were able to grow under aerated and shaken conditions, initially in flasks but subsequently in large traditional bioreactors. (By this method it is possible to produce important secondary metabolites with potential commercial value; Table 8.1).

While it has been possible to produce many secondary metabolites using plant cell culture, only two secondary metabolites – shikonin and paclitaxel (Taxol) – have thus far been produced on a commercial scale. It has been difficult to achieve even moderate yields of most target compounds.

In contrast, the use of plant cell culture for recombinant protein production has become an area of considerable success, producing antibodies, enzymes, hormones, growth factors and cytokines. However, to date, no recombinant proteins have been produced commercially using plant cell cultures. Most of these studies have used suspension cultivation of plant cells as previously discussed in Chapter 4.

The next major advance in plant cell culture was to achieve the complete reversal of this process by causing these individual plant cells to go through a developmental programme from individual plant cells to tissues, to organs and finally to entire plants. In this way it has become possible to clone plant cells.

Rapid, large-scale clonal propagation of many plant species including trees is now feasible. Small tissue explants of many species can be aseptically removed from the parent plant and artificially maintained and increased in number by suitable control of the medium. The process can be rapid and produces high-quality, uniform plants. Outstanding examples of this technology have been the recent successful cloning of oil-palms and coffee plants from callus tissues producing unlimited numbers of stable types. This area of micropropagation not only allows rapid propagation or mass production of identical clones of plant species but also has the following uses:

(1) elimination of viruses and other pathogens
(2) storage of essential germ plasma instead of conventional seeds
(3) embryo rescue

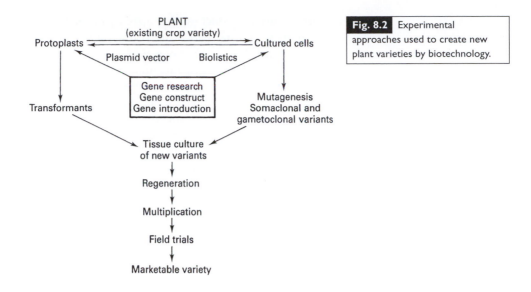

Fig. 8.2 Experimental approaches used to create new plant varieties by biotechnology.

(4) production of haploids by anther and ovary culture (gametoclonal variants), useful for cereals.

It is now possible to take plant cells and subject them to the battery of manipulative techniques long practised in industrial microbiology, for example, mutation, strain selection and process development. Thus the genetic diversity of plants may be altered without the normal sexual process of fertilisation, by production of haploid, triploid and tetraploid cells, by the use of protoplast fusion between different species and even genera, and by transformation, i.e. transferring DNA from one plant cell (or even another type of organism) into the cells of another. The techniques of recombinant DNA technology are now practically available to the plant technologist (Fig. 8.2).

Protoplasts can be produced from most plant cells by digesting away the cell wall and maintaining the protoplasts in a suitable osmotic medium. Many types of protoplasts can be induced to reform cell walls and to divide to form cell colonies. Some plants, including potato, pepper, tobacco, tomato, etc., can be fully regenerated from protoplasts. Full regeneration for important cereal crops is not yet possible. Some protoplasts may be fused with other species, allowing a novel mixing of genetic traits.

With tissue culture of callus or large structures, regeneration mainly leads to uniformity of plants. In contrast, regeneration from single plant cells or protoplasts can often be accompanied by minor or extensive changes in the final plant phenotype. This has been termed *somoclonal variation* and is widely used as a means of crop improvement, in particular with respect to yield and disease resistance (Fig. 8.2).

Plant genetic engineering

The basic principles of genetic engineering have been outlined in Chapter 3 and encompasses the identification of the relevant gene(s) and their transfer into the chosen plant species by means of a vector or by other vectorless means. The first practical system for genetically manipulating plants occurred in 1983 using the ability of the bacterium *Agrobacterium tumifaciens* to transfer part of its Ti (tumour inducing) plasmid into the host genome (DNA). *Agrobacterium tumifaciens* is a natural, soil-borne plant pathogen that is able to generate tumorous growth in plants. The bacterial cells contain a large plasmid, the Ti plasmid, which bears tumour-inducing genes in a region of the plasmid called T-DNA. It has been possible to eliminate the tumour-inducing genes from the T-DNA region and insert foreign or transgenes into the plasmid. Subsequently, the transgenes in the bacterial plasmid DNA can be integrated into the protoplasts of the chosen plant genome. Transformants can be identified by selection methods, adult plants reconstituted from the transfected cells and the new genetic material transmitted as a Mendelian trait. Nowadays, the Ti plasmid-derived vector is used routinely in laboratories throughout the world for transforming dicotyledon crop plants. This method was originally unsuitable for most monocotyledon crop plants such as maize, wheat, rice, etc. However, new plasmids have been genetically engineered that allow the *Agrobacterium* method to be used to transfer genes into cereal crops such as rice. Successful gene transfer into the monocotyledon crop plants was first achieved by biolistics or the 'particle gun', which was used to bombard plant cells with DNA (gene)-coated particles. In this way the microprojectiles penetrated the cell walls and delivered the DNA into the nucleus. The intact cells could be regenerated into whole plants (Fig. 8.2). Other vectorless transmission methods include:

(1) electroporation – where cells are placed in a solution of transgenes; a strong electric field is then applied that affects the permeability of the membrane surrounding each cell and allows the penetration of the transgenes

(2) an aqueous solution of transgenes and fine crystals of silicon carbide is shaken together and the tiny puncturing of the cell membrane allows transgene entry. In each case a proportion of the transgenes will be inserted into the cell's DNA.

By these methods it is now possible to introduce advantageous new traits into almost any plant species, and most agricultural crop plants and many tree species have been manipulated (Table 8.2).

Tumour-inducing plasmids have also been used for inserting 'antisense genes' in order to negate the functions of specific plant genes concerned with an undesirable phenotype. Such genes are produced by reversing the orientation of a gene in relationship to its promoter. The transcripted product cannot be translated into a normal protein thus inhibiting that function within the plant.

What are the current main goals for the application of genetic engineering to plant agriculture? In essence genetic engineering releases the plant breeder from two major constraints:

(1) limits imposed by interspecific barriers

(2) lack of precision inherent in traditional breeding methods.

Presently genetic engineering methods allow the introduction of single gene characteristics into plant cells, and this later should extend to

Table 8.2	Important crop characteristics undergoing genetic modifications

Pest resistance.

Resistance to viral, bacterial and fungal diseases.

Oil, starch and protein modification to provide sustainable supplies of raw materials for biodegradable plastics, detergents, lubricants, paper making and packaging; also improvements in baking and brewing qualities.

Herbicide tolerance to enable certain crop varieties to tolerate specific herbicides and, in many instances, reduce the number of herbicide applications to achieve effective weed control.

Plant architecture and flowering including plant height, flowering time and flower colour.

Reduction in seed losses through shedding at harvest time.

Modifications in fruit and tuber ripening and storage research on potatoes are likely to reduce the dependence on the use of anti-sprouting compounds applied to stored tubers.

Increased tolerance to environmental stresses, including cold, heat, water and saline soils.

Increase in the ability of certain plants to remove toxic metals from soils (bioremediation), e.g. from mining wastes.

The elimination of allergens from certain crops, e.g. rice.

The enhancement of vitamins, minerals and anti-cancer substances.

The production of pharmaceutical substances, e.g. anti-coagulant compounds, edible vaccines.

Source: from Dale (2000)

multiple genes and indeed whole biochemical pathways. The main introduced improvements in commercial application include:

(1) improved resistance to specific herbicides
(2) improved resistance to insect pests and microbial diseases
(3) improved post-harvest characteristics.

Improved resistance to specific herbicides

The killing of plant weed species by the application of selective herbicides gives a growth advantage to commercial crop plants. Such compounds have been designed to disrupt the growth of certain weed species without affecting the particular crop plant. The annual global herbicide market is in excess of US$6 billion. However, there is increasing opposition to the continued use of such chemical compounds from environmental and human health considerations. Herbicide-tolerant crop plants have now been produced by genetically engineering genes resistant to specific herbicides. This has been seen as a way of producing more effective, less costly and more environmentally compatible weed control.

There is now a wide range of genetically modified herbicide-tolerant (GMHT) agricultural crops, such as cotton, maize, sugarbeet, canola, etc., being grown especially in the USA. For example, much of the soybean grown in the USA and Argentina is genetically modified to tolerate the herbicide glyphosate (Round Up®). This herbicide disrupts amino acid metabolism in plants by blocking the action of one enzyme 5-enolpyruvyl-shikimate-3-phosphate synthase (EPSPS) and is thus toxic to both weeds and crops. Genetically modified herbicide-tolerant plants were developed by incorporating the EPSPS gene from a bacterium that eludes binding by glyphosate, which can kill the dicotyledon weeds and leave the herbicide-resistant crop unharmed. In a similar manner GMHT crops are tolerant to the herbicide glufosinate, which disrupts glutamine synthesis and leads to the accumulation of toxic levels of ammonia. In maize, tolerance has been achieved by inserting a synthetic phosphinothricin N-acetyltransferase (*pat*) gene similar to a bacterial enzyme. Genetically modified herbicide-tolerant crops have been very popular with farmers *and* seed companies, simplifying weed management and helping to conserve fertile topsoil. Weed control is an indispensable aspect of modern agriculture. Are GMHT crops harmful or beneficial to the farmland environments? Large farm-scale evaluations are now in progress.

Improved resistance to insect pests and microbial diseases

Historically, the use of chemical pesticides has led to dramatic improvements in production levels of agriculture and forestry. Their continued widespread use is the dominant reason why fewer people can now produce more food at less cost than previously. The pesticide market is dominated by synthetic chemicals and will undoubtedly remain so. However, consumers are becoming increasingly concerned about food quality and possible carry-over of pesticide residues into food products. What are the alternatives to chemical pesticides? All organisms have their own specific diseases and predators. Biological control involves the use of microorganisms applied in the field, usually foliar, to control pests. However, biological pest control has not proved to be as effective or economical as chemical control. Problems associated with the use of biocontrol to manage pest problems include: slow, delayed and/or inadequate activity; a restricted pest-control spectrum; inconsistent activity across different environments; and high costs involved in production and processing of biological control agents (BCAs).

The most successful BCA is *Bacillus thuringiensis*, a spore-forming bacterium containing crystalline protein inclusions. The proteins are highly toxic to insect pests but specific in their activity. They have been widely used for over 30 years against *Lepidoptera* (caterpillar) pests. The commercial folial application of these biopesticides is usually as formulations of spores and crystalline inclusions of disrupted *B. thuringiensis* and they are applied at 10–15 g per acre or about 10^{20} molecules per acre. *Bacillus thuringiensis* (*Bt*) toxins have a considerable world market.

Transgenic plants expressing insecticidal proteins from *Bt* were first commercialised in 1996, and many companies have since been involved in developing *Bt* crops. *Bacillus thuringiensis* has become a major insecticide because genes encoding *Bt* toxins have been engineered into important crops such as cotton and maize on a cumulative area >80 million ha by 2005. Such crops have benefited growers economically, reduced the use of other chemical insecticides, and in the case of maize have lowered the incidence of toxic mycotoxins (such as aflatoxins and fumonisms) by reducing insect damage that makes the maize more susceptible to the mycotoxin-producing fungi. Studies have also shown that *Bt* cotton led to long-term regional pest suppression.

In the early stages of the worldwide use of *Bt* crops some scientists, regulators and environmentalists expressed concern that their use would inevitably lead to resistance development to *Bt* toxins. This has not materialised. Preventing insect pests from acquiring resistance to *Bt* toxins produced by transgenic crops has been a major challenge for agriculturalists and a range of realistic field and molecular methods have been devised (see Bates *et al.* 2005 for full details).

Microbial diseases, in particular fungal and viral, remain one of the major factors limiting crop productivity worldwide, with continuing huge losses set against large cash inputs for pesticide treatment. Global estimates of losses due to plant diseases in 1987 were approximately US$90 billion. Much improved resistance to viruses by the integration of genes for viral coat proteins has now been achieved in several crop plants, particularly rice. These approaches could well be the most advantageous aspects of all plant biotechnology. The necessary widespread use of insecticides, fungicides and pesticides for crop protection undoubtedly has damaging effects on the environment, and consequently it is imperative to improve the control of pests and diseases by genetic and other rational alternative means.

Improved post-harvest characteristics

Losses during storage and transport of some crops can be as high as 40% in the USA and Europe, and as high as 80% elsewhere. While a great deal of this loss will be due to diseases and pests, with soft fruits and vegetables there can be bruising, heat and cold damage, over-ripeness, off flavours and odours, etc. Most of these physiological changes result from endogenous enzyme activity. Can such activity be genetically stopped or slowed down? In the tomato the enzyme polygalacturonase breaks down cell wall constituents leading to softening of the fruit during ripening. This process is independent of colour development. In normal conditions if the tomato is left to ripen on the vine and develop full colour, the softening process is also occurring thus creating an easily bruised and damaged fruit on shipment. By inhibiting the polygalacturonase enzyme by antisense genes the tomato can remain on the vine until mature and be transported in a firm solid state. The Flavr Savr GM tomato has been engineered by Calgene in the USA with improved flavour and keepability and is now marketed in the USA. The current annual market for fresh tomatoes is US$3.5 billion. Such principles will now be used in a wide variety of soft fruits. Other studies are considering ethylene synthesis/inhibition as a means of controlling fruit and flavour maturation.

Genetic manipulation of ornamental plants and floriculture involving flower and leaf colour, abundance of flavours, perfume and shape are now major targets for the decorative plant industries, especially in Germany, Australia and the USA (Table 8.3).

Transgenic crops worldwide

There are now over 20 countries worldwide planting transgenic crops, with soybeans, cotton, maize and canola as the main types. Whereas herbicide tolerance and improved resistance to insect pests and microbial diseases have been the major applications, there is now an enhanced level of activity

Table 8.3	Floriculture traits in development
Desired trait	Developmental stage
Drought, cold tolerance	R&D
Blue carnation	On market since 1996
Blue rose	Market approval expected in 2008
Fragrant rose	R&D
Delayed senescence	R&D

Source: adapted from Patera (2007)

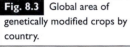

Fig. 8.3 Global area of genetically modified crops by country.

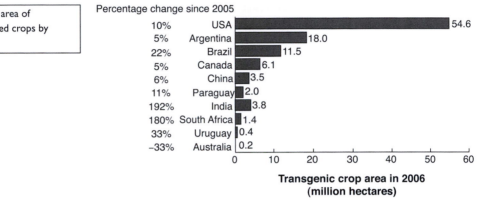

in the USA for approvals for product quality. The USA is by far the dominant grower of GM crops followed by Argentina, Brazil, Canada, China and, more recently, Paraguay and India (Fig. 8.3). There are strong indications that major expansions in GM crops areas are yet to come, particularly in Asia, Latin America and parts of Africa. Worldwide, between 2000 and 2005 there was a doubling of land devoted to GM crops and also the value of these crops was estimated in excess of US$50 billion. Well over 60 countries are now involved in GM plant research and development.

Unfortunately, the European Union (EU) continues to support a restrictive policy on GM crops, and as a consequence there is a steady exodus of valuable scientists to other countries. It is only to be hoped that the EU will eventually support an orderly regulatory framework harmonised with the rest of the world.

While the current GM crops are substantially benefiting the production cost reduction to the farmer, novel GM crops with direct consumer benefits are now appearing or are in advanced stages of development (Table 8.4). Of special interest are nutritionally enhanced foods, e.g. vitamin-enriched cereals, vegetables and fruits, low-calorie sugars, healthy oils and others.

In many parts of the developing world, such as India, other South East Asian countries and Africa, billions of people have inadequate levels of essential vitamins (especially vitamin D) and minerals (iron) in their staple diet. This can result in severe anaemia, immune deficiency, blindness,

Table 8.4	Potential uses of transgenic plants relevant to consumers and the food industry	
Plant	Modification	Advantage
Tomato and other plants	Delayed ripening	Easier transport for fruits: improved quality
Tomato	Increased chitinase	Less post-harvest spoilage
Maize	Control over starch structures	Fewer requirements for starch conversions
Maize, canola, etc.	Control over lipid profile	Oils that promote human health
Legumes	Suppression of protease inhibitors	Increased digestibility
Soybeans	Suppression of lipoxygenase	Improved flavour
Various plants	Modification of enzyme activity	Increased antioxidants
Peanuts	Elimination of allergens	Less allergenicity
Rice	Increased provitamin A	Increased vitamin A supply

Source: adapted from Johnson-Green (2002)

impaired intellectual development and death. Attempts to rectify these deficiencies make use of supplements, food fortifications and improved dietary diversity, e.g. increased availability of vegetables and fruits. However, such educational programmes and vitamin supplements need annual budgets and networks for delivery, which sadly can foster dependency.

Could biofortification of staple crops, such as rice, by GM technologies be a worthwhile approach? Such a concept has been extensively and meaningfully explored by expressing β-carotene (provitamin A) in rice. A new variety of rice 'golden rice 2', which incorporates a phytoene synthase from maize (the original GM golden rice 1 used daffodil phytoene synthase) accumulates a much higher level of provitamin A and it is considered that it could supply up to 50% of the essential daily requirement of vitamin A. It also contains elevated levels of digestible iron. The term golden rice derives from its colouring due to its content of β-carotene.

The producing company Syngenta is part of the Humanitarian Golden Rice Network, which has obtained free licences for humanitarian use of the necessary technology for golden rice for a large number of companies and universities that have pioneered the overall process. For rice breeders and farmers the costs will be minimal. This must be viewed as a new humanitarian face of GM crops. But still the GM opponents seek to block it!

Genetically modified crops engineered to improve agricultural productivity, where environmental stresses such as drought, heat, soil salinity and flooding reduce or destroy crops, are widely being developed and will help to ensure increased food security.

The development of GM crops is knowledge and resource intensive, and is more often viewed as the product of multinational corporations. In contrast, in poorer developing nations public-funded research is the only way to achieve their development. While public research institutes developing GM crops should be most relevant to local needs it does pose unique challenges for gaining regulatory approvals that have been formulated in wealthy Western economies. As it presently stands it can cost millions of

Table 8.5 | Approximate annual world production of some plant-derived agricultural products

Sector	Product	Tonnes
Food and feed	Cereals	1.8 billion
	Sugar	120 million
	Crude starch	1.0 billion
Materials	Harvested wood	1.6 billion
	Paper	200 million
	Cotton	16 million
Chemical	Plant oils	43 million
	Natural rubber	4 million
Others	Tobacco	4 million

Source: adapted from Organisation for Economic Co-operation and Development (1992)

dollars to obtain regulatory approval for a single novel trait change in a commercial crop (see Cohen, 2005 for a fuller discussion of this complex area of GM crops).

Scientific research worldwide has repeatedly demonstrated that GM (biotech) crops and foods are safe for human and animal consumption. Examination of the ethics, morality and safety of GM crops and foods will be considered later.

The proportion of plant agricultural production directed towards non-food uses has now passed 20% in many developed countries, e.g. cotton, tobacco, natural rubber and, of course, wood.

The first stages of the plant biotechnology revolution have now arrived and are being assessed by a somewhat sceptical and unprepared public. Successful commercial products will need to meet a genuine market need. The approximate annual world production of some agricultural products (many of which have already been subjected to genetic manipulation) is shown in Table 8.5.

The correlation and coordination of the vast quantities of information molecular researchers are generating will involve a substantial effort in bioinformatics. This will be essential to link all operations in crop development, on the molecular constitution of plants, and on the interactions between molecules. While genomics has dominated plant research in the last two decades, plant proteomics has now come of age.

As will be discussed later, there has been much unjust opposition to plant genetic engineering by a vocal minority, especially in Europe. To argue that this new technology is not required in the food affluent Western countries does great disservice to the vast majority of people in the developing world. Sustainable agriculture will not be possible in many developing countries without the use *and* availability of creative plant genetic engineering. There is not a choice – it is obligatory. The constrictions now envisaged by these 'full-stomachs' sceptics will damage the full development of this scientific area and will, undoubtedly, in the near future, lead to unprecedented suffering in developing countries.

Pharming: pharmaceutical crops

Pharmaceutical recombinant protein production by means of transgenic animal, bacteria and yeast cells has demonstrated the commercial success of this approach. Production methods are complex and currently not fast enough to meet existing demand. As a result, many companies worldwide have been exploring the possible use of whole plants as production vehicles for recombinant proteins on the basis that there would be higher yields, less expense and ultimate reductions in product prices. Production of such plant made proteins (PMP) is now referred to as *pharming*. There are three stages in the pharming process.

(1) Identify a particular gene that codes for a specific, desired pharmaceutically active protein, isolate the gene(s) and insert into the genetic framework of the chosen crop plant. This transgene can potentially come from a different plant species, an animal or human or a microorganism.
(2) The genetically engineered plants are grown and the plant acts as a mini-factory synthesising the pharmaceutical protein.
(3) The crop is harvested and the protein extracted, purified and subject to normal commercial distribution. In some cases it has been proposed that the plant material could be consumed directly.

Hundreds of pharmaceutical crops are currently at research and development level but none has yet achieved commercial acceptance. What are the main target drugs? Of particular interest are hormones, antibodies, blood thinners, coagulants, insulin and contraceptives. Plant-derived vaccines to cholera, rabies, hepatitis B, human immunodeficiency virus, malaria and influenza have been proposed and researched.

Maize has been the most utilised vehicle for pharming with other candidates being soya, rice, potato, tobacco and others.

The major problem is that pharming cannot ensure 100% containment of the transgene and the crops, and many disadvantages have already been identified:

- transgenes could escape by way of pollen and contaminate non-pharmaceutical crops
- seed left in the soil after harvesting could establish volunteer pharmaceutical plants
- regulatory mistakes have generated bad publicity and have been seized upon by GM protesters.

Clearly the use of crop plants, such as maize, has been a poor industrial decision because of potential cross-contamination in grain elevators and food processing. Could such crops be grown on isolated islands far from normal food crop situations? Better still should non-food crops such as tobacco be the adopted process vehicle? Much interest is now focused on plant species, such as duck weed and mosses, that could be grown indoors with high containment using photobioreactors and are not of food interest.

The commercial potential of pharming is immense but the lack of foresight on GM hostility by the biotechnological/pharmaceutical companies is disturbing.

8.3 | Forest biotechnology

Throughout the world there is an escalation in demand for wood-derived products, and many major regions such as Europe, India and Japan are now in deficit. This will be further compounded by increased pollution, such as 'acid rain', and the huge losses now occurring in the rain forests of South America and Asia by indiscriminate felling. Worldwide forests are diminishing while the demand for their products, such as pulp, and for paper industries, construction, fuel and other requirements, is increasing. Forest experts have calculated that the approximate 3.9 billion hectares of global forests will not for much longer be able to support the current annual demand of 3.4 billion cubic metres of timber; 90% of this comes from natural forests. Traditional breeding programmes will not solve this increasing demand. Forest trees have not had the research and management that cultivated crops, such as coffee, citrus, rubber, coconut and others, have received, and are more often viewed as self-regenerating resources that need little cultivation. This is in sharp contrast to most other plant crops, which have been tailored to accommodate human needs through extensive breeding programmes. Furthermore, resulting from their long generation times, there is a paucity of information on tree genetics, and modern plant breeding strategies may not be truly relevant.

However, biotechnology will play an important role in achieving an increase in production as well as bringing major improvements to the quality of the trees. Tissue culture technology such as micropropagation, somatic embryogenesis (induction of single cells or cell aggregates to develop into embryo-like structures from which a shoot and root develop), selection of somoclonal and gametoclonal variants and gene transfer are being developed to improve forests (Fig. 8.2). Trees have long generation times and, as a consequence, genetic improvements will be slow. Loblolly pine has been transformed by *Agrobacterium tumefaciens* and this may allow gene transfer techniques similar to those used with other plant species.

Targets for tree improvement are well recognised: apical dominance; wood quality (fibre length, lignin content, texture); disease, pest and herbicide resistance (especially for fruit trees); and nutrient use. While herbicide and insect-resistant crops are becoming available, the genes involved have yet to be characterised. Future focus will involve functional genomics applying microarray technology to define differentially expressed genes.

Increased yield is the prime target of all forestry sectors with emphasis on shorter cycle times. It is well recognised that tree productivity correlates with solar input and temperature; thus a forest the size of Sweden in Brazil would satisfy current global wood needs. If high-yielding forests can be achieved by selective breeding programmes it could lead to a doubling of present-day plantation productivity (estimated at 1.5 million cubic meters per year) while halving the land area required. If commercial wood

Table 8.6 | The potential impact of biotechnology in forestry

Industry demands	Biological/biotechnological challenges
Enhanced growth rate and decreases in rotation time.	Tree genomes are larger.
	Long generation times.
Feedstock suited to harvesting and handling capacity (straight trunks, short limbs).	Some desirable traits genetically complex.
	Uniformity already achievable by cloned forestry.
Uniformity of feedstocks.	Price of feedstock critical.

Product/technology benefits	Deliverable by 2020
Increased yield.	Correlation of genetic markers and desirable traits.
Shorter generation times.	Methods for mass-propagation of superior germ plasm.
Pest resistance.	
Enhanced cold and drought resistance.	Environmentally acceptable systems for testing and deployment of genetically modified trees.

Source: Robinson (1999)

production could be confined onto a smaller landbase and achieve a sustainable system, natural forests could then be left for biological diversity and public amenity. Table 8.6 identifies some potential impacts of biotechnology on forestry. Environmental studies have shown that planting energy crops such as short rotational coppice (SRC) is beneficial to wildlife with more insect and bird species recorded around the willows than equivalent arable and grasslands throughout the year. A major hurdle for forest biotechnology is technological, especially understanding the biology of most commercial trees. Compared with most agricultural crops, tree biology is in its infancy. Most of the global funding in forest biotechnology is being channelled into universities for basic research. Most of this is governmental support with some variable contributions from industrial companies. There is little evidence of investor input. The science and technology of genetically manipulating tree genes has lagged behind crops such as corn, cotton, etc. The first tree genome, *Populus trichocarpa*, the poplar tree, has recently been worked out and this should lead to increased impetus in this area. However, there are major costs involved in transformation studies, together with integration into breeding programmes and subsequent field trials.

Most trees take decades to reach maturity, and replacing harvested trees is a long-term proposition. Genetic manipulation could be the key to bridge the time gap that traditional tree breeding cannot achieve. Some GM trees are now ready to plant! However, the environmental opponents of GM trees have already set in motion 'what if?' scenarios of doom and disaster.

Their main concern is tree pollen, which can travel great distances and in great volumes, creating massive potential for gene transfer to nearby and distant trees, with the potential problems of cross-breeding. The sheer scale of pollen gene flow dynamics with trees creates a major challenge in assessing the environmental impact of a transgenic tree. Whereas seasonal agricultural crops have a limited period of seed and pollen mobility, trees produce seeds and pollen for many years before they are harvested. Biocontainment zones suitable for transgenic food crops would not prevent the escape of seeds and pollen from transgenic trees. Consequently it may prove difficult to reassure the public that the promised rewards of GM forest biotechnology outweigh fears of the unknown.

However, the proponents of forest biotechnology believe that ultimately GM trees will achieve the early promises, especially producing fast-growing trees maturing in 10–15 years instead of 20–30 years, and producing trees that do not produce blossoms, seed or pollen. In this way cross-fertilisation would not occur and the debilitating tree-pollen allergies prevalent worldwide could be reduced. However, reproductive sterility in trees remains in its infancy.

Forest biotechnology will take patience and time to achieve its ultimate goals.

Trees as energy crops

Short rotation coppice crops, especially willow and poplar, can produce wood chips that can be used to co-fire power stations where they are mixed with coal thereby using a renewable source and reducing carbon dioxide emissions. Giant grasses (up to 3–4 m tall), such as *Miscanthus*, switchgrass and reed canary grass, are also considered as solid energy crops, which can be used whole to produce heat and electricity direct through combustion. Similarly, all of these crops can be viewed as *cellulose crops* where the cellulose and hemicelluloses can be reduced to sugars by acid hydrolysis and then fermented to produce ethanol. Lignin, a major component of plant cell walls, which gives wood its strength, is the second most abundant natural polymer on Earth. This amorphous and insoluble aromatic material is not susceptible to hydrolytic attack, unlike hemicellulose and cellulose (the most abundant natural polymers on earth). However, a small group of mushroom-type fungi called 'white rot fungi' can selectively degrade lignin and are important in forest decay both in living and dead trees. The molecular biology of these fungi is now being extensively researched. Extensive worldwide efforts are underway to devise enzymatic technology to economically break down the complex lignocellulose for ethanol synthesis. The ability to use tree cellulose for ethanol energy formation would dramatically influence forest biotechnology. Energy crops are 'carbon neutral' since plants/trees fix atmospheric CO_2 by photosynthesis and when the biomass is burned the CO_2 is released back into the atmosphere; thus, recycling the CO_2.

Chapter 9

Animal and insect biotechnology

9.1 | Introduction

Animal agriculture in the form of cattle, pig, sheep, poultry and fish farming represents a major aspect of food production worldwide. While many of these animals are produced for their meat alone, others contribute to human nutrition by way of milk and egg production, and yet others produce products such as wool and leather. In the developed world animal production is highly intensified and technologically driven. Animal production will reflect quality of feed, availability and need of growth hormones, pesticides, antibiotics and vaccines, good animal husbandry and welfare, and increasingly selective breeding, molecular biology, embryo manipulation and gene transfer.

As with plant agriculture early animal breeders sought to identify worthwhile properties in animals and to perpetuate them into future offspring. Selective breeding aims to increase the frequency of a large number of genes that work together with the remainder of the animal's genes or genome to produce the desired phenotype (selective breeding pre-dates our understanding of genes and the science of genetics). Between 1945 and 1993, selective breeding increased milk production of the average dairy cow by a factor of three. Further, when we consider the huge variety of dogs it should be remembered that they are all one species, capable of easily interbreeding, and the present varieties have arisen by carefully controlled selective breeding programmes. For many farm animals conventional breeding has already achieved high-producing animals, but it is apparent that the increases in productivity possible by this means now seem to be approaching a plateau. To sustain an ever-increasing world population ways must be achieved to meet this increasing demand for animal products.

Selective breeding is a painfully slow process and, especially with larger animals with long gestation periods, can take many years to establish desired phenotypic changes. However, the advent of recombinant DNA technology and its application to animal breeding programmes could greatly increase the speed and range of selective breeding.

Table 9.1	The reasons for producing genetically modified animals

- To help scientists to identify, isolate and characterise genes in order to understanding more about their function and regulation.
- To provide research models of human diseases, to develop new drugs and new strategies for repairing digestive genes ('gene therapy').
- To provide organs and tissues for use in human transplant surgery.
- To produce milk that contains therapeutic proteins; or to alter the composition of the milk to improve its nutritional value for human infants.
- To enhance livestock improvement programmes.

Source: adapted from Straughan (1999)

Table 9.2	Anticipated changes involving transgenic animals

Efficiency of meat production	Wool quality and quantity
Improved quality of meat	Disease resistance in animals
Milk quality and quantity	Production of low-cost pharmaceuticals and biologicals
Egg production	

9.2 | Genetic manipulation and transgenic animals

There are many important scientific reasons for proceeding with programmes of genetic manipulation of animals (Table 9.1). On a purely scientific basis genetic modifications will allow an improved understanding of how genes function in the animal system, and by means of animal models it may be possible to gain insight into certain human diseases (e.g. cancer) and to develop medical solutions. The ability to repair defective genes (i.e. gene therapy) is being extensively researched with animal models. In the context of this chapter, attention will be given to how genetic manipulation in several forms can be beneficial in enhancing livestock improvement and to the production of therapeutic proteins, eg. in the milk of lactating animals. Some of the main opportunities where these new technologies can be envisaged within animal breeding programmes are listed in Table 9.2.

Pro-nuclear infection

How can novel DNA be incorporated into animal genomes and then stably inherited by the offspring? The overall strategy of creating a transgenic animal is similar to that used to develop a transgenic plant. As in all cases, it is necessary to isolate the desired DNA sequence that codes for the desired protein together with an understanding of promoter, terminator and regulatory regions of the gene. The linearised DNA is then ready for transfer.

| Table 9.3 | Sequences necessary to establish transgenic animals |

- Identification and construction of foreign gene (genetic engineering).
- Microinjection of DNA directly into the pronucleus of a single fertilised egg.
- Implantation of these engineered cells into surrogate mothers.
- Bringing the developing embryo to term.
- Proving that the foreign DNA has been stably and heritably incorporated into the DNA of at least some of the newborn offspring.
- Demonstrating that the gene is regulated well enough to function in its new environment.

At the present time the most successful method for gene transfer into livestock is by microinjection into the pronucleus of fertilised eggs. Microinjection techniques make use of finely constructed glass needles, which allow the injection of purified DNA into the fertilised eggs of the chosen species: a process known as transfection. The eggs are then surgically transferred into hormonally synchronised surrogate mothers (Table 9.3). Unlike mice and pigs, litter size is limited to one or two in sheep and cattle and, therefore, large numbers of animals have to be employed as recipients for the microinjected eggs. Transgenic pigs, sheep and cattle, and other animals, have now been obtained although the frequency of success is only about 1% compared with 2–5% in mice. This low efficiency of the technology will continue to exert some limitation to wider acceptance. However, with fish the eggs are fertilised externally and thus eliminate many of the complicated techniques required in mammals to harvest ova, fertilise them and then introduce the embryos into foster mothers. Successful fish transgenics can be as high as 70%.

The ultimate goal of animal breeders will be to introduce specific economically important traits into commercial livestock. However, the knowledge of the mechanisms regulating gene expression in most higher animals is limited, and this limits the ability to construct transgenic animals.

Regrettably, the much acclaimed process of genetic engineering as a means of enhancing livestock production has largely remained unfulfilled. There have been limited successes with projects aimed at improving feed efficiency and increasing lean muscle mass, but most international efforts have been directed to the production of compounds mainly for human medical application. Again, only limited studies have been concerned with the improvement of an animal's ability to resist disease.

Mastitis in lactating dairy cattle is the most costly disease in animal agriculture worldwide, resulting in lost profits in the US dairy industry alone of c. US$2 billion per year. Not only are there massive losses in milk production but also debilitating effects on animal well-being, and this is the major reason for culling or death in dairy cattle. The bacterium *Staphylococcus aureus* causes up to 30% of clinical mastitis cases and is difficult to control by application of antibiotics, which have poor penetration throughout the milk gland. *Staphylococcus aureus* in vitro is strongly inhibited by the antibiotic lysostaphin, and a recent study has tested the feasibility of protecting cows through genetically engineering a gene for lysostaphin production into cows. The gene was transfected into fibroblasts from Jersey fetuses, which served as nuclear donor cells. Activation followed by embryo culture produced blastocysts, which were then transferred into cows. A small number of calves were born and survived into adulthood. The transgenic cows expressing lysostaphin in their milk were resistant to *S. aureus* infection of the mammary glands. The early results confirm the feasibility of using genetic engineering to introduce beneficial genes into cattle and that such transgenes could be a major improvement on the economics of dairy farming *and* on animal well-being.

The health benefits of long chain *n*-3 fatty acid or omega fatty acids, which are mainly found in fish oils, are now well appreciated and they are regularly added to many foods such as milk. Meat products contain large quantities of *n*-6 fatty acids and small quantities of omega fatty acids. Diets with high ratios of *n*-6/*n*-3 fatty acids are now considered to contribute to many human diseases such as coronary heart disease, arthritis, diabetes and cancer. It is now known that the high ratio of *n*-6/*n*-3 fatty acids in meat is derived from the grain in animal feed, which is rich in *n*-6 fatty acids because they lack an *n*-3 fatty acid desaturase gene. Transgenic pigs have been developed that express a humanised gene, *fat-1*, which encodes an *n*-fatty acid desaturase. Such transgenic pigs produced high levels of *n*-3 fatty acids from *n*-6 fatty acids and their tissues have a significantly reduced ratio of *n*-6/*n*-3 fatty acids. Good news for healthier eating.

A novel and commercially realistic use of transgenic animals is the production of human proteins/pharmaceuticals in transgenic lactating animals. Transgenic constructs that allow the mammary glands of lactating animals to secrete high-value human proteins are now possible and could be the first truly commercial use of transgenic animals for product formation. The animals will in fact become bioreactors producing pharmaceutical products previously only produced in culture by transgenic microorganisms. Gene constructs for human factors IX or α-1 antitrypsin (some haemophiliacs lack a blood-clotting agent called factor IX) have been successfully inserted into the sheep genome and while expression levels are still low, factor IX is present and the trait is heritable. The potential of transgenic animals to secrete a wide range of commercially valuable healthcare products is almost unlimited and may be realised in the future. Pharmaceutically used transgenic sheep will not be allowed to enter the human food chain thus removing possible public outcry concerning the consumption (cannibalism) of the human gene inserts.

Recombinant proteins produced in animals typically have altered glycosylation patterns when compared with native proteins. It is now recognised that it is difficult for transgenic animals to produce 'nature identical' proteins in their milk. In cows, sheep and goats the oligosaccharide decoration on proteins will contain N-glycolylneuraminic acid monomer, which is virtually absent from native human proteins. The high level of protein produced in milk (g/l) overextends the glycosylation capacity of the mammary glands. Indeed, only in rabbits and chickens are the oligosaccharides more human-like (containing *N*-acetylneuraminic acid).

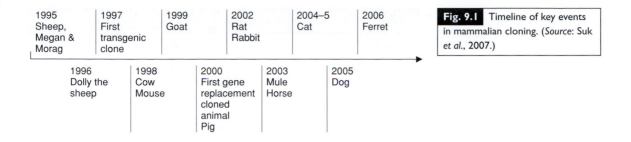

Fig. 9.1 Timeline of key events in mammalian cloning. (*Source:* Suk *et al.*, 2007.)

Recent concerns have been raised by regulatory authorities on potential immunogenicity. Should immunogenicity of milk-produced proteins prove to be a generic problem then the long-term future of this method of transgenic production could be in doubt. As yet, no drug produced in a transgenic farm animal has reached the marketplace.

Somatic cell nuclear transfer (SCNT)

In the 1950s scientists removed the nuclei from frogs' eggs and replaced them with somatic nuclei from embryos and succeeded in raising adult frogs. This was then followed by serial transplantations using the nuclei from the transplanted embryos for more transplantation. Consequently, all the embryos could be considered to have identical nuclei; this was originally termed *nuclear cloning*, but is now known as *somatic cell nuclear transfer* (SCNT). In the 1990s, Dolly the sheep was created in Scotland from a nucleus derived from an adult ewe inserted into an enucleated oocyte (Fig. 9.1). This subsequently led to huge public interest and debate fuelled by exaggerated media coverage, on the possible 'cloning' of human beings. The debate continues.

There are two aspects to the SCNT process. A ewe is induced to super-ovulate and the eggs collected. By means of a micropipette the cell nucleus (DNA) is siphoned out leaving an enucleated cell, but with a small residual amount of mitochondrial DNA in the cytoplasm. Meanwhile, tissue has been removed from the udder of an adult ewe, the individual cells then cultured axenically on a plate dish and subsequently induced into a resting phase by limited starvation. A single cell, containing a full set of chromosomes, is picked up by a micropipette and transferred into the space between the empty egg and the cytoplasmic outer lining. An electric current is applied and fusion occurs. The resulting embryo or clone is cultured and then transferred into a surrogate mother and in *c.* 21 weeks a lamb is born. The potential values of SCNT are listed in Table 9.4.

A wide range of farm animals have now been exposed to this technology with mostly successful results. However, the process of SCNT is quite inefficient (1–5% success rate), and expensive, which implies that for the foreseeable future its use in agriculture will be limited to insurance against loss of prize animals to disease or death before they have had opportunity for reproduction. While some breeders may resort to SCNT to create elite animals, by far the majority of meat, milk and other products will still be derived by existing methods.

Table 9.4	Potential application of somatic cell nuclear transfer

- Production of genetically identical laboratory animals.
- In animal breeding, producing multiple copies of supreme animals that could be utilised in animal farming.
- Providing more reliable ways of producing transgenic animals with less wastage.
- Helping scientists to identify the genetic contribution to different animal diseases and to find genetic solutions.
- Genetic conservation: storing frozen semen and embryos is expensive, could skin biopsies and other cells be used for long-term storage?

Source: adapted from Straughan (1999)

There are now several successful examples of equine cloning. Cloning could prolong lines of superior horses when the founders are no longer fertile, enable reproduction of castrated male horses (geldings), and perhaps allow better understanding of equine physiology. Most critics consider that it is now unlikely that cloned foals will be accepted into long-established breed registers such as the Jockey Club.

It is now considered that some populations of cloned animals have an attenuated lifespan compared with their conventional counterparts, e.g. Dolly the sheep died somewhat earlier than expected. This has been attributed to premature ageing or senescence, and to accumulation of abnormalities in gene expression in their tissues. More specifically, it is believed to arise because the process of nuclear transfer used to create cloned animals misses one of the two essential independent steps involved in the reprogramming of cell nuclei (for a detailed explanation, see Fulka *et al.*, 2006).

9.3 | Genetically engineered hormones and vaccines

The pituitary gland of animals secretes growth hormones that can have major influence on how an animal grows and, in lactating animals, on milk production. In the 1980s, the gene responsible for bovine growth hormone (somatotropin; BST) production was successfully isolated and transferred into bacterial cells to produce large quantities of BST. When cows were injected with *c.* 30 mg BST there was significant increase in milk production (10–30%) but continued increased yields depended on regular injections. Such improvements in milk production could lead to fewer animals producing the same volume of milk. There is no evidence of increased concentrations of BST in the milk or that the constituents of milk are in any way altered. Comparable studies with genetically engineered pig somatotropin (PST) have shown that body fat can be reduced by up to 80% and feed efficiency increased by 20%. The approval of BST by the US Food and Drug Administration in November 1993 represented the first biotechnology derived pharmaceutical to be commercialised for animal agriculture in the USA.

Bovine somatotropin is the first genetically engineered product in agriculture that has been intensively examined for its economic impact. This is due mainly to the vast importance of milk to most Western economies and the positive product image of milk for human health. Animal welfare is also of major current concern.

From a scientific point of view BST has been clearly demonstrated to be a safe product and is now permitted in many countries, in particular in the USA where it is marketed by Monsanto under the tradename *Posilac*. Many consumer organisations continue to oppose the use of this method. In Europe the European Commissioners have recommended a continuation of the earlier ban for a further five years on reasons that are more politically based than for health and safety reasons. In Europe, struggling to control overproduction of milk, is a milk-boosting hormone really needed? Furthermore, the large numbers of small dairy farmers who might go out of business have considerable political impact.

From an animal welfare consideration there is now evidence that pigs transgenic for PST suffer skeletal and joint problems, while cows have increased mastitis. Some would consider that BST and PST were the wrong biotechnology derived products to lead the way for public acceptance of new biotechnology. The public viewpoint of this biotechnology product is that it has been profit-driven and not need-driven. Much has been learned from this product that may be applicable to the introduction of other new biotechnology products in agriculture.

Animal vaccine production has been developed against many microbial diseases and uses methods described in a later chapter. Animal diseases represent a major cause of suffering in all forms of animal farming, and if disease could be reduced or eliminated then animal welfare as well as yields would improve. By improving the health of the animals (e.g. in intensive farming), the number of animals required to give the same final yield could be reduced.

A new equine DNA vaccine against West Nile virus, a serious and highly infectious disease of horses, is now nearly at final regulatory approval in the USA.

The poultry industry has to contend with the threat of many diseases. The most important is caused by the protozoan, *Eimeria*, which lives within the intestine of the bird. All of the 30 billion chickens raised annually throughout the world must be protected by the application of anti-coccidial drugs. However, parasite drug resistance is becoming a major problem. Using attenuated strains of the parasite that were limited in their capacity to reproduce in the host, a new vaccine, Paracox 5, has been developed in the UK, which allows the host chicken to safely develop a natural immunity to attack. Over 1.3 billion chickens have now been vaccinated and Paracox 5 is now the largest selling attenuated vaccine ever developed against a protozoan parasite.

Rinderpest or cattle plague has historically caused repeated economic and social disasters worldwide resulting in vast destruction of cattle, disrupting agriculture and rural livelihoods, and often causing terrible famines and starvation. It is highly contagious and has been the cause of many historical pandemic outbreaks, and was even used as the first major agrobiological weapon in ancient times.

A successful vaccine was first developed in the 1950s, by repeated passage through infected bovine kidney cells (RK) in suspension cultures. The virus required a large number of passages to become attenuated for cattle application. Global eradication of the disease is now being put into operation: this will be the first animal virus disease to be eradicated and be second only to smallpox eradication. The whole of the Asian and African continents will be targeted. Because of the huge number of serum samples that were required to be analysed worldwide, a simple, high-throughput competitive ELISA suitable for sera from all cattle species was successfully developed.

The production of genetically engineered animal vaccines has been a major, if somewhat unheralded, success story in biotechnology. Numerous vaccines have been developed for specific cattle, pig, poultry, sheep and fish diseases. The commercial success is considerable, though not dramatic, and it has led to much reduction in animal hardship. A new genetically engineered vaccine against rabies is now being scattered in chicken heads in many parts of Europe where rabies is endemic in the wildlife. The future for this type of disease prevention is immense.

9.4 | Animal organs for human patients

In the last few decades medical skills have permitted a wide range of human organ transplants, such as kidneys, heart, lungs and liver. However, throughout the world there are massive waiting lists with donors falling far short of demand. Can suitable animal organs be a serious option? Two international companies, together with many research institutions, have been striving to meet the demand by tailoring pigs so that their organs could save human lives. Analysts believe the market could be worth US$5 billion for solid organs alone with at least the same again possible from cellular therapies, e.g. transplantable cells that could produce insulin for the treatment of diabetes.

Previous attempts at transplanting animal organs into humans have been unsuccessful because of rejection by the human immune system. The human immune system recognises that the animal organ is 'foreign' and sets in motion a 'hyperacute' rejection. An important reason for this rejection can be related to an enzyme present in all animals but not in humans, α 1,3 galactosyl transferase, which adds a sugar to the surface of all animal (pig) cells. It is this sugar that is recognised by the human immune system and causes a rapid allergic response.

The intense recent excitement on animal organs for transplants relates to the birth of piglets in which the transferase enzyme has been deleted from their genome. Enzyme deletion can only be achieved in single cells, and the piglets have been produced by cloning from these single cells just as Dolly the sheep was created. These present studies are an essential step forward but not the final solution. It is believed that at least three more genes will need to be deleted to deal with all stages of rejection.

Apart from rejection, scientists will have to be concerned about infection, since pigs carry viruses that could potentially cause human disease or epidemics. However, pig cells have already been used in various experiments with humans, with no signs of porcine retroviruses. Much still needs to be done but this is undoubtedly a major step forward for animal/human transplants. Ethical considerations will also be a source of much debate.

9.5 | Genetically modified insects

Insects are the largest and most varied group of organisms on the planet, and are the cause of many serious diseases of man, animals and plants. There is an extensive range of chemical pesticides used to control insects in the human and agricultural environment, while in plant agriculture plants have been genetically manipulated to resist specific insect infestations.

Genetic engineering of certain insect species has been an obvious area of research, and especially in the USA there have been many meaningful studies. There has been considerable work on mosquitoes and kissing bugs to counteract human diseases such as malaria, dengue fever and Chagas disease, engineering of parasite-resistant honeybees, and silkworms that produce stronger silk. Limited field trials have been permitted in the USA for agricultural pests, i.e. roundworm (nematodes), mites (arachnids) and bollworm (insects).

In area-wide insect control programmes a technique called sterile insect technique (SIT) has been used successfully to suppress economically important insect species. This technique involves mass production of the target species, sterilisation by irradiation and sustained release over entire regions of vast numbers of the sterilised insects (usually a hundred times more than native species), which quickly reduce the native populations through infertile matings. Such SIT programmes are now widely practised especially for organic fruit and vegetable production, since it avoids use of chemical pesticides. However SIT is expensive and a new approach is now being considered using a transformation system that allows genetic engineering of many different types of insects. In particular, a transgenic system that causes embryo-specific lethality after transmission to the progeny could possibly replace irradiation and produce more competitive sterile insects. Regulatory issues concerning GM insects are still awaited!

The recent developments that involve genetic modification of animals, i.e. the direct manipulation of an animal's genetic make-up and also the technology of nuclear transfer, have been set out in this chapter. The ethical, moral and social issues related to these new technologies have been the subject of considerable debate and will be fully discussed in a later chapter.

9.6 | A look to the future

When compared with biomedical research there is a great paucity of public interest in basic research on animals, which has lead to a shortage in research and the necessary expertise. Research by biotechnology companies on diseases of animals can be very expensive and it is difficult for animal

Table 9.5	Criteria required for successful rapid methods
They should be fast, accurate and reliable.
Be simple to operate and have low running costs.
Have readily available and stable reagents.
Have minimal labour requirements.
High degree of sensitivity and specificity.

producers to see financial benefits, since food animals are commodity products with low margins. Yet, when we consider the massive recent cullings of poultry, cattle and pigs associated with highly contagious microbial diseases in Asia and Europe, could this have been moderated by vaccination or efficient early diagnosis?

A continuing lack of meaningful guidelines in Europe and the USA on genetic manipulation of especially food animals does not encourage investors to support animal biotechnology enterprises. Sales of biotechnology-based products amount to approximately US$3–5 billion per year, for use in animal health products! In contrast to food animals, companion animals (or pets) contribute well in excess of US$30 billion annually in the USA to veterinary costs, e.g. veterinary oncology, orthopaedics, ophthalmology, etc. While embryonic stem (ES) cell therapy, reproductive cloning and xenotransplantation in human research are creating considerable ethical and moral controversies, could they be applied to health problems with pets where the moral and ethical difficulties would be of less concern?

9.7 | Diagnostics in plant and animal agriculture

In traditional analytical methods applied to plant and animal agriculture, be it chemical or microbiological, the primary aim has been to isolate or separate out the analyte from the complex chemical milieu of the sample. Such methods normally require an operator of considerable chemical analytical experience, and are time consuming and expensive. However, new methods based on biotechnologically derived techniques are revolutionising many aspects of agricultural analysis, not only by being able to equal the sensitivity of the established methods but also by being able to carry out many determinations *in situ* without the need for complex isolation procedures. Furthermore, these methods are usually cheaper, more easily adapted to automation and are more rapid. Often too they can be performed by relatively unskilled operators (Table 9.5).

In the present context, the impact of three new biotechnologically derived rapid methods, immunoassays, DNA probes and biosensors, will be examined in the context of plant and veterinary diseases and physiological monitoring of animals. In almost all cases these new rapid methods were first developed with the massive human healthcare market in mind, where economic rewards were obvious, with huge sales anticipated in

Table 9.6 Successful and anticipated uses of rapid diagnostic methods for animal diseases

Companion animals	Feline leukaemia, canine heartworm, rheumatoid arthritis.
Poultry	Screening of avian reovirus; coccidiosis, salmonellosis, respiratory infections.
Large animals	Trichinosis, mastitis, leukaemia, brucellosis, rinderpest, trypanosomiasis, swine fever, foot-and-mouth disease virus.

hospitals, surgeries, and for home care and monitoring. The veterinary market has also been a highly profitable activity, while in plant agriculture the new methods are increasingly being used.

Immunoassays in general, but specifically those using monoclonal antibodies, are widely recognised for their commercial success in clinical and veterinary diagnostics. Indeed, these diagnostic tests make up a major part of new biotechnological products presently on the market. Immunoassays differ from other analytical methods in that the high technology resides in the molecules rather than the apparatus. Nucleic acid probe technology is based on the principle of hybridisation of complementary sequences of DNA or of DNA and RNA. The respective nucleotide strands must have exact, corresponding sequences of nucleotide bases for exact hybridisation or alignment to occur; thus a given strand can hybridise only with its complementary strand. This high level of specificity has now been directed to identify microorganisms in complex mixtures – the DNA probe or hybridisation assay.

Using these diagnostic methods it is now possible to detect microbial diseases in animals at very low levels of infection in body fluids or tissues, and to be able to isolate such animals before they become infectious. A wide range of animal diseases can now be more easily monitored by 'user friendly' diagnostic kits applied by the veterinarian or the farmer. Early diagnosis can be an essential prerequisite for containment and elimination of infectious diseases (Table 9.6).

One of the largest areas of application for diagnostic kits is in measuring fertility hormones in animal blood or milk, e.g. progesterone, oestrogen sulphate, equine gonadotrophin, etc. Illegal use of growth hormones and antibiotics can also be monitored. Several hundred different diagnostic kits are now available worldwide.

Immunochemical technology using monoclonal antibodies is now widely used for the analysis of pesticide residues in foods, and for toxic microbial products such as mycotoxins. Specific plant diseases can now be detected in a crop at very early stages and appropriate treatment applied earlier. Such methods can also be used to analyse the phytosanitary quality of seed products for sale and to certify that potatoes, bulbs, fruit trees and ornamental plants are disease-free. These methods now allow more efficient crop breeding and international trade. Genetic fingerprinting now allows easy differentiation between plant varieties.

Several pre- and post-harvest problems are of major concern in food production, distribution, processing and subsequent storage and handling. It has been estimated that globally 30–60% of total food produced is lost during these processes. The main problems include pests and diseases, senescence in fruits and vegetables, chemical and biochemical degradation of fruits, vegetables, dairy and meat products, and microbial spoilage. Rapid screening tests are now increasingly used to monitor food from field to table for quality and safety. Rapid diagnostic methods must also be advantageous should there be any possible chemical or microbiological contamination of crops and the general food supply by bioterrorism.

The cost of microbial diseases to world plant production is estimated at US$50 billion annually. However, present estimates consider that only a relatively small part of this would be suitable for the use of immunodiagnostics. It is now not difficult to develop antibodies specific to known fungal, bacterial and viral disease. A wide range of rapid diagnostic kits are now commercially available, especially for the high-value horticultural markets.

Intensive agricultural practices are achieving ever-more reduced returns at an increasingly detrimental cost to the environment. Genetic engineering offers the potential for improvements for a wide range of agricultural practices, but global acceptance must respond to socio-economic, environmental and safety issues. Are such issues real or have they been excessively exaggerated deliberately by the press? Agricultural biotechnology may not be a panacea for problems with future world food supplies, but if applied correctly and judiciously it can give real improvements in the quality of life on a global scale.

Chapter 10

Food and beverage biotechnology

10.1 | Introduction

A major challenge to creating a sustainable future for the world's populations will be to secure adequate food supplies for the majority. By 2030 it has been estimated that the size of urban populations will be at least twice that of rural, agricultural-based populations. The growth of urbanisation, together with ensuing environmental degradation, is already causing serious losses in the availability of productive agricultural land. Furthermore, worldwide climate changes and increasing civil strife continue to make accurate predictions of future food supplies difficult. What role can traditional and new biotechnology play in achieving food sustainability?

Food production is the largest worldwide industry, and in industrialised nations the expenditure on food can account for at least 20–30% of household budgets. However, whereas food is in general in excessive production in most parts of the world, scarcity and insufficient production exists in Africa, Central China and most parts of South America. The food industry has evolved through specialist trades or occupations, e.g. butchers, bakers, confectioners, etc., to national and multinational organisations involved in the manufacture and distribution of food on a worldwide scale. With the improvement in means of transportation, foods are available on a worldwide basis, and developments in food preservation methods give independence from seasonal availability.

In essence, the food industry now serves the function of supplying society with high-quality, wholesome foods, all the year round, and at a distance, in time and location, from the place of primary production.

The food chain has its origins in production agriculture with the planting of the seed or the rearing of animals, and concludes with the utilisation of the food products by the consumer. Apart from fruits and vegetables, most food raw materials, e.g. cereals, meats, etc., will require some degree of processing. The link between the products of the farm and the consumer is the food processing industry, whereby relatively bulky, perishable raw agricultural products are transformed into shelf-stable, convenient and palatable foods and beverages.

Biotechnology has a long history of practice in food production and processing, and can be viewed as a continuum involving both traditional breeding techniques and the latest techniques based on molecular biology. The new biotechnology techniques will especially create possibilities of rapidly improving the quantity and quality of foods available. Furthermore, the application of these techniques will not result in food that is inherently less safe than that produced by conventional systems. The application of new biotechnology to produce foods and food ingredients has become a subject of considerable public interest, at consumer, public policy and scientific levels. Negative images of GM products in large segments of the population, especially in Europe and parts of USA, continue to prevail.

Food biotechnology is concerned with the integration of both modern biological knowledge and techniques and current bioengineering principles in food processing and preservation. This will achieve an elevation of the scientific and technological basis of industrial food processing and preservation to that presently achieved in other advanced biotechnological industries, e.g. antibiotic production. In the next decades, we will witness the optimal integration of the production of agricultural materials, their processing into foods and subsequent utilisation. Food science and food technology have been the mediators between production and consumption.

In present-day developed food markets, the question will be what do consumers desire with respect to physiological needs as well as their social, cultural and religious needs? Truly a reversion of the classical bottom-up paradigm.

The challenge is to recognise the potential of biotechnological techniques to fulfil the food requirements of today's society both for developed and developing nations. Food biotechnology encompasses a wide range of options for improved quality, nutrition, safety and preservation of foods. Clearly, no single biotechnological advance will revolutionise the food industry, while economics, customer acceptance and regulatory rather than scientific hurdles will have a major influence on the range and spread of food biotechnology applications. Modern biotechnological techniques will have considerable importance in influencing trends in the food market: cost, preservation, taste, consistency, colour, safety and, above all, health aspects.

The food and beverage industries are very different from the pharmaceutical industry; their products are cost and marketing driven rather than technologically driven. Research and development in most of the food and beverage industries is usually less than 1% of sales, is very process-oriented and enjoys little patent protection. Since most food and drink products are high-volume, low-cost items, it is inevitable that market research has become more significant than basic research. Some products such as organic acids, amino acids and gums now increasingly used by the food and drinks industry are in the middle price range, while only a few really high-priced products will have a viable future (e.g. sweeteners and flavourings).

Table 10.1 | Biotechnology at all levels of the food chain

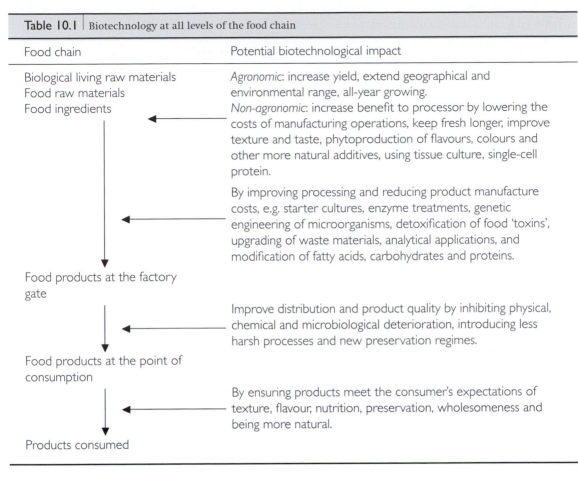

Food chain	Potential biotechnological impact
Biological living raw materials Food raw materials Food ingredients	*Agronomic*: increase yield, extend geographical and environmental range, all-year growing. *Non-agronomic*: increase benefit to processor by lowering the costs of manufacturing operations, keep fresh longer, improve texture and taste, phytoproduction of flavours, colours and other more natural additives, using tissue culture, single-cell protein.
	By improving processing and reducing product manufacture costs, e.g. starter cultures, enzyme treatments, genetic engineering of microorganisms, detoxification of food 'toxins', upgrading of waste materials, analytical applications, and modification of fatty acids, carbohydrates and proteins.
Food products at the factory gate	
	Improve distribution and product quality by inhibiting physical, chemical and microbiological deterioration, introducing less harsh processes and new preservation regimes.
Food products at the point of consumption	
	By ensuring products meet the consumer's expectations of texture, flavour, nutrition, preservation, wholesomeness and being more natural.
Products consumed	

Source: from Boulter (1986)

The food and beverage industries are high in terms of turnover and labour employed and are very diverse, ranging from small individual producers to giant multinationals.

Supplying food to consumers on a global scale is a major task, which engages not only politics but must involve sound scientific knowledge provided by a multitude of scientific disciplines.

The impact of biotechnology on the food and beverage industries can be anticipated in two directions:

(1) *agronomic*, i.e. increased plant and animal yields, extended growth range and environments, from which the farmers will mainly benefit
(2) *non-agronomic*, i.e. improving plants and microorganisms to provide benefits to the food producer, retailer or consumer (Table 10.1).

New developments in biochemical engineering could also be of advantage to those industries using mechanical (e.g. grinding), physical (e.g. membrane separation, cooking) and chemical (e.g. hydrolysis, salting) methods.

Table 10.2 Some traditional fermented/processed foods and ingredients created by biotechnology methods

Category	Fermented product			
Alcoholic beverages	Beers	Wines	Spirits	
Food	Cheese	Sauerkraut	Flavours	Biopolymers
	Bread	Soy sauce	Organic acids	Sweeteners
	Vinegar	Pickles	Amino acids	Mushrooms
	Yoghurt	Enzymes	Vitamins	

10.2 | Food and beverage fermentations

Fermented foods and beverages have a significant role in all societies, and result from the action of microorganisms or enzymes on a wide range of agricultural materials with associated desirable biochemical changes giving significant organoleptic improvements to the final product. As a result of the fermentation process the product is usually more nutritious, more digestible, has improved flavour and is toxicologically and microbiologically safer.

Fermented foods and beverages derived from plant and animal materials are an accepted and essential part of the diet in almost all parts of the world, involving a wide diversity of raw materials as substrates, using technology from the most primitive to the most advanced, and achieving an astounding range of sensory and textural qualities in the final products. Fermented foods include breads, cheeses, yoghurts, sauerkraut, soy sauce, tempeh, mushrooms, etc., while fermented beverages include alcoholic beers, wines, saké, brandy, whisky, and non-alcoholic tea, coffee and cocoa. (For a fuller awareness of this extensive subject *Fermented Foods of the World: A Dictionary and Guide* by Campbell-Platt (1989) should be consulted) (Table 10.2). While most of these fermentations remain at the level of village or household arts, others have achieved massive commercial application and play a significant part in most national economies. All such fermentations have been or remain classified as indigenous, native to a country or culture, and most were developed before recorded history. However, the very roots of modern biotechnology are to be found in these traditional fermentations. How these fermentations first came about is a question that cannot be completely answered.

Climate and available raw materials have influenced the types of food and beverage fermentations that were geographically developed, and such products continue to form an enduring part of the cultural background of a civilisation. It must be remembered that many of the world's populations are vegetarian, not necessarily by choice, but rather for mainly economic reasons. While a very important reason for the development of such fermentations was to preserve the basic organic components from spoilage, of equal or greater importance were the resulting changes in organoleptic, physical and nutritional characteristics of the relatively bland starting materials, resulting in products of enhanced flavour, improved

		Importance	
World production rate	Region	Major	Minor
High	Europe	Dairy, beverages, cereals, meat	Legumes, starch crops
	North America	Beverages, dairy, meat	Fish, legumes, starch crops
	Africa, south of Sahara	Starch crops, cereals, beverages	Dairy
Medium	South America	Beverages, dairy	Legumes
	Middle East	Dairy	Legumes, meat
	Indian subcontinent	Cereals, legumes	Meat
	East Asia	Fish, legumes	Dairy
	South East Asia	Fish, legumes	Dairy
Low	Oceania	Dairy	Legumes
	North Africa	Dairy	Legumes

Table 10.3 Production of classes of fermented foods by geographical region

Source: from Campbell-Platt (1989)

vitamin content and, in some vegetable products, a meat-like texture *and* flavour. The nutritional value of these fermentations, in particular to the populations of the developing world, is inestimable and modern fermentation practices (e.g. brewing, cheese-making, etc.) are providing increased control, consistency of production and, above all, ensuring improved product safety. Food fermentations represent a cornerstone of a civilised society, in which raw food materials are processed to make them safe, to have lasting properties and to make them palatable.

For most of these fermentations the procedures were developed in ignorance of the role of microorganisms. The original artisans unwittingly controlled and directed microbial activity by purely empirical methods, but most often achieved consistent end-products. The Egyptians, Sumarians and Babylonians produced alcoholic beverages from barley; sour-dough bread from rye occurred in Europe in 800 BC; while accounts of fermented dairy products are found in early Sanskrit and Christian works. It is only in relatively recent times that the microbial nature of most of these fermentations has been recognised, and while some fermentations have been shown to have a relatively simple microbiology, others possess a complexity of microbial involvement that may never be fully unravelled.

Fermented foods can be divided into nine groups: beverages, cereal products, dairy products, fish products, fruit and vegetable products, legumes, meat products, starch crop products and miscellaneous products. The relative importance of these fermentations in geographical areas is shown in Table 10.3. These fermentation products represent the largest financial sector of all biotechnologies and represent a major aspect of the gross national product of developed nations. Almost 90% of all revenues from biotechnology come from the food and beverage sectors. Too often we laud modern biotechnological innovations and overlook the continued presence of the long-standing traditional biotechnology-based industries. However, in almost all sectors of traditional fermentations, new-biotechnology is becoming increasingly exploited.

Some of these fermentations will be examined in more detail, and reference made where relevant to the impact of modern biotechnology techniques on their present and future production.

Alcoholic beverages

Alcoholic beverages occur throughout the world in many different forms and tastes. The types of beverage produced in any particular region or country almost entirely reflect the crops grown. Thus, the cooler regions of Europe, Scandinavia, Poland and Russia will produce and consume beers and lagers from barley, while the southern warmer climate of Spain, Greece, Italy and France will have much higher production and consumption of wines derived from grapes. Alcoholic beverages and potable spirit industries worldwide represent one of the most economically stable sectors in modern-day commerce. Demands on economics and need to increase conversion efficiencies or productivity are all driving forces in the search for new and improved technologies. The main objective is to produce a controlled quantity of alcohol in the liquid to be harvested after the fermentation.

The starting material normally comprises either sugary materials (fruit juices, plant sap, honey) or starchy materials (grains or roots), which need to be hydrolysed to simple sugars before the fermentation (Table 10.4). When these substrates are incubated with suitable microorganisms and allowed to ferment, the end-product is a liquid containing anything from a few per cent up to 16% or more of alcohol, with an acid pH and depleted in nutrients for most contaminating microorganisms; these factors combine to give the product a certain degree of biological stability and safety. The alcoholic beverages can be drunk fresh but normal practice for many requires a period of storage or ageing, leading in many cases to improved organoleptic properties. Further distillation will increase the alcohol strength and produce spirits of many types, e.g. whisky, brandy, vodka, gin, rum, etc., which can contain between 40 and 50% ethanol (Table 10.5). Cordials and liqueurs are sweetened alcohol distillates derived from fruits, flowers, leaves, etc.

The most regularly used fermenting organism is the yeast *Saccharomyces cerevisiae* or one of its closely related forms. This yeast is now used for brewing beer and lager, for producing distilled beverages, for many forms of baking and in most modern wine productions. The present form of *S. cerevisiae* may well have arisen by selection during the evolution of brewing and wine production. It is also most probably the first microbe to have been harnessed for human benefit. The art of making alcoholic beverages by fermentation must have been discovered many times in history for such beverages occur in many different forms the world over. This organism can assimilate and utilise simple sugars, such as glucose and fructose, and metabolise them to ethanol. It has a high tolerance to ethanol.

Saccharomyces cerevisiae was the first eukaryote to have its complete genome sequenced and this will undoubtedly lead to new applications in brewing and baking together with novel uses. The process details of

Table 10.4 Substrates for selected alcoholic beverages (non-distilled)

Substrates	Beverage	Country	Saccharifying agent
Starch (barley and other cereals)	Ale Lager	Belgium; W Germany; Canada; Australia; worldwide (industrial countries)	Barley malt Barley malt
Barley, rye, rice, beet	Kvas	Former USSR	Barley and rye malt
Millet	Busa Braga Thumba	Former USSR (Crimea) Romania India	
Rice	Arak Busa Pachwai Saké Sonti	India, SE Asia Turkestan, SSR India Japan India	*Mucor* spp. *Aspergillus oryzae*
Rice (red)	Ancu Hung-Chu	Taiwan China	*Rhizopus* spp.
Sorghum	Kaffir beer Merissa	Malawi Sudan	Sorghum malt *Aspergillus* spp. *Mucor rouxii* *Bacillus* spp.
Sweet potato	Awamori	Japan	Not required since sugar is present in the substrate
Agave spp. (sap)	Pulque	Mexico	
Apple (juice)	Cider	UK, France, N America	
Grape (juice)	Wine	Temperate: N and S hemispheres	
Honey	Mead	UK	
Pear (juice)	Perry	UK, France	
Palmyra (juice)	Toddy	India, SE Asia	
Palm flower-stalk juice	Tuwak	Indonesia	

wine and beer production are briefly examined here since their production represents major worldwide biotechnological industries.

Wines

Historically, wine is a European drink, and although other parts of the world, such as the USA, Australia and South Africa, are now large producers, France, Italy and Germany still produce over half the total world output of approximately 10^{10} litres annually. Historically, the Greeks and Romans

Table 10.5 Potable alcohol production from sugars or starch containing raw materials

Sugar	Product	Starch	Product
Molasses	Rum cognac	Barley	Whisky
Agave	Tequila	Maize and rye	Bourbon whiskey
Pear	Pear brandy	Potatoes and barley	Aquavit
Cherry	Kirsch	Potatoes, rye and wheat	Vodka
Plums	Slivovice	Rice	Chinese brandies

preferred wine to beer and with the spread of Christianity across Europe, wine was used as a symbol of the 'blood of Christ'.

Most commercial wines use the wine grape *Vitis vinifera*, and cultivars of this species have been transported throughout the world to establish new wine-producing areas. Soil quality can have an important and subtle effect on the eventual quality of the wine. Red wine is formed when black grapes are crushed and fermented whole. In contrast, if the skins are removed from black grapes or when white grapes are used, white wine is the final product. Hundreds of different wines are recognised in the many producing areas of the world. Rosé wine results from some limited contact with the skins of black grapes, dry wine is the end-product of complete sugar utilisation while sweet wine will still retain some residual sugars.

Harvesting time of the grapes is judged largely by artisan skills, and the grapes, containing 15–25% sugar, are then crushed mechanically or by treading of feet. The juice (now termed *must*) is the substrate for the truly biotechnological stage of the production. Since the must will contain many contaminating yeasts and bacteria it is usual practice to add SO_2 to control or abolish this natural fermentation capacity. In large-scale wine production the must is partially or completely sterilised, inoculated with the desired strain of yeast, *Saccharomyces cerevisiae* var. *ellipsoideus*, and subjected to controlled fermentation in suitable tanks or bioreactors. The dryness or sweetness of the wine will depend on the degree of sugar conversion, glycerol levels, secondary infections, etc.

Fermentation conditions such as time and temperature will depend on the type of wine desired. After fermentation, the wines are run into storage vats or tankers where the temperature quickly drops, precipitates form and subtle chemical changes take place. Many wines undergo a spontaneous secondary bacterial (*Leuconostoc* spp.) or malolactic fermentation, converting residual malic acid to lactic acid. The final alcoholic content of wines ranges between 10 and 16%.

Modern scientific research now supports the view that moderate wine consumption is associated with lower coronary heart disease mortality. As Louis Pasteur stated 'Wine is the most healthful and most hygienic of beverages'.

Fortified wines, such as sherry, port and vermouth, are wines to which additional alcohol is added after fermentation, raising the alcohol level to about 20%.

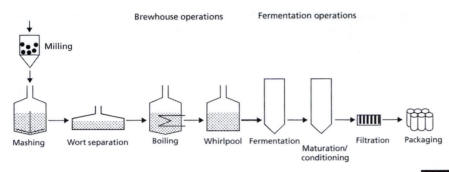

Brewhouse operations   Fermentation operations

Milling

Mashing   Wort separation   Boiling   Whirlpool   Fermentation   Filtration   Packaging

Maturation/
conditioning

Fig. 10.1 The brewing process, showing the split between the brewhouse and fermentation operations.

Beers

The earliest record of brewing was inscribed in cuneiform characters on clay tablets in Sumaria (present day Iraq) at least 6000 years ago. However, it is quite possible that primitive forms of brewing existed many thousands of years earlier. Beer can be defined as 'a drink obtained by the alcoholic fermentation of an aqueous extract of germinated cereal with addition of hops'. Beer is a relatively poor medium for bacterial growth, largely due to its low pH, content of antiseptics such as carbon dioxide, alcohol, hop extracts and its low temperature of storage. Pathogens cannot live in beer thus making it safer to drink than water in many countries. Because of its complex biochemical content, beer is almost impossible to analyse.

Beers, ales and lagers are produced mostly from starchy cereals such as barley. Additional carbohydrate sources, known as adjuncts, are normally added in varying proportions. In practice, there are five major steps in the manufacture of beers from grains: malting, mashing, fermentation, maturation and finishing (Fig. 10.1).

Malting

Dried barley is soaked or steeped in water and then spread out on the malthouse floor or in revolving drums, where the seeds germinate with the formation of starch-degrading (amylase) and protein-degrading (protease) enzymes. The germinated seeds are then killed by kilning (slow heating to 80°C) while still retaining most of the enzyme activity (*malt*).

Mashing

In this stage the malt is mixed with hot water (55–65°C), and the starches and proteins break down to produce dextrins, maltose and other sugars, protein breakdown products, minerals and other growth factors (the *wort*). This is the medium for the beer fermentation. Hops may be added prior to the fermentation to give characteristic flavour and some antiseptic properties.

Fermentation

The wort is transferred to open bioreactor systems and inoculated with pure strains of yeast. In Britain a top-fermenting *Saccharomyces cerevisiae* is used at 20–28°C to produce beers, ales or stouts. In continental Europe a bottom-fermenting yeast *Saccharomyces uvarum* ferments the wort at a lower temperature (10–15°C) to produce lager. Light or low-alcohol beers are usually derived from lagers, which contain fewer fermentable substrates and consequently less alcohol production and fewer calories. Such styles of beers have become very popular in North America and the UK.

The fermentation of glucose is anaerobic and can be summarised by the following equation:

$$C_6H_{12}O_6 \rightarrow 2C_2H_5OH + 2CO_2$$

	glucose	ethanol	carbon dioxide
Theoretical yield	180 g	92 g	88 g

Maturation and finishing

Beer is usually matured in casks at 0°C for several weeks to improve flavour, settle out the yeasts and remove haze. Bottled or canned beers are usually pasteurised at 60–61°C for 20 minutes. The alcohol content of beer is usually between 4 and 9%; with ales it is somewhat higher.

While European type lagers and beers are now produced worldwide, the traditional beer in India and Asia is rice beer and in Africa, sorghum beer. Sorghum beer is a very crude material rich in solids and vitamins and is, in fact, a valuable source of nutrition to those who drink it. Approximately 1.2 billion hectolitres (1 hl = 100 l) of beer are consumed annually worldwide. Without doubt, beer is the most consumed alcoholic beverage.

Traditional applied genetics, together with protoplast fusion and recombinant DNA technology, are constantly improving the yeast strains used in these fermentations. In particular, there has been a vast upsurge in genetic engineering knowledge of *Saccharomyces cerevisiae*. A new commercial brewing yeast has been developed and approved using recombinant DNA techniques.

Spirits

Spirits refer to any volatile, inflammable liquid sustained by distillation whatever the raw material (Table 10.5). Spirits for human consumption, or *potable spirits*, are the distillates of alcoholic liquids, the alcohol in which has been formed by the fermentation of sugars derived from grape juice, sugar-cane, etc. or from saccharified materials such as specially prepared cereals, e.g. malted barley.

Whisky has been produced in Scotland for hundreds of years and is a continuing biotechnology success story. It is known as the 'Water of Life' or in Gaelic 'Uisge Beatha' (Gaelic is the branch of Celtic spoken in the Highlands and Islands of Scotland). Whisky outsells every other spirit in world markets.

Distillation

Whisky is the spirit distilled from a mash of cereals. Malt whisky is distilled twice in large copper pot stills (Fig. 10.2). The first distillation separates the alcohol from the fermented liquid and eliminates the residue of the

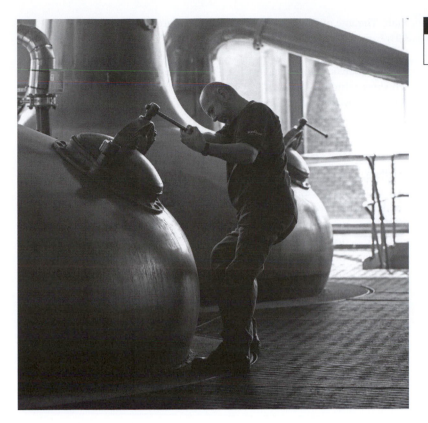

Fig 10.2 The Macallan pot still. (*Source*: courtesy of the Edrington Group.)

yeast and unfermentable materials – this is known as *low wines*. This is then passed into another still and distilled for a second time. Grain whisky uses the patent Coffey still, which is a continuous operation, as opposed to the pot still.

Maturation

Both malt and grain whiskies must be matured after distillation. The raw spirit is filled into casks of oak wood, which is permeable to air passage and allows evaporation to occur and eventually creates a mellow whisky. Normally, malt whisky takes longer to mature than grain whisky and may often be left in the cask for up to 15 years or even longer. The process of maturation is influenced by cask size, strength of stored spirit, and temperature and humidity of the warehouse.

Whisky is one of the most famous exports from Scotland and can be produced in the Lowlands, Highlands and Islands, creating different styles and tastes. The historical significance of whisky to Scotland can be seen by the great Jacobite uprisings of the eighteenth century, which bore the slogan 'no salt tax, no *malt*-tax, no union'.

A 'single' malt whisky derives from malted barley, water and yeast from one distillery only, and while the word 'single' refers to a single distillery, the finished product will contain whisky from lots of different barrels from that distillery. Barrels of different ages and styles will be mixed to form the malt. The age of the label refers to the youngest whisky in the mix, e.g. if 99% comes from 12-year-old whisky and only 1% from 10-year-old it will be labelled 10-year-old whisky.

Most whiskies produced are used to make well-known brands of blended whiskies, which account for 98% of all Scotch whisky sold in world markets. A blended whisky is a collection of single malt whiskies from one or more distilleries mixed with whisky made from another grain such as unmalted barley or maize, which makes for a rounded flavour.

Coffee, tea and cocoa

In Asia, India, Africa and South America, non-alcoholic fermented beverages are derived from coffee, tea and cocoa plants. These beverages have gained worldwide approval and high commercial value. Tea is derived from the enzymic action released after the crushing of the leaves, while for coffee and cocoa, the pulp surrounding the beans is removed in part by a natural fermentation with bacteria, yeast and fungi, which is critically important for full flavour and aroma development. The dried products, tea leaves, and coffee and cocoa beans, can then be shipped throughout the world and the final beverage formed by the addition of water. Little is known about the exact microbial contribution to these fermentation processes. The processes are still empirical with little exact science. Huge quantities of these products are consumed worldwide and form the economic basis of several multinational companies.

Dairy products

The manufacture of cultured dairy products represents the second most important fermentation (after the production of alcoholic beverages), accounting for over 20% of fermented foods/drinks produced worldwide. The origin of the development of dairy products, such as fermented milk, butter and cheeses, is lost in antiquity. Such fermentations are related to areas with high numbers of lactating animals, cows, goats and sheep, and Europe is the major world area of production (Table 10.3). Worldwide, fermented dairy products account for about 10% of all fermented food production. It is now known that these fermentations result largely from the activity of a group of bacteria called lactic acid bacteria. Fermentation by lactic acid bacteria results in preservation and transformation of milk, and has been used unknowingly for thousands of years. In the past, these fermentations arose directly from the natural occurrence of lactic acid bacteria, but gradually it was recognised that a portion of a previously successful 'ferment' when added to milk gave better results. Nowadays, an inoculum (a pure starter culture) of selected bacteria is generally added to the milk to be fermented. The modern worldwide dairy industries owe much to the development of pure starter cultures, good fermentation practices and strict adherence to hygienic protocol. In the USA alone, these bacteria are involved in the manufacture of food products with an annual value of US$20–30 billion.

The lactic acid bacteria can have many beneficial effects in the foods in which they grow.

(1) They have an inhibitory effect (*bacteriocins*) on many undesirable bacteria while they themselves are generally harmless; in this way they preserve the milk.

(2) They produce highly acceptable texture and flavour modifications in the milk.

(3) Reputedly, they have beneficial health effects on intestinal microflora (probiotics).

When growing in milk, these beneficial bacteria break down lactose to lactic acid. However, many other reactions can occur, depending on the composition of the substrate, types of additives and mode of fermentation. These can result in many other metabolites being formed, giving distinctive flavour and appearance to the milk products, e.g. buttermilk, sour cream, yoghurt and the vast range of cheeses.

One of the largest activities of the dairy industry is cheese production. The earliest known reference to cheese was in 1800 BC. Cheese is made by separating the casein of milk from the liquid or *whey*. Over 900 individual types of cheese are recognised; yet they could all be prepared from any given batch of milk by proper control of the fermentation and by correct selection of the promoting microorganisms.

The discovery of the role of the animal rennet is believed to have arisen from the use of animal stomachs by nomadic sheep herders for carrying liquids. When milk was transported in this way, it would become heated by the sun, soured by naturally occurring bacteria and contaminated with enzymes (rennet) from the stomach lining. The consequence of this inter-action would be the transformation of the milk into solid curds and liquid whey. The curds were then eventually drained, salted and could be used later – an early example of basic food preservation.

In Europe the Romans were the first to really document this process using sheep or goat's milk. Cow's milk was a very much later innovation. The first industrial production of calf rennet essence or enzymes was in Denmark in 1874. Current world production is now in excess of 30 million litres per year.

Cheese production from milk is essentially a dehydration process in which the milk protein (casein) and fat are concentrated between 6 and 12 times. The common, basic steps in most cheese productions are:

(1) acidification of the milk by the conversion of the sugar lactose into lactic acid by the lactic acid bacteria

(2) coagulation of the casein by a combination of proteolysis and acidification.

Proteolysis is started by the rennet (chymosin enzyme) (animal or fungal origin) and the coagulated caseins form a gel, which entraps any fat present (Fig. 10.3).

The separated curd is cut into blocks, drained and pressed into shapes, matured and made into cheeses. The details of cheese production are very complicated and involve many individual strains of bacteria and in some cases filamentous fungi (camembert, blue cheese), special milks, selected additives and differing process techniques, which cannot be covered here.

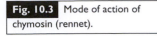

Fig. 10.3 Mode of action of chymosin (rennet).

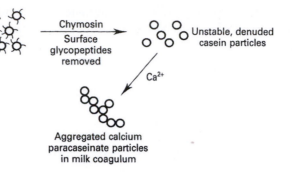

However, an important recent biotechnological innovation in cheese production has been the use of recombinant DNA techniques for chymosin production *and* commercial use. In the 1960s it became apparent that there would be an increasing shortage of animal-derived rennet, and subsequently several substitutes have been developed. At present there are six sources of commercial rennet: three from animals (veal calves, adult cows and pigs); and three fungal sources. The fungal sources are almost identical in function to the animal chymosins and account for approximately one-third of world cheese production – particularly in the USA and France. However, they can on occasion cause yield reductions and poor flavour when compared to animal chymosins.

Within the last decade genetically modified microorganisms have been produced that can yield identical chymosin to the animal chymosin. Several industrial companies have now produced pure animal-derived chymosin by such methods and these products are now available worldwide. In the UK at least 95% of chymosin is genetically engineered. The enzyme behaves in exactly the same manner as normal calf chymosin, it has fewer impurities and its activity is more predictable. Contrary to some pessimistic forecasts, recombinant chymosin has been well received by the public and also by the Vegetarian Society. Expert tasters cannot detect any difference between cheeses made using recombinant chymosin and calf chymosin. Its commercial success is ensured. The production of calf chymosin by genetically modified microorganisms is shown in Fig. 10.4.

The flavour of raw cheese, such as Cheddar, is bland and the texture rubbery. It is the period of ripening or maturation, when other microorganisms such as bacteria and fungi can have pronounced effects, which causes the development of distinctive flavours and aromas as well as major textural changes (Table 10.6). World cheese markets now exceed US$36 000 million annually.

The second major group of dairy products are the yoghurts. They are major foods consumed worldwide and represent one of the fastest growing food products in the food industry. Claims are now being made that live yoghurt bacteria can exist transitorily in the human gut with benefits to the digestive and other systems.

Traditionally, yoghurt is fermented whole milk; the process uses a mixed culture of *Lactobacillus bulgaricus* and *Streptococcus thermophilus*. The characteristic flavour compound, acetaldehyde, is produced by *Lb. bulgaricus*

Table 10.6	Principal types of cheeses

Unripened cheeses
Low fat (cottage cheese)
High fat (cream cheese)

Ripened cheeses
Hard cheese (internal ripening)
   Ripened by bacteria (Cheddar and Swiss cheese)
   Ripened by mould (Roquefort and other blue cheeses)
Soft cheeses (ripening proceeds from outside)
   Ripened by bacteria (Limburger)
   Ripened by bacteria and moulds (Camembert)

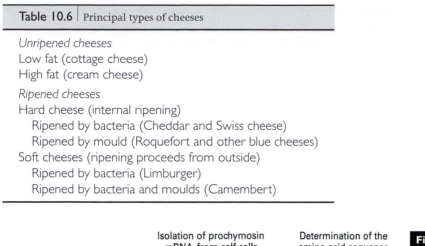

Fig. 10.4 Production of calf chymosin by genetically modified microorganisms.

while the *St. thermophilus* generates the fresh acid taste by the conversion of lactose to lactic acid. Both bacteria produce extracellular polymers that give the characteristic viscosity of the product. Incubation is at 30 or 45°C. Set yoghurt is packed into the container after inoculation and allowed to ferment in the container. Frozen yoghurt is gaining increasing popularity as an alternative for ice cream.

Microbial growth in the intestine

The human intestine contains ten times as many microbial cells as there are human cells in the whole body. The gastrointestinal (GI) tract accommodates 10^{12} bacterial cells per gram for each 200 g of gut content. Some bacteria resident in the gut can cause serious gastrointestinal disorders, e.g. *Escherichia coli* and *Clostridium difficile*. Thankfully, the great majority of GI microorganisms are harmless or beneficial, helping to prevent infections, supporting a healthy gut lining and especially promoting normal immune development. There is continuing research interest to unravel the mechanisms of these living 'probiotic' ('for life') microorganisms, but their mode of action is still not known in any detail.

Probiotics

Probiotics can be considered as live microorganisms that have a beneficial effect on human and animal health by influencing qualitatively and quantitatively the composition and/or metabolic activity of the microbial flora of the GI tract. Of special current interest is the influence on the immune status. It is considered that they may function by repairing a deficiency, reconstituting the normal GI tract microflora that would exist under natural conditions but that may have become damaged by various factors such as diet, medication, stress or other environmental influences.

Probiotics can be produced as powders, tablets, capsules or liquid suspensions. They are extensively used in certain animal/poultry feeds with definite productivity yield gains. Recently, there has been a major increase in sales of so-called bioyoghurts that use specific live intestinal bacteria, mostly strains of *Lactobacillus* and *Bifidobacterium*, as starter cultures. While Europeans have embraced probiotic yoghurts and drinks, in the USA there is still a deep-rooted perception that all bacteria have negative effects. However, the US market is slowly becoming aware of their benefits!

The aim of the probiotic supplement is to establish an actively metabolising population of probiotic bacteria in the GI tract. Such bacteria do not appear to colonise the GI tract so it is essential that they are consumed regularly to compensate for washout.

Dietary supplements, such as lactulose, inulin and fructo-oligosaccharides are compounds that have beneficial stimulatory effects on probiotic microbial growth and are termed *prebiotics*.

Vegetable fermentations

In various ways throughout the world, fruits and vegetables can be preserved using salt and acid – the acid being derived largely from bacteria in the form of lactic acid. Of particular Western interest is the fermentation preservation of cabbage to give sauerkraut and the pickling of cucumbers and olives.

In sauerkraut production shredded cabbage is packed anaerobically with salt – the salt reducing the water activity and promoting the leakage of sugars from the cabbage leaves (Fig. 10.5). Subsequently, lactic acid bacteria proliferate, releasing lactic acid, lowering the pH and preventing the growth of putrefying bacteria. Accurate control of temperature (7.5°C), salt concentration (2.25%) and the anaerobic state will produce excellent, long-lasting sauerkraut – a nutritious, tasteful food. Large-scale production of sauerkraut can be traced back in Germany to the year 800 AD. Much research is in progress to produce sauerkraut with lower salt concentrations.

In cucumber and olive fermentations, especially in Greece and Spain, the fermentations are carried out at much higher salt concentrations (5–8%) but the microbial sequences are relatively similar to sauerkraut fermentation.

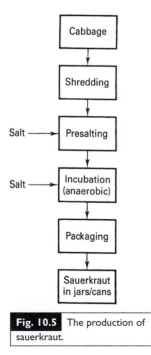

Fig. 10.5 The production of sauerkraut.

Cereal products

In almost all parts of the world cereals are produced and are the main class of food consumed by humans; a considerable proportion of these cereals will be fermented into solid foods or into alcoholic beverages.

Bread in its many local forms is the principal fermented cereal product and has been known since Roman times. The bread market is worth at least US$3 billion a year worldwide. In Europe, wheat and rye are two widely used cereal flours and are usually mixed with water or milk, salt, fat, sugar and other varied ingredients, together with the yeast *Saccharomyces cerevisiae*. As the fermentation proceeds the dough rises owing to the formation of carbon dioxide. The expansion and stretching of the dough, particularly with wheat, is due to the unique extensible and elastic protein, gluten. In this way the dough rises and retains its shape on oven baking.

Early forms of bread were unleavened and similar to modern naan breads. It is believe that contamination of such flat bread mixtures by natural yeasts yielded the first 'risen' breads, which were much more palatable. The Romans are believed to have introduced leavened bread to Western Europe.

Bread texture is affected by fats, emulsifiers and oxidising agents, while the speed of bread making (of commercial importance) is affected by fats, oxidising and reducing agents and soya flour. While the yeast enzymes have an important role, additional enzymes, e.g. amylases, are added to assist mixing, fermentation, baking and eventual storage characteristics of the bread. Modern biotechnology will increasingly supply improved enzymes to bring even greater control over this complex process.

Overall the fermentation achieves three primary objectives: leavening (carbon dioxide production), flavour development and texture changes in the dough. At the end of the fermentation process the risen dough is baked in an oven giving a final product free of living microorganisms and with an extended shelf-life.

Modern applied genetics seeks always to improve the quality of the yeast organism, leading to improved activity, better flavour and improved texture of the product. A genetically engineered *Saccharomyces cerevisiae* with improved fermentation properties has been produced and passed all regulatory requirements for safety. However, as yet, the producer company has not put it into commercial operation!

In other parts of the world, *sourdough breads* use the yeast *Candida milleri* and *Lactobacillus sanfrancisco* for the fermentation stage, while *Streptococcus* and *Pediococcus* species are used on the Indian subcontinent to ferment mixtures of cereal and legume flours to produce *idli* and *popadoms*. Rice is widely used in Asia during legume and fish fermentations. In South America *corn bread* from the cereal maize is a staple food.

New strains of baking yeasts are regularly being developed (not yet by recombinant DNA technology) and most research is directed to improving the technology of bread making and the preservation of the final product, especially by packaging innovations.

The soybean *Glycine max* is the main legume used for fermentation and products derived are of particular importance in diets in East Asia, South East Asia and India. Fermentation improves digestibility of the beans by

Table 10.7 Per capita annual consumption of fermented foods prepared from *Aspergillus* moulds in Japan (1981)

Food	Yeast/per capita	Total production/year
(1) Soy sauce	10.1 litres	1 200 000 kilolitres
(2) Miso	4.9 kilograms	572 000 tonnes
(3) Saké	12.3 litres	1 445 000 kilolitres
(4) Mirin	0.6 litres	260 000 kilolitres
(5) Shochu	2.2 litres	30 000 kilolitres
(6) Rice vinegar	2.5 litres	305 000 kilolitres

Japanese population 117 850 000 (1 October 1981)
Source: from Yokotsuka (1985)

breaking down anti-nutritional factors and compounds that cause flatulence in the intestine. In Indonesia cooked soybeans are fermented with the fungus *Rhizopus oligosporus* and the product, *tempeh*, is fried in oil and eaten as a snack or in soups. Over 250 000 people are involved in the production of tempeh in Indonesia. There is a growing interest in this product in Europe and the USA.

The major fermentation of soybeans is in the production of *soy sauce* and *miso*. The production of *soy sauce* has three phases – the *koji*, the *moromi* and *maturation*. The koji is a solid substrate fermentation in which cooked soybeans and wheat flour are fermented with *Aspergillus oryzae* to break down starches, proteins and pectins. The moromi is a liquid/slurry fermentation under anaerobic conditions with *Candida* and *Pediococcus* as the fermentation microorganisms. Maturation gives the final full flavour spectrum.

Table 10.7 gives details of Japanese consumption of soy sauce and related soybean fermented products. The Asiatic countries enjoy a rich range of legume and rice fermented products with high annual per capita consumption.

In all of the discussed food and beverage fermentations specific microorganisms play an indispensable function in achieving the final product. Starter cultures are now used in all these fermentations and bring control and greater uniformity to the end-product(s). In most processes the microorganisms become part of the food and are consumed intact. In others such as wine, beer, vinegar and soy sauce, the cells are removed by filtration or centrifugation to eliminate turbidity. (For a fuller appreciation of fermented foods, see Campbell-Platt (1989) and Wood (1998)).

10.3 | Microorganisms as food

In the 1950s, agriculturalists and nutritionists were becoming concerned that in the near future traditional sources of protein, such as cattle, pigs and poultry, would not be adequate for the increasing world demand. In essence, they envisaged a global shortage of protein foods resulting in extensive protein malnutrition, as was being seen in some developing

Table 10.8	The time required to double the mass of various organisms		
Organism	Time required to double biomass
Bacteria and yeasts	20–120 minutes
Moulds and algae	2–6 hours
Grass and some plants	1–2 weeks
Chickens	2–4 weeks
Pigs	4–6 weeks
Cattle (young)	1–2 weeks
Humans (young)	3–6 months

countries with the childhood diseases of kwashiorkor and marasmus. As a result, several international organisations, including the World Health Organization (WHO), the Food and Agriculture Organization (FAO) and the United Nations Children's Fund (UNICEF), considered how this protein deficiency could be alleviated and one of many proposals was to examine the possible use of microbial-derived protein as a food supplement or as an animal feed source to substitute for protein-rich cereals.

Thus began one of the most creative periods in the history of microbial fermentation technology, largely involving bacteria and yeasts utilising 'cheap' (at that time) petroleum by-products such as methanol, ethanol, methane and *n*-alkanes as well as waste organics as sources of carbon and energy for microbial growth. The product was called *single-cell protein* (SCP). While protein quantity and quality were the goals of SCP production the microbial biomass also contained carbohydrates, fats, vitamins and minerals. Single-cell protein was originally considered as a potential protein supplement for humans and as a feed for animals. Because humans have a limited capacity to degrade nucleic acids, it was soon realised that additional processing would be required because microorganisms have high DNA/RNA contents. Single-cell protein for animals could serve as a replacement for fishmeal and soymeal.

Microorganisms produce protein much more efficiently than any farm animals (Table 10.8). The protein-producing capacities of a 250 kg cow and 250 g of microorganisms are often compared. Whereas the cow will put on 200 g of protein a day, the microbes, in theory, could produce 25 tonnes in the same time under ideal growing conditions. However, the cow also has the unique ability to convert grass into protein-rich milk. No rival method has ever been developed. The cow has been described as 'a live, self-reproducing and edible bioreactor'. The challenge was then set to produce economically large quantities of protein-rich microbial biomass utilising modern fermentation/bioreactor technology. The potential advantages of using microorganisms for protein production are listed in Table 10.9.

SCP derived from high-energy sources

Prior to the dramatic escalation of oil prices by the oil-producing nations in the 1970s, there was a wide range of SCP fermentation processes being

| Table 10.9 | The potential advantages of using microbes for SCP production |

- Microorganisms can grow at remarkably rapid rates under optimum conditions; some microbes can double their biomass every 0.5–1.0 hours.
- Microorganisms are more easily modified genetically than plants and animals; they are more amenable to large-scale screening programmes to select for higher growth rate, improved amino acid content, etc., and can be more easily subjected to gene transfer technology.
- Microorganisms have relatively high protein content and the nutritional value of the protein is good.
- Microorganisms can be grown in vast numbers in relatively small, continuous-fermentation processes, using relatively small land area and are also independent of climate.
- Microorganisms can grow on a wide range of raw materials, in particular low-value wastes, and some can also use plant-derived lignocellulose.

developed utilising gas-oil, methanol, ethanol, methane or n-alkanes. Even at that time the wisdom of using high energy-potential compounds for food production was being questioned by many scientists. How right they were! Most oil and gas companies had large gluts of petroleum by-products and consequently had large research and production facilities devoted to SCP production.

Methane as an SCP source was extensively researched, but there were too many technical difficulties to warrant exploitation. The use of n-alkanes as a substrate for SCP was studied in many countries but several established processes ceased operation because of suspected health hazards resulting from the presence of carcinogens in the SCP. While ethanol had many advantages as a substrate for SCP the current focus on ethanol use is now overwhelmingly towards biofuel.

For many years methanol offered great economic SCP interests. A large-scale (75 000 l) fermentation plant for producing the methanol-utilising bacterium *Methylophilus methylotrophus* was constructed by ICI, UK. The ICI SCP protein (named 'Pruteen') was developed to be used exclusively for animal feeding. The ICI Pruteen plant was the only process of the kind in the Western world, but could not operate economically at the then current methanol prices and went out of operation. In the Soviet-bloc countries, many methanol plants were operational, due in part to chronic shortages of animal feed, excess production of methanol, lack of foreign currency to buy alternative animal feeds such as soy meal and, above all, a disregard for economic planning. At its peak in Russia, there were several SCP plants on stream or being planned with production capacity of 300 000–600 000 tonnes per annum.

The vast range of studies carried out in the 1960s and 1970s on the potential use of methanol and related compounds as substrates for SCP processes certainly pushed bioreactor technology to its limits for cheap bulk-product formation. The aerobic process for Pruteen production was the world's largest continuous bioprocess system. The stringent economics required in these processes led to extensive use of airlift bioreactor design. Furthermore, the massive volume and expense in harvesting and preparing the final production forced many economies of scale and of downstream processing.

SCP from waste organic materials

The materials that make up waste organics should normally be recycled back into the ecosystem, e.g. carbohydrate wastes, sugars, starch, whey, molasses; lignocellulosic waste, straw, bagass, oil- and date-palm, as well as animal manures. It was proposed that many of these wastes could be transformed into edible protein for animals and, possibly, human consumption. Over the years, there have been many feasibility studies carried out worldwide, but only two approaches have achieved acceptance as worthwhile contributions to human protein consumption: Quorn™ myco-protein and edible mushroom production.

Quorn™ myco-protein

The use of abundantly available waste starch and sugars as a source of raw material for an SCP process was considered in the early 1960s by Lord Rank (then the chairman of the Rank Hovis McDougall (RHM) group of companies) to be a feasible and worthwhile project to alleviate the then anticipated world protein famine. Under the direction of the late Professor Gerald Solomons, a 'starch into protein' process was commenced, which ultimately was to become the only successful SCP process developed entirely with human consumption as the primary aim. Three criteria were considered for this proposed food:

- it must be 'delicious' to eat
- the final product, the substrate and all possible intermediates used in the process must be safe to eat
- above all, the final food presented should be highly nutritious.

Because the final product would require to be textured, bacteria would be unsuitable and filamentous fungi became the obvious choice. While starch was the best available substrate it was considered that for good controlled fermentation it would be necessary to use a soluble carbohydrate (glucose) produced by the hydrolysis of starch; after much experimentation the fungus finally chosen was *Fusarium venenatum* and this was followed by an extensive fermentation programme that ultimately led to the development of a novel continuous process.

In the early studies, the myco-protein mycelial biomass was produced in a 300 l stirred tank bioreactor. This allowed for extensive safety testing of the product over a period of 12 years, which demonstrated that myco-protein could be consumed by test animals and human volunteers, without any observable harmful effects. Following government approval it was then possible to plan large-scale production and an agreement was developed

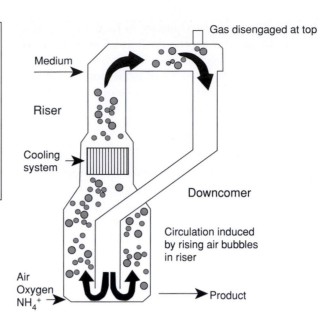

Fig 10.6 Diagrammatic representation of the Quorn™ pressure cycle fermenter used by Marlow Hoods at Stokesly, UK, for the production of mycoprotein in continuous flow culture. Carbon dioxide evolution rate to control medium flow offers the advantage that carbon dioxide evolution is measurable on-line, so that finer, more regular adjustments to the flow rate can be made.

between RHM and ICI (Marlow Foods) to commission a 40 000 l airlift (pressure cycle) bioreactor (Fig. 10.6). At a later date two 150 000 l pressure cycle tower bioreactors were designed and operated. While glucose concentration was initially selected to control medium flow rate, in the continuous system carbon dioxide evolution rate, which can be measured on-line, is now used instead.

Under optimum growing conditions mycelial doubling time is between 3.5 and 4.1 h allowing the production of 300 to 350 kg biomass per hour. The biomass is then subjected to a heat treatment (c. 68°C for 30–45 minutes) to reduce RNA content of the biomass. The resultant RNA monomers leak out of the cells, together with some proteinaceous and other cell components. The fungal biomass can then be heated to 90°C and concentrated by centrifugation, and the resultant paste can then be shaped by food processing technology into forms suitable for final products, e.g. mince, sausages, burgers and steaks.

Quorn™ provides a low-calorie (80 kcal per 100 g) food, which lacks animal fats and cholesterol and is low in saturated fats and high in dietary fibre. Quorn™ is marketed as a healthy food choice rather than a vegetarian product. Quorn™ is marketed throughout Europe and now the USA and is the only source of myco-protein for human consumption currently available.

Edible mushroom production

The world has an immense lignocellulosic sustainable biomass resource. As discussed elsewhere in this volume, intense efforts are in process worldwide to utilise lignocellulose for energy generation. However, one of the most economically viable processes for the conversion of these lignocellulosic

Table 10.10 | World production of cultivated edible and medicinal mushrooms in different years

Species	1981 Tonnes	1981 %	1990 Tonnes	1990 %	1997 Tonnes	1997 %
Agaricus bisporus/bitorquis	900.0	71.6	1420.0	37.8	1955.9	31.8
Lentinulas edodes	180.0	14.3	393.0	10.4	1564.4	25.4
Pleurotus spp.	35.0	2.8	900.0	23.9	975.6	14.2
Auricularia spp.	10.0	0.8	400.0	10.6	485.3	7.9
Volvariella volvacea	54.0	4.3	207.0	5.5	180.8	3.0
Flammulina velutipes	60.0	4.8	143.0	3.8	284.7	4.6
Tremella spp.	–	–	105.0	2.8	130.5	2.1
Hypsizygus spp.	–	–	22.6	0.6	74.2	1.2
Pholiota spp.	17.0	1.3	22.0	0.6	55.5	0.9
Grifola frondosa	–	–	7.0	0.2	33.1	0.5
Others	1.2	0.1	139.4	3.6	518.4	8.4
Total	1357.2	100.0	3763.0	100.0	6158.4	100.0

wastes (such as wood and straws) is the cultivation of edible basidiomycete mushrooms.

The cultivation of edible mushrooms is one of the limited examples of a microbial culture in which the cultivated fungus, i.e. the macroscopic, highly developed mushroom structure, is used directly as a human food. A wide range of edible mushrooms are now cultivated throughout the world (Table 10.10) for human consumption. This solid-substrate fermentation is now one of the most challenging and technically demanding of all vegetable cultivations known to man. On a worldwide basis, mushroom growing is one of the fastest growing biotechnological industries. China is the world's leading mushroom producer with 10.4 million tonnes in 2003.

The cultivation of the common white mushroom, *Agaricus bisporus*, has expanded worldwide and the USA continues to be the world's largest producer. However, mushrooms traditionally grown in the Far East, such as *Lentinula edodes* (the Shiitake mushroom) and *Pleurotus* spp. (the oyster mushroom), are now expanding into other areas of the world, largely because of their unique flavours and textures and recognised medicinal qualities.

Mushroom production is, in principle, a fermentation process. In the case of *Agaricus*, the substrate for growth is fermented straw, while for *Lentinula* it is wood. For *Agaricus* cultivation the straw is composted with animal manures and other organic nitrogen compounds over a period of one to two weeks, and the final product is a unique substrate suitable for the rapid growth of the *Agaricus* inoculum. There is no standard pattern for compost formulation, being based only on the availability and price of the raw materials and supplements in the particular growing region. The nature of the substrate and its pre-treatment – more than all other aspects of growing – determine the method by which specific mushrooms are grown. When the mushroom mycelium has grown throughout the prepared compost

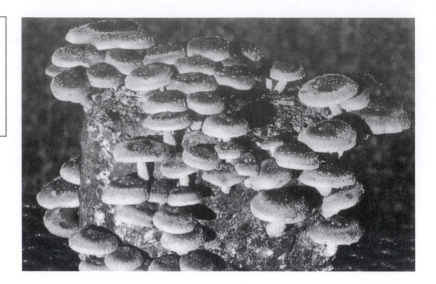

Fig. 10.7 *Lentinula edodes* cultivation on sawdust blocks. Since the plastic bags were removed at a later stage of mycelial development, most of the mushrooms appear on top. (Photograph courtesy of Dr Myra Chu-Chou.)

(usually contained in large wooden boxes), the environmental conditions of temperature and humidity are altered, and subsequently the large mushroom structure rapidly forms in large numbers or 'flushes'. These are then harvested by hand cutting, and approximately seven to ten days later another crop will appear. Usually up to four crops are produced before the process is terminated. The cultivations of *Volvariella* and *Pleurotus* are again straw-based but have a much simpler procedure.

Lentinula edodes is the second most cultivated mushroom in the world and has been cultivated for over 2000 years. Currently, over 90% of its production occurs in Japan, but cultivation extends to China, Korea, Singapore, Taiwan, Sri Lanka and, more recently, into the USA and Europe. The traditional method of cultivation has been to inoculate wooden logs (1.8 m × 0.15 m) with spore inoculum or mycelial plugs, allow the logs to stand for up to nine months to achieve colonisation by the fungus, and then, during subsequent early summer and autumn periods, the mushrooms will grow out and be harvested. This seasonal production is augmented by drying mushrooms to achieve all-year-round consumption. The fungus derives its total nutrition from the lignocellulose of the log.

More recently, a new method of cultivation has been developed in which deciduous sawdust is mixed with cereal supplements and compressed into large plastic bags – artificial log production. The bags are sterilised and then inoculated aseptically with the pure fungus culture and, after a period of vegetative growth, are induced to produce the mushroom (Fig. 10.7). This controlled form of cultivation is leading to a wider geographical range of commercial cultivation not only for *Lentinulas* but also for many other cultivated mushroom species. *Lentinulas edodes* and other Asiatic mushroom species have a long history of therapeutic use, and extensive industries have been developed to utilise their products in the treatment of many human illnesses. Such mushrooms are termed *medicinal mushrooms*. Finally, after mushroom production, the spent substrate can be used as animal food or as a biofertiliser.

Table 10.11	Use of enzymes in food processing	
Industry	Enzymes	Expenditure (million US$)
Brewing	α-amylase, β-amylase, protease, papain, amyloglucosidase, xylanase	30
Dairy	Animal/microbial chymosins, lactase, lipase, lysozyme	90
Baking	α-amylase, xylanase, protease, phospholipase A and D, lipoxygenase	20
Fruit and vegetable processing	Pectinesterase, polyglacturanase, pectin lyase, hemicellulases	18
Starch and sugar	α-amylase, β-amylase, glucoamylase, xylanase, pullulanase, isomerase, oligoamylases	120

10.4 | Enzymes and food processing

Enzymes are indispensable in modern food processing technology. Enzymes are an essential part of most food and beverage fermentation and while most of the enzymes will be derived from participating microorganisms, increasingly processes are being improved by the direct addition of exogenous enzymes (Table 10.11). There will be an increasing production of food enzymes using rDNA biotechnology. Chymosin has been the front runner for this new technology and its use now exceeds 80% of the market in the USA and Canada. The accepted use of chymosin or other enzymes by rDNA technology is based on the following: enzyme preparations are free of any bioprocessing and purification steps, and viable rDNA biotechnology-driven microorganisms are not present in the final preparation. Improvements are increasingly apparent in enzyme availability, purity and cost, which will benefit and improve the quality of foods available to consumers. Examples close to commercialisation include lactase for lactose hydrolysis, α-amylase and amyloglucosidase for high-fructose corn syrup, and acetolactate decarboxylase for beer ageing and diacetyl reduction.

The role of exogenous enzymes to facilitate or even replace mechanical processes is well demonstrated in fruit and vegetable processing, while in industrial starch transformation chemical processing has yielded almost completely to enzyme processing.

A major development that will revolutionise the use of enzymes in the food industry involves the near elimination of water from enzyme reaction media. Thus, hydrolytic enzymes can be reversed so that with no metabolic energy input the same enzymes that degrade biomolecules can now synthesise them. A wide range of food-related compounds have now been produced by this novel approach and include polyglycerol esters (emulsifiers), chiral flavour esters and oligopeptides, and structural polymers.

The new concept of protein engineering will facilitate the design or alteration of food enzymes at a molecular level, allowing minor

Table 10.12 | Worldwide production of amino acids

Production (tonnes per year)	Amino acid	Preferred production method	Main use
800 000	L-Glutamic acid	Fermentation	Flavour enhancer
350 000	L-Lysine	Fermentation	Feed additive
350 000	D, L-Methionine	Chemical synthesis	Feed additive
10 000	L-Aspartate	Enzymatic catalysis	Aspartame
10 000	L-Phenylalanine	Fermentation	Aspartame
15 000	L-Threonine	Fermentation	Feed additive
10 000	Glycine	Chemical synthesis	Food additives, sweeteners
10 000	L-Cysteine	Reduction of cystine	Food additives

Source: from Eggeling, Pfeffarte and Sahm (2001)

modifications or the design of completely novel enzyme catalysts. An important application has involved the enzyme phospholipase A2 currently used as a food emulsifier. There is little doubt that the process of protein engineering coupled to gene cloning technology will be extensively applied to many enzymes used in food processing, allowing greater accuracy and selectivity of action.

Enzymes will also be extensively used in the design of novel and functional foods. Particularly in Japan there has been considerable research into oligosaccharides, designer fats and special food fibre ingredients. Much effort is now being directed to the role of nutrition and the ageing process. The affluent, ageing populations of the West will wholeheartedly support such research efforts!

10.5 | Amino acids, vitamins and sweeteners

Amino acids are extensively used in the food and beverage industries as flavour enhancers, as seasonings or as nutritional additives. The pharmaceutical industry also has a high demand for amino acids in infusions and in special dietary foods. However, the largest market for amino acid use is in animal feed additives. Amino acid synthesis by fermentation is a major part of modern biotechnology with the market doubling every ten years.

World production levels for food use are in excess of 1.6 million tonnes per year, with Japan commanding a major proportion of the US$2 billion market. Glutamic acid and lysine are two amino acids produced by large-scale (500 m^3) fermentation processes involving the bacteria *Corynebacterium glutamicum* and *Brevibacterium flavum* respectively (Table 10.12). Some amino acids are still chemically synthesised, e.g. glycine and DL methionine. Monosodium glutamate is extensively used in the food industry as a flavour or sensory enhancer.

Table 10.13	Traditional and alternative sweeteners
Product	Relative sweetness
Sucrose	1.0
HFCS[a] (55%)	1.4
Cyclamate	50
Aspartame	150
Saccharin	300
Thaumatin	3000

[a] HFCS: high fructose syrup

Extensive mutant selection has produced microorganisms that over-produce and excrete these primary metabolites, while DNA technology is further improving production capabilities. Amino acid production is an outstanding example of the integration of many different technologies, which now includes metabolic engineering.

Vitamins are usually used as dietary supplements, e.g. ergosterol (provitamin D), riboflavin, B_{12}, etc., while vitamin C (ascorbic acid) is mostly used as a food ingredient: annual production is about 40 000 tonnes. While some vitamins are chemically synthesised many are now produced by means of selected microorganisms.

In most societies there is a considerable need for sweeteners to accompany food intake. The consumption of sweeteners in the USA and Europe is approximately 57 kg of sucrose equivalent per capita. Up to the late 1960s, sweeteners were mainly cane and beet sugar, and sucrose. In the 1970s, enzyme technology created a new class of sweeteners derived from starch (see earlier chapter for high-fructose syrups). Saccharin, which is chemically derived, has been widely used as a sweetener for many years but is now being increasingly challenged by new, natural, low-calorific sweeteners, while biotechnological methods have been used to develop one of the most important additions to this market, aspartame. Aspartame (trade name Nutra-sweet) is used extensively in many low-calorie 'diet' soft drinks. Thaumatin, a protein extracted from berries of the plant *Thaumatococcus danielli,* is the sweetest compound known (Table 10.13). It is marketed extensively in Japan and now Europe and considerable effort is being made to produce the protein in genetically engineered microorganisms.

Sweeteners find extensive markets and applications in soft drinks, confectionery, jams and jellies, ice cream, canning, baking, fermentation, pickles and sauces, and meat products – truly an immense market that will benefit from biotechnological innovations.

The most expensive component in the synthesis of aspartame is the amino acid phenylalanine, which is now produced on a large scale by fermentation methods. Extensive toxicological studies were necessary before aspartame was permitted to be marketed. All new biotechnologically derived food products must undergo a programme of regulatory approval similar to that demanded for new pharmaceuticals. Approval for aspartame took ten years.

10.6 | Organic acids and polysaccharides

Citric acid is widely used in the food-related industries in fruit drinks, confectionery, jams and preserved fruits and also in the pharmaceutical industry. Over 100 000 tonnes of citric acid are manufactured annually by fermentation processes involving the fungus *Aspergillus niger* and molasses as substrate. Citric acid was originally produced from low-grade citrus fruits, but now 95% of world production of citric acid is by fungal fermentation. The fermentation can be as static liquid surface cultures in trays, or in deep-tank, large-scale bioreactors (100 m³). Citric acid is used in foods to enhance the flavour, to prevent oxidation and browning, and as a preservative. Lactic acid can be produced by fermentation (40%) or by chemical synthesis (60%) and is used largely as an acidulant. Other organic acids include gluconic, itaconic and propionic acids. Bulk production of lactic acid is now being associated with aspects of biofuel production.

Many microorganisms can produce copious amounts of polysaccharides when surplus carbon sources are available in their environment. Some of these polysaccharides accumulate within the cell and act as storage compounds (glycogen), while others known as exopolysaccharides are excreted by the cell and are mostly the microbial polysaccharides of commercial interest. Such polysaccharides may remain associated with the cell as capsules or slime, or may dissolve in the medium. They are used mainly to modify the rheology (i.e. flow characteristics) of solutions by increasing viscosity and are commonly used as thickeners, gels and suspension agents. They can stabilise food structures and improve appearance and palatability.

Xanthan produced by the bacterium *Xanthomonas campestris* is a large polysaccharide (10⁶ daltons) and is the most important commercial microbial polysaccharide with current production at *c.* 20 000 tonnes per year. Other bacterial species produce pullulan, scleroglutan, curdlan and cellulose. All are produced in batch, aerated, stirred tank bioreactors.

10.7 | Rapid diagnostics

It is a major requirement of all food processes to supply a product free of dangerous microorganisms and microbial toxins. A wide array of traditional, time-consuming procedures has routinely been applied to identify, control, reduce or remove such contaminants. Major food pathogens include *Listeria, Salmonella* and *Campylobacter,* while the bacterial endotoxins and the fungal mycotoxins are the principal toxins considered.

Developments in biotechnology now permit a complete reshaping of many of these testing protocols by the application of antibody detection systems and DNA and RNA probe technology. These procedures are much shorter in time, generally cheaper and often do not need highly skilled operators. By means of these new technologies there will be major improvements in safety standards in the food supply.

The use of immunoassays in the food industry is a recent development but is rapidly becoming an accepted analytical tool. The enzyme-linked immunosorbent assay (ELISA) based on a 96-well microtitration plate is the most widely used format by the food scientist. It is extremely versatile in that a wide range of handling methods can be used, from manual operation to completely automated assays. Time and labour savings offered by ELISAs over conventional assays can be considerable. The detection of *Salmonella* bacteria in foods is a very complex procedure and can take up to five days using traditional enrichment procedures. By means of immunoassay procedures this can be done in as little as one day. Similarly, the mycotoxin aflatoxin requires many hours of extraction, purification and concentration for accurate traditional chemical identification. However, using affinity columns containing the specific antibodies to the toxin, the whole process of extraction and quantification can be carried out within 30 minutes.

Food immunoassay procedures are now available for many potential food analytes, e.g. trace residues, mycotoxins, antibiotics, hormones, bacterial toxins, etc. With the increased development and availability of such diagnostic procedures in user-friendly kit form new options will be available for food safety control, which will achieve obvious benefits to manufacturer, consumer and regulatory authorities.

10.8 | Bioprocess technology

In food biotechnology, fermentation is the main means of producing a wide range of products, and the basic concepts of bioprocess technology have been considered in Chapter 4. Improved bioprocess technology in food production will increase productivity, lower costs, improve nutrition and reduce environmental damage presently occurring in many food processes.

10.9 | Public acceptance and safety of new biotechnology foods

The public to some extent has a *negative* attitude to excessive manipulation of foods and demonstrates marked hostility, in particular, to genetic engineering of foodstuffs. This highly controversial topic is discussed in much more detail in Chapter 15.

The food industry is highly conservative and slow to welcome technological change. The ultimate full acceptance of new biotechnology in the food sector will depend on many interacting factors, e.g. economics, consumer acceptance, regulatory procedures and the types of technology. Biotechnology has a great ability to increase productivity by decreasing costs per unit of output, or by increasing yields per unit of output. Biotechnology will increase the vertical integration of agriculture and the food industry. At present new biotechnology is having a greater impact in developed nations. It is to be hoped that these new approaches can also be brought to the advantage of the developing nations where food needs are greatest.

As with all advances in food technology, it must always be remembered that food is to be eaten and that it must be good to eat.

Chapter 11

Biotechnology and medicine

11.1 | Introduction

During the twentieth century there have been the greatest gains in health in most parts of the world due to dramatic reductions in infant mortality, eradication of life-threatening diseases, such as smallpox, and considerable improvements in life expectancy in developing and industrialised countries. In the past, life for most people was coarse, lacking in adequate nutrition, poor housing and, above all, short in years. With the advent of improved sanitation and better living conditions, together with the availability of vaccinations and antibiotics, there has been, for many, a vast improvement in health status. However, health status still differs widely among nations and by geographical region. For instance, life expectancy is less than 50 years in some sub-Saharan African countries but over 75 in established industrialised countries. The wealthiest economies appear to be the healthiest. A crucial factor related to life expectancy is access to safe water! In much of the developing world, simply drinking water is a high-risk exposure.

Undoubtedly, the real gains in health over the last century can be attributed mainly to the impact of public health and disease prevention rather than to medical interventions. Public health can be primarily distinguished from clinical medicine by placing emphasis on the prevention of disease rather than the curing, and having a main focus on populations and communities rather than the individual patient. It is essential to continue to develop a public health approach that will protect populations and create prevention strategies for groups and not just for individuals. Biotechnology has, and continues to play, a major part in establishing programmes for achieving clean drinking water and waste treatment technology.

Nowadays in industrialised societies, infectious diseases are no longer the main threat to life but rather it is the chronic diseases (cancer, cardiovascular disease, Alzheimer's disease, etc.) that plague our increasingly ageing population. Much of the increased life span achieved in the last 50 years has not prolonged youth but extended dotage. The late John F. Kennedy said in the 1960s: 'It is not enough for a great nation to have added new years to

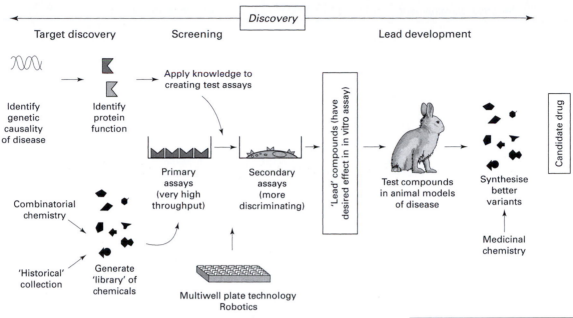

Discovery

Target discovery   Screening   Lead development

Identify genetic causality of disease

Identify protein function

Apply knowledge to creating test assays

Combinatorial chemistry

Primary assays (very high throughput)

Secondary assays (more discriminating)

'Lead' compounds (have desired effect in in vitro assay)

Test compounds in animal models of disease

Synthesise better variants

Candidate drug

Medicinal chemistry

'Historical' collection

Generate 'library' of chemicals

Multiwell plate technology Robotics

Fig. 11.1 Biotechnology drug discovery path. The process starts with genomics-driven discovery of a target gene and hence proteins, and with the generation of a diverse set of chemicals from combinational libraries or from collections of chemicals accumulated within a company. The chemicals are assayed for their ability to block (or sometimes enhance) the target protein's action. (*Source*: from Bains and Evans, 2001.)

life. Our objective must be to add new life to those years.' Addressing the new problems of an ageing population will be a major challenge to modern medicine and biotechnology.

Chronic diseases will most probably not have a single, identifiable genetic cause but rather arise from a complex, cascading series of biological events interacting with environmental factors. As indicated by Edward Golub (a former professor of immunology) 'the era of biology of specificity may rapidly be drawing to a close [. . .] we are entering the era of the *biology of complexity*!' Consequently, biotechnology will increasingly be directed at maintaining normal human functions and a high level of personal health.

The impact of pharmaceuticals on human healthcare is an area where biotechnological innovations are likely to have the earliest commercial realisation. The long-standing awareness within the health-related industries of biological and biochemical innovations has led to these industries being heavily involved in biotechnological research, particularly molecular biology. Furthermore, since health-related products are generally high value, the financial return warrants extensive research investment. Indeed, the majority of 'new' biotechnology investment over the last 30 years has been in healthcare and especially in the discovery of new drugs. However, the considerable time required to develop a modern pharmaceutical product must not be underestimated, and long periods of toxicological testing are necessary before the national regulatory bodies will grant approval for marketing. The cost of achieving this approval can be many millions of pounds, and the product must have a high sales potential to warrant this investment. Many potentially worthwhile products will not appear on the market because it is not in the financial interest of the producing companies to meet such vast costs of gaining approval (Figs. 11.1 and 11.2).

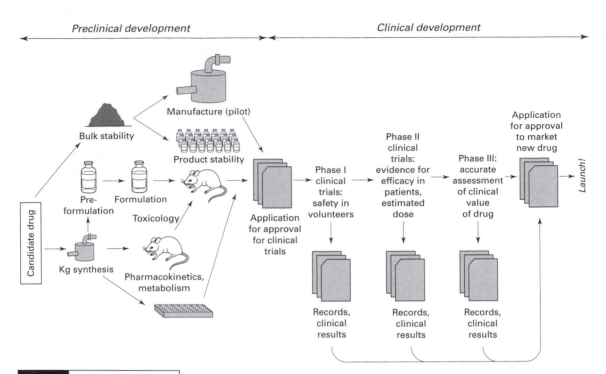

Preclinical development   Clinical development

Candidate drug

Kg synthesis → Pharmacokinetics, metabolism

Pre-formulation → Formulation → Toxicology

Bulk stability → Manufacture (pilot)

Product stability

Application for approval for clinical trials

Phase I clinical trials: safety in volunteers

Phase II clinical trials: evidence for efficacy in patients, estimated dose

Phase III: accurate assessment of clinical value of drug

Application for approval to market new drug

Launch!

Records, clinical results   Records, clinical results   Records, clinical results

Fig. 11.2 Drug development path. The compound is formally tested for metabolism, toxicity, bioavailability and other pharmacological properties, traditionally in animals but increasingly in in vitro model assays. Successful compounds are then entered into an escalating series of clinical trials, producing systematic and extensive records, which are used in the submission for permission to market the product as a drug. (*Source*: from Bains and Evans, 2001.)

New medical treatments based on new biotechnology are appearing almost daily in the marketplace. These include: (a) therapeutic products (hormones, regulatory proteins, antibiotics); (b) prenatal diagnosis of genetic diseases; (c) vaccines; (d) immuno-diagnostic and DNA probes for disease identification; and (e) genetic therapy. This is the largest commercially developed area of new biotechnology with massive present and future markets and can only be selectively examined here.

11.2 | Pharmaceuticals and biopharmaceuticals

The vast bulk of pharmaceutical drugs presently on sale are synthetic chemicals derived either directly by chemical synthesis or by chemically modifying molecules derived from biological sources. Biopharmaceuticals are considered as recombinant protein drugs, recombinant vaccines and monoclonal antibodies (for therapeutic roles). Biopharmaceuticals are becoming increasingly relevant in biological applications but are still only a small part of the pharmaceutical industry. However, there can be little doubt that the techniques of molecular biology/genetic engineering will become a dominating factor of drug discovery, design and development. Biotechnology will also accelerate screening, speed of bioassays and production of new drugs, and also explain more accurately how drugs act in the human system. Biotechnology will almost certainly vastly reduce the huge costs presently incurred in product development of new drugs (e.g. costs of discovery, development, scale-up, clinical trials and regulatory paperwork).

Table 11.1	Some economically important antibiotics	
Antibiotic compound	Producer microorganism	Activity spectrum
Actinomycin D	*Streptomyces* sp.	Anti-tumour
Asparaginase	*Erwinia* sp.	Anti-leukaemia
Bacitracin	*Bacillus* sp.	Anti-bacterial
Bleomycin	*Streptomyces* sp.	Anti-cancer
Cephalosporin	*Acremonium* sp.	Anti-bacterial
Chloramphenicol	*Cephalosporium* sp.	Anti-bacterial
Daunorubicin	*Streptomyces* sp.	Anti-protozoal
Fumagillin	*Aspergillus* sp.	Amoebicidal
Griseofulvin	*Penicillium* sp.	Anti-fungal
Mitomycin C	*Streptomyces* sp.	Anti-tumour
Natamycin	*Streptomyces* sp.	Food preservative
Nisin	*Streptococcus* sp.	Food preservative
Penicillin G	*Penicillium* sp.	Anti-bacterial
Rifamycin	*Nocardia* sp.	Anti-tuberculosis
Streptomycin	*Streptomyces* sp.	Anti-bacterial

11.3 | Antibiotics

The discovery in 1929 by Alexander Fleming that a fungus called *Penicillium notatum* could produce a compound, penicillin, selectively able to inactivate a wide range of bacteria, without unduly influencing the host, set in motion scientific studies (carried out by the groups led by Howard Florey and Ernest Chain at Oxford) that profoundly altered the relationship of humans to the controlling influence of bacterial diseases. Indeed, antibiotics changed forever the world in which we live. From these, and later, studies emerged the fungal antibiotics penicillin and cephalosporin, and the actinomycete antibiotics streptomycin, aureomycin, chloramphenicol, tetracyclines and many others. Many bacterial diseases have largely been brought under control by the use of antibiotics. Pneumonia, tuberculosis, cholera and leprosy, to mention only a few, no longer dominate society and, at least in the developed parts of the world, have been relegated to minor diseases. Griseofulvin, an antibiotic active against fungi, has brought great relief to those infected with debilitating fungal skin diseases such as ringworm. Fleming and Florey were later to become Nobel Laureates.

Antibiotics are antimicrobial compounds produced by living microorganisms, and are used therapeutically and sometimes prophylatically in the control of infectious diseases. Over 4000 antibiotics have been isolated but only about 50 have achieved wide usage (Table 11.1). The other antibiotic compounds failed to achieve commercial importance for reasons such as toxicity to humans or animals, ineffectiveness or high production costs.

Antibiotics have been extensively used in medicine since about 1945 with the arrival of penicillin. New antibiotics soon extended the range of antimicrobial control, and antibiotics are now widely used in human and veterinary medicine and (to a lesser extent) in animal farming, where some antibiotics have been shown to increase the weight of livestock and poultry. Antibiotics can also be used to a limited extent to control plant diseases and to act as insecticides.

Antibiotics that affect a wide range of microorganisms are termed *broad spectrum*, for example, choramphenicol and the tetracyclines, which can control such unrelated organisms as *Rickettsia, Chlamydia* and *Mycoplasma* species. In contrast, streptomycin and penicillin are examples of *narrow-spectrum* antibiotics, being effective against only a few bacterial species. Most antibiotics have been derived from the actinomycetes (filamentous bacteria) and the mould fungi.

The production of antibiotics has undoubtedly been a highly profitable part of the pharmaceutical industries in the industrialised world. The world market for antibiotics and anti-fungals was worth over US$26 billion in 2001 and is the most valuable segment of the total pharmaceutical market (*c.* US$200 billion). Due to biotechnology innovation, as world sales of antibiotics increase their production costs have decreased.

In 1992, the cephalosporins (products derived from cephalosporin C and penicillins G or V) were one of the largest business sectors in the global pharmaceutical market with sales at US$8.3 billion. The present processes are highly efficient and have been achieved with little knowledge about the genetics of the producing organisms. This was, in part, due to the lack of an obvious sexual cycle, which limited crossbreeding experiments. However, new techniques such as protoplast fusion and gene transfer technologies are leading to the development of new strains with higher productivity, improved stability and possible new products. These improvements have all resulted in continued decreases in overall costs of production. At present all antibiotic fermentations involve centrally stirred tank reactors run under aerobic batch conditions. Modifications in production processes may well follow on from the novel fermenter designs that are gaining wider industrial acceptance.

Because of the increasing knowledge of the biosynthetic pathways in microorganisms it is increasingly possible to involve genetic manipulation directly, rather than to rely mostly on mutation and natural selection. The three major applications of genetic manipulation technology to antibiotic production are:

(1) strain improvement programmes
(2) producing novel antibiotics by gene insertion
(3) engineering microbial strains and enzymes relevant to the production process.

It is regrettable to note that most studies on antibiotics have been concerned with diseases prevalent in the developed nations. Many diseases of developing countries, including many major tropical diseases, have received little attention from the major pharmaceutical industries. In part this may be due to the high level of technology, including specially trained personnel, that is normally associated with antibiotic research and development. More probably, the reason lies with the economics of developing new drugs for countries with limited financial resources. Let it be hoped that the advances in biotechnology may make it possible to follow a more enlightened pathway to develop the antibiotics necessary to combat the massive specific disease problems of the developing nations. Biotechnology may well make it possible to economically produce *orphan drugs* – drugs with specific needs but small profit return.

A disquieting observation has been the gradual evolution of drug resistance in many bacteria. As soon as antibiotics began to kill bacteria, bacteria began to evolve and change to disarm antibiotics. The possibility of this acquired resistance being transmitted to another species of bacterium is now real. For example, gonorrhoea (a venereal disease) resistant to treatment with penicillin is now present in 19 countries. It is recognised that the resistance factors are located on plasmids within the bacterium and because of this can be more easily transmitted between organisms. The very core of gene transfer technology derives from this phenomenon. Antibiotic resistance in many well known diseases is steadily increasing and must cause serious concern in our society. For example, tuberculosis (TB), a former scourge of nations, had been nearly eradicated but is now increasingly being diagnosed in Western countries! Hospitals are now infested with antibiotic-resistant bacteria such as methicillin-resistant *Staphylococcus aureus* (MRSA). Microorganisms can become resistant to antibiotics by way of several mechanisms. The exchange of genetic material between bacteria occurs frequently, not just between like species but between diverse groups of bacteria. This consequently constitutes a global pool of resistant genes, which are easily spread between different bacterial populations in humans, animals and the environment.

The very large market for antibiotics in animal feeds and food preservation is now under considerable reappraisal. Without doubt, the addition of relatively small amounts of certain antibiotics (for example, bacitracin, chlortetracycline, procaine penicillin, etc.) in the feed of livestock and poultry led to the production of animals that were healthier, grew more rapidly and achieved marketable weight faster. However, there is now little doubt that the incorporation of medically important antibiotics into feed has led to increased spread of drug-resistant microorganisms, increased shedding of dangerous *Salmonella* bacteria in animal dung, and the transfer of antibiotic residues into human food.

As a consequence of the dangers of using antibiotics of human relevance in animal feed, there has been a massive effort to produce antibiotics specifically for animal feed incorporation, so replacing the medically used antibiotics. Thus antibiotics of low therapeutic potency in humans or with an insufficient spectrum of activity are now more regularly used in animal nutrition.

While antibiotics continue to have a major role in the fight against microbial infections, antibiotic resistance is now a disturbing concern for humankind. The cause of this lies mainly with the medical profession, with over-zealous prescribing and inappropriate applications of antibiotics for viral infections. There is, belatedly, more effort to educate doctors and the public on the inappropriate use of antibiotics. Sadly, there are still many countries that are not enlightened and continue to use antibiotics indiscriminately. Microbial populations do not respect national boundaries.

Since the mid-1990s, the main large pharmaceutical companies and the biotech industry have invested heavily in exploiting genomics to find new antibiotic molecules. While many new antibacterial strategies have been created, the discovery of new antibiotics has been extremely poor. This, combined with changing corporate priorities and regulatory issues, has seen the large pharmaceutical companies abandon antibiotic discovery programmes.

Undoubtedly, the clinical need for new antibiotics will always be present and it is possible that smaller biotechnology companies may exploit this special area. The ethics of the large pharmaceutical companies withdrawing from this area of medicine for purely financial reasons must be questioned.

11.4 | Vaccines and monoclonal antibodies

Vaccines

According to the World Health Organization, each year more than 17 million people die from infectious diseases, preponderantly in the developing world. Human ingenuity has permitted humankind to protect itself against many infectious diseases through vaccination – a process that has been successful for more than a century. Central to the survival of humans and animals is the immune system. There is probably no area of biomedicine that has a greater potential for affecting human health than studies of the immune system, a critical component in the body's defence against disease assault. The immune system is composed of a series of organs, cells and molecules distributed throughout the body that can function in concert: the innate (or non-specific) immune system and the acquired (or specific) immune system. The immune system provides a protective mechanism through which the body defends itself against invading organisms. The basic unit of immune function, the lymphocyte, is undoubtedly the most studied of all eukaryotic cells. Undoubtedly, immunology is at the centre of biomedical science, but yet remains a subject of great complexity.

During the last 20 years we have witnessed the unravelling of the bewildering processes of immune response in human and animal systems. When a foreign molecule (e.g. a microorganism) enters an animal system a remarkable chain of reactions is set in motion, which, if successful, will result in the inactivation and exclusion of the invading microorganism. This molecular response can in some cases remain in the animal system for many years, giving complete or partial immunity against that type of microorganism. As discussed earlier, the foreign molecule is the *antigen*, which can elicit a counteracting response, the *antibody*, from the host system.

In general, antigens are proteins, or proteins combined with other substances such as sugars, though polysaccharides and other complex molecules may also act as antigens. In the disease process, antigens usually reside on the surface of the invading microorganism and trigger the body's defences against it. In this way antibodies are the essence of immunity against disease.

Antibodies are made by special cells throughout the body and it is now recognised that individual animal species, including humans, can produce unbelievable numbers of different antibodies. The antibody-producing cells recognise the shape of particular determinant groups of the antigen and produce specific antibodies in order to neutralise and eliminate the foreign substance. Thus the human body has sufficient antibodies to combat not only the vast array of microbial invasions that can occur but also an unlimited range of synthetic chemicals. In short, the mammalian system can bind and inactivate almost any foreign molecule that gets in. However, should a particular antigen challenge not be dealt with adequately, then the invading microorganism can rapidly multiply and create imbalance, illness and perhaps death in the susceptible host. Antibiotics constitute the most rapidly growing class of human therapeutics and the second largest class of drugs after vaccines.

The ability to stimulate the natural antibodies by vaccines has long been known. Vaccines are preparations of dead microorganisms (or fractions of them), or living attenuated or weakened microorganisms, that can be given to humans or animals to stimulate their immunity to infection. In this way they mimic infectious agents without the pathogenic consequences and elicit in the body protective immune responses. When used on a large scale, vaccines have been a major force in the control of microbial diseases within communities. The major goals of vaccine research are to identify and characterise the individual antigens of infectious agents that elicit protective immune responses and to define the components in the immune response that induce protection.

Historically, vaccines have been relatively low cost with a course of paediatric vaccines (e.g. measles, mumps, etc.) in the 1980s costing a few dollars while, more recently, the pneumococcal vaccines cost $c.$ US$200. The whole scenario of vaccine manufacturing has changed radically over the past 30–40 years. In the 1960s there were large numbers of companies licensed for vaccine manufacture, but the introduction of strict good manufacturing practice regulations to vaccine production and increased problems of liability caused massive escalation in overall costs. Consequently, in more recent times, world vaccine manufacturing has become dominated by five companies: Chiron, GlaxoSmithKline, Merck, Sanefi-Pasteur and Wyeth. Vaccines have long processing times and are difficult and expensive to produce (Fig. 11.3).

While the worldwide market for vaccines in 2006 was $c.$ US$10 billion this compares badly with single healthcare blockbuster drugs, which, in some cases, can be at least US$3 billion annually. However, changes are now taking place due to the worldwide concern regarding a possible influenza pandemic and the arrival of new vaccines such as the vaccine for preventing cervical cancer, which is projected at US$750–1 billion annually. Furthermore, the US Project Bioshield programme has been a significant source of vaccine production growth with the US Government spending hundreds of millions of dollars on vaccine stockpiling to protect against anthrax and smallpox and other potential terrorist-generated diseases.

Keeping up with the demand for new vaccines to respond to possible epidemics, natural or man-made, could well overwhelm the already

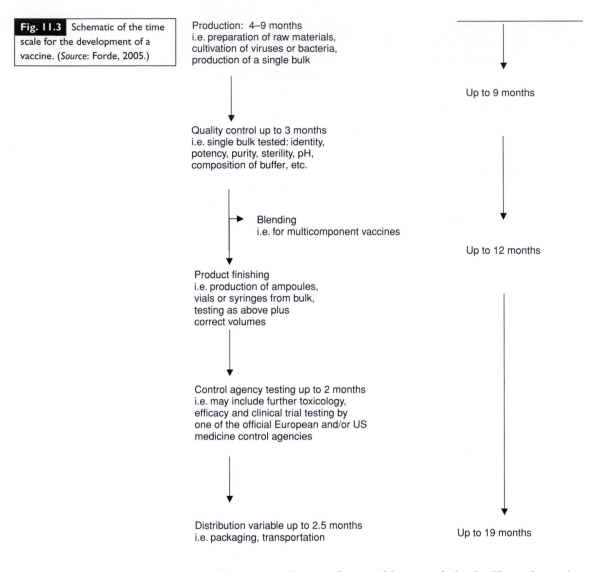

Fig. 11.3 Schematic of the time scale for the development of a vaccine. (*Source*: Forde, 2005.)

Production: 4–9 months
i.e. preparation of raw materials,
cultivation of viruses or bacteria,
production of a single bulk

Up to 9 months

Quality control up to 3 months
i.e. single bulk tested: identity,
potency, purity, sterility, pH,
composition of buffer, etc.

Blending
i.e. for multicomponent vaccines

Up to 12 months

Product finishing
i.e. production of ampoules,
vials or syringes from bulk,
testing as above plus
correct volumes

Control agency testing up to 2 months
i.e. may include further toxicology,
efficacy and clinical trial testing by
one of the official European and/or US
medicine control agencies

Distribution variable up to 2.5 months
i.e. packaging, transportation

Up to 19 months

stretched-to-capacity manufacture of these prophylactics. The main vaccine-producing companies have increased capacity either by acquisitions or by building new facilities. As a consequence, many small biotechnology companies are entering this new lucrative market especially with novel approaches to vaccine production.

At the present time humankind is under severe threat of the spread of viral diseases, e.g. human immunodeficiency virus (HIV), mosquito-borne West Nile virus, severe acute respiratory syndrome (SARS) and a possible highly virulent influenza pandemic on a scale similar to the fatal outbreaks in 1918, 1957 and 1968.

Vaccines have been developed against many microbial diseases. However, the success and persistence of the antimicrobial effect varies widely between types of vaccines. Vaccines have eliminated smallpox from the world and polio from the Northern hemisphere and have greatly reduced measles, rubella, tetanus, diphtheria and meningitis in many countries, saving countless millions of lives. Vaccines still remain the most cost-effective intervention available for preventing death and disease. However, there is a great disparity in their availability throughout the world. Reducing these differences between countries must be answered in the future. Vaccines must also be found for acquired immunodeficiency syndrome (AIDS), malaria, tuberculosis, dysentery and other respiratory and diarrhoeal diseases. In excess of 30 million people will die of TB in the next decade, while the AIDS pandemic is causing devastation in many parts of the world, especially on the African continent.

Vaccine production is a high-cost, low-volume production system that encompasses many basic principles of biotechnology. Scale-up, in particular, is a constant problem when concerned with viral diseases that need to be produced from animal or human cell cultures. New advances in fermenter technology are rapidly revolutionising this work and should greatly increase vaccine production in the near future.

The scientific and ethical difficulties associated with vaccine development and application must not be underestimated. The positive effects of a successful vaccination programme on public health issues can have dramatic outcomes as seen with the eradication of smallpox. In contrast to most medically applied compounds, vaccines are normally given to healthy individuals to prevent disease and not to sick individuals to cure them. A clinician is concerned with the health of the individual patient whereas public health authorities are concerned with the health of the general public. Vaccines are extremely sensitive products both for the public and for the medical establishment. It has long been recognised that for most vaccines there can be a minor to severe side-reaction for a small number of patients. Consequently, vaccines must be of a high efficacy and very low risk to be medically accepted.

New methods of antibody production are now being considered. In current practice antibodies are obtained from immunised animals, but this is usually a tedious and time-consuming operation. At the end of the various extraction and purification stages the antibodies are usually weakly specific, available only in small batches and of variable activity. Attempts to culture antibody-secreting cells have been unsuccessful, since such cells neither survive long enough nor produce enough antibodies in culture to become worthwhile sources of antibodies. Furthermore, such systems normally produce mixtures of different antibodies (polyclonal antibodies).

The production of vaccines to combat human and animal diseases represents an immense market that has been extensively developed by the pharmaceutical industries. At present vaccine quality and efficacy range from excellent to unsatisfactory.

In viral-derived diseases, vaccines are being developed by recombinant DNA technology against the influenza virus, polio virus, hepatitis B virus, herpes virus and more recently the AIDS virus. Successful vaccines in these important world diseases could mean massive commercial gains for the producing companies. The biggest opportunities exist for diseases such as AIDS or herpes, where neither a vaccine nor a cure is yet available.

Extensive studies are also in progress with certain bacterial vaccines, as well as vaccines for parasitic diseases. Malaria still remains the most

Table 11.2	Monoclonal antibody markets
(1) Cancer diagnosis and therapy
(2) Diagnosis of pregnancy
(3) Diagnosis of sexually transmitted diseases
(4) Prevention of immune rejection of organ implants
(5) Purification of industrial products
(6) Detection of trace molecules in food, agriculture and industry

prevalent infectious disease in the world; this complex and demanding problem could well be overcome in the very near future.

Monoclonal antibodies

A significant new development in medically related biotechnology has been the ability to produce monoclonal antibodies. A major advance of this technique is that when antibody-producing cells are immortalised and stabilised the secreted antibodies will always be the same from that particular cell line, and can be fully characterised to assess their suitability for different applications. In this way suitable antibodies can be produced and scaled-up (either as ascites tumours in mice or by various forms of fermentation technology) in large quantities, allowing much greater standardisation for diagnostic applications. Monoclonal antibodies are now finding wide applications in diagnostic techniques requiring highly specific reagents for the detection and measurement of soluble proteins and cell surface markers in blood transfusions, haematology, histology, microbiology and clinical chemistry, as well as in other non-medical areas (Table 11.2).

In particular, monoclonal antibodies have found ready application in in vitro diagnostic products that do not need such rigorous safety testing. Diagnosis can be achieved for many diseases including human venereal diseases, hepatitis B and some bacterial diseases. Recognition of molecular diversity in disease is required for the development of targeted therapies. Monoclonal antibodies can also be used in pregnancy testing.

Harnessing the immune system to treat chronic infectious diseases or cancer is a major goal of immunotherapy. Therapeutic monoclonal antibodies used today are genetically engineered molecules designed to ensure high specificity and functionability. In some cases the monoclonal antibodies are loaded with toxic chemicals or radionucleotides, while others are designed to function naturally.

On a commercial scale monoclonal antibodies are being produced in 100-litre airlift fermenters, by encapsulation in 100-litre fermenters and in perfusion chambers using lymph from live cattle.

The twentieth century has witnessed tremendous advances in the diagnosis, understanding, prevention and cure of many infectious diseases. The success of global vaccination programmes and the discovery and development of antibiotics falsely induced microbiologists and clinicians to consider that microbial infections were conquered. That is no longer the case with the arrival of new diseases such as AIDS and bovine spongiform encephalopathy (BSE), the rapid spread of antibiotic resistance, and diseases that were believed to be under control have re-emerged. As Louis Pasteur stated: 'Messieurs, ce sont les microbes qui avant le dernier mot.'

11.5 | Biopharmaceuticals/therapeutic proteins

The vast majority of pharmaceutical products are small-molecule compounds derived either from synthetic chemical processes, from naturally occurring sources (plants, microorganisms) or combinations of both. Such compounds are used to regulate essential bodily functions or to combat disease-causing microorganisms. Increasing attention is now being directed to the body's own regulatory molecules, which occur normally only in very small concentrations and have predominantly defied modern methods of extraction or synthesis. Limited quantities of some of these compounds have historically been derived from organs of cadavers and from blood banks. Genetic engineering is now increasingly being recognised as a practical means of providing some of these scarce molecules in unrestricted quantities. In practice, this involves inserting the necessary human-derived gene constructs into suitable host microorganisms or mammalian cells that will produce the therapeutic protein (biopharmaceutical) in quantities related to the scale of operation. Not only is it now possible to produce these biopharmaceuticals in a form identical to that normally occurring in the human body but also to design meaningful improvements in activity, stability or bioavailability. Such products will also be free of the dangerous contaminants that have occasionally arisen from extraction of cadavers, e.g. the degenerative brain disease Creutzfeldt–Jacob disease (CJD) has been associated with early human growth hormone extractions.

The successful development of biopharmaceuticals requires:

(1) advanced biochemical/biomedical research to identify and characterise the native compounds
(2) skilled molecular biology and cloning technology to identify the relevant gene sequences and insert them into a production mammalian or microbiological host
(3) bioprocess technology to grow the organisms and to isolate, concentrate and purify the chosen compounds
(4) clinical and marketing expertise.

Table 11.3 indicates some of the main biopharmaceuticals approved for marketing worldwide between 1982 and 2006. At least 100 recombinant proteins are now used in therapy and a further 500 are at various stages of development. Top selling biopharmaceuticals in the USA are shown in Table 11.4.

However, the use of these protein-type pharmaceuticals has several restrictions, which will limit their use and size of market. As proteins they are unstable and poorly absorbed from the gastro intestinal tract – consequently they have to be given parenterally by a medically trained person. Thus, their main use will be for acute rather than chronic

Table 11.3 Some of the 200 biopharmaceuticals approved in the USA and EU over the last 25 years

Product	Therapeutic indication
Recombinant blood factors, e.g. Factor VIII	Haemophilia A
Recombinant thrombolytics and anticoagulants, e.g. tissue plasminogen activator	Myocardial infarction
Recombinant hormones, e.g. insulin, human growth hormone	Diabetes mellitus, growth disturbances in children and adults
Recombinant growth factors, e.g. erythropoeitin	Anaemia
Recombinant interferons and interleukins, e.g. Interferon-α, Interferon-β	Hepatitis B, C and various cancers
Recombinant vaccines, e.g. Hepatitis B	Hepatitis B
Monoclonal antibodies, e.g. Herceptin, ProtaScint	Breast cancer, prostate adenocarcinoma
Recombinant enzymes, e.g. Myozyme	Pompe disease
Nucleic acid-based products, e.g. Macugen	Macular degeneration

Source: www.fda.gov; www.eudra.org/eu_house.htm; www.phrma.org

Table 11.4 Top-selling biopharmaceuticals in the USA

Product (indications)	Company	2006 sales (US$ millions)
Enbrel (arthritis, psoriasis, ankylosing spondylitis)	Amgen, Wyeth, Takeda	4.4
Aranesp (anaemia)	Amgen	4.1
Rituxan/MabThera (non-Hodgkin's lymphoma)	Biogen Idec, Genentech, Roche	8.9
Herceptin (breast cancer)	Genentech, Roche	8.1
Human insulins (diabetes)	NovoNordisk	2.5
Avastin (colon cancer)	Genentech, Roche	2.4

Source: adapted from Lawrence, S. (2007) *Nature Biotechnology* **25**, 380–382

conditions. Some proteins may also cause allergic reactions in the patient with long-term therapy.

A wide range of cellular forms including bacteria, yeasts, mammalian and human cells have been used for heterologous protein expression. Transgenic animals and plants can also be used as expression vehicles. When a transgene is introduced into a recipient animal, the expression of the gene product can occur in the milk, blood or urine of the animal.

With the advent of gene technology it is now possible to produce human therapeutic proteins in large quantities and high purity. As such, recombinant human proteins can now be used in rational therapy using the body's own substances, which will not be immunogenic. The major differences between classic small-molecule drugs and biopharmaceutical/therapeutic drugs are summarised in Table 11.5. The DNA sequences coding for the therapeutic proteins can also be modified by direct mutagenesis allowing further changes in protein structure. This is called *protein engineering* and the mutated proteins are termed *muteins*.

Table 11.5	Comparison of therapeutic proteins and small-molecule drugs
Large complicated molecules	
Heterogeneity	
Produced by genetically modified living cells	
Complex mode of action mediated by large surface area	
Complicated production and purification	
Relatively unstable	

Source: Schellekens (2004)

The first human gene sequences encoding important therapeutic proteins cloned into microorganisms were insulin, human growth hormone (somatostatin) and interferons.

By way of gene technology it has become possible to produce human proteins in large amounts and high purity, which can allow in some cases a rational therapy with the body's own proteins where they can function for substitution, amplification or inhibition of physiological processes. Some examples of recombinant therapeutic drugs are given here.

Insulin

Throughout the world there are millions of people who need regular intake of insulin to overcome the lethal effects of diabetes. Insulin extracted from pigs and cattle has long been the source of worldwide usage, and it is now believed that some of the unfortunate side-effects that have occurred with continued long-term use of insulin could be due to additional contaminating compounds present in the animal insulin. Recombinant human insulin appears not to have such problems and is increasingly having the largest market share of sales. Production is unlimited and free from market shortage of animals and all the problems associated with previous production methods.

Somatostatin

The growth hormone, somatostatin, has been extremely difficult to isolate from animals; half a million sheep brains were required to extract 0.005 g of pure somatostatin. By cloning the human gene for somatostin into a bacterium, this same amount of hormone can be produced from nine litres of a transgenic bacterial fermentation. One child in 5000 suffers from hypopituitary dwarfism resulting from growth hormone deficiency and the easy availability of this biopharmaceutical will have immense benefit to these child sufferers. The annual world market is estimated at US$100 million.

However, a potentially massive market could arise from the increasing evidence that this growth hormone can increase muscle formation in normal individuals and is now being exploited by some athletes. There are also claims that regular administration of the hormone can improve quality of life in the aged!

Interferons

In 1957, two British researchers discovered substances produced within the body that could act against viruses by making cells resistant to virus attack. Most vertebrate animals can produce these substances, known as interferons, and many animal viruses can induce their in vitro synthesis and become sensitive to them. Why, then, have the interferons not become the 'penicillins' of virus infections? Primarily, this is because only minute amounts of interferon are produced within cells, and it has proved unbelievably complicated to extract and separate them from other cellular proteins.

Human interferons are glycoproteins (proteins with attached sugar molecules) and are believed to play a part in controlling many types of viral infections, including the common cold, as well as having potential in controlling cancer. However, the scarcity of these compounds has consistently hampered efforts to understand the extent of their effectiveness.

There are many different types of interferons characteristic of individual species of animals; mouse interferons will respond to mouse cells but not human cells, and vice versa. Furthermore, different tissues from the same species appear to produce different interferons. Thus interferon for human studies must be derived from human cells, and it has been here that the blockage to production has occurred. Most early human interferon production was carried out in Finland using leucocytes from blood, and the small amounts of interferon produced this way were used for limited clinical tests throughout the world.

So far, studies have shown that interferons can confer resistance to some virus infections, and are involved in the body's natural immune reactions even in the absence of viruses. However, much of the current interest in interferons arises from their ability to inhibit cancer in experimental animals. Interferons present a new approach to cancer therapy because they appear to attack the cancer cells by inhibiting their growth, and that of any viruses involved in the cancer process, and they can also stimulate the body's natural immune defences against the cancer cell. Although the limited clinical studies of these compounds have indicated considerable potential in cancer therapy, the restricted supplies have severely hampered conclusive experimentation; this must await greater availability of interferons.

Two sources of interferon are currently available. The first is from human diploid fibroblasts growing attached to a suitable surface and the interferon produced is widely considered to be the safest available. The second source is from bacteria in which the gene for human fibroblast interferon has been inserted into a plasmid in such a manner that interferon is synthesised and can be extracted and purified.

Lymphokines

Lymphokines are proteins produced by lymphocytes (part of the body's immune system) and are considered to be crucially important to immune reactions. They appear to have the capability of enhancing or restoring the immune system to fight infectious diseases or cancer. Interleukin-2 at present offers the greatest potential and is now produced by genetic engineering, and consequently more readily available on the market.

With each of these important compounds it has been possible to achieve a level of realistic pharmaceutical drug delivery only because recombinant DNA technology enabled the synthesis of large quantities of the product.

The production of human vaccines by recombinant methods has been quite successful and should allow for new approaches to diseases without existing remedial treatments. Recombinant hepatitis B virus has gained regulatory approval and has high market sales.

Presently, all biopharmaceuticals are produced by way of genetically engineered mammalian cell or microbial fermentations. However, with the development of transgenic animals, it has become possible to produce certain human proteins of biopharmaceutical potential, including tissue plasmogen activator, blood clotting factors, etc., in the lactating glands of several animal species, such as the mouse, sheep, cow and pig, and to be able to express the products in the milk of the animal. These products can then be more easily extracted and purified. A further feature of this process is that it is accomplished in a mammalian system, which can confer on certain human proteins the complex structural modifications required for full biological activity. Such modifications cannot be achieved in microbial systems. As yet no commercial production is in operation, and awaits improvements in yields and final regulatory approval. Undoubtedly this will become a major source of production of certain complex human proteins. There is no apparent adverse effect on the animal, which continues to produce milk in the normal way.

Haematopoietic growth factors

Recombinant erythropoietin is used therapeutically mainly in renal anaemia but also tumour anaemia, and was the first recombinant therapeutic protein to achieve US$1 billion sales worldwide. It is regrettably used by some athletes to boost performance.

Granulocyte colony stimulating factor stimulates proliferation and differentiation of neutrophil precursor cells to mature granulocytes, and is primarily used as an adjunct in chemotherapy of cancer to offset neutropenia or the destruction of white blood cells by the toxic chemotherapeutic agents.

A US company can now produce human haemoglobin in the blood of transgenic pigs, which could serve as a human blood substitute. Such transgenic haemoglobin could capture a massive market. Each year worldwide, 70 million units of human blood are transfused at a cost of US$10 billion. This transgenic haemoglobin would be free of human pathogens, such as HIV, and would not need typing or matching before transfusion because it is not composed of red blood cells. Much yet requires to be done before this becomes a reality.

11.6 | Pharmacogenetics

Pharmacogenetics is the study of the variations in a patient's response to drugs due to hereditary traits that may explain individual differences in the efficacy of drugs and in the occurrence of adverse drug reactions. Pharmacogenetics is a term often associated with the application of genomics in drug discovery. In practice these terms are associated with the dividing of patients or populations into groups on the basis of their biological response to drug treatment using a genetic test. This is now an interdisciplinary area involving medicine, informatics, cell and molecular biology, genomics, epidemiology and pharmacology. From these studies should evolve:

- discovery of better drugs and the determination of disease mechanisms
- improvement of drug safety and efficacy.

11.7 | Molecular biology and human disease

Since the beginning of the Human Genome Project and subsequent developments in proteomics and metabolomics there has been a remarkable upsurge in deciphering the molecular basis of complex human diseases. New in vitro molecular diagnostic tests (nucleic acid probes, microarrays, etc.) are now quantitatively measuring response to therapy, and can monitor disease progress and predict recurrences. Central to the success of these diagnostic procedures is the correct identification of suitable human biomarkers.

Human biomarkers have long been utilised in medicine and have evolved over time from simple, single physiological (heart rate, blood pressure) or laboratory (cholesterol, white blood cells) parameters to highly complex imaging modalities or multimarkers in genome/proteome panels. Any measurement that can predict a person's disease state or response to a drug treatment can be called a biomarker. DNA-based biomarkers are already being incorporated into routine patient management. In many ways this molecular diagnostic approach supports a future market for personalised medicine. Revenue from molecular biomarker-related products and services is expected to exceeed US$2 billion by 2009.

The overall field of medical diagnostics generated *c*. US$29 billion of which over 80% was related to identification of infectious diseases and the rest made up of assays related to genetic diseases, predictive testing, cancer and paternity testing. A vast range of such testing kits is now available over the counter. Over 500 companies now have molecular diagnostics as a part or all of their business. Molecular diagnostics have brought technical advances with improvements in sensitivity, speed and selectivity.

While in vitro diagnostic tests dominate the medical market, in vivo systems are being developed. However, unlike in vitro systems, in vivo products will have to undergo extensive, time-consuming clinical trials to prove their safety in use.

11.8 | Diagnostics in developing countries

Infectious diseases continue to devastate the developing world. Diagnostics are crucial for identifying the presence and cause of disease at both the individual and the population level. In developing countries there is a lack of diagnostic tests that can be performed at low-infrastructure sites. Without these tests healthcare workers are unable to differentiate between diseases with similar visible symptoms (i.e. fevers) and to be able to apply the correct treatment, monitor the effects of intervention (whether preventative or therapeutic) and to assess levels of drug resistance or recurrence of existing diseases.

Current available diagnostic equipment is mostly inadequate for serving health needs in most developing countries. Commercial companies have mostly shown a lack of willingness to commit to the development of accurate and affordable molecular-based diagnostic tests for infectious diseases in the developing world. Most existing diagnostic systems have been formulated for industrial countries and are generally inappropriately complex in operating and manpower skills and costs, to be utilised in developing countries. There is great need for massive funding to speed up the development and delivery of diagnostic solutions to the disease problems of the developing world.

The Bill and Melinda Gates Foundation sponsored the Global Health Diagnostic Forum, which issued the report titled *Improved Diagnostic Techniques for the Developing World* (www.nature.com/diagnostics).

In this report the contributors have identified the acute need for new diagnostic tools, the potential impact of new diagnostics for people in the developing world and the specific performance requirements of these tools.

11.9 | Gene therapy

Undoubtedly, the most far-reaching and controversial area of genetic engineering of humans is gene therapy. Gene therapy can be considered as any treatment strategy that involves the introduction of genes or genetic material into human cells to alleviate or eliminate disease. The aim of gene therapy is to replace or repress defective genes with sequences of DNA that encode a specific genetic message. Within the cells, the DNA molecules may provide new genetic instructions to correct the host phenotype. However, to bring this about the exogenous genes must first achieve passage to the diseased cells. Herein lies the main and continuing difficulty. To date, gene therapy has been used to treat several thousand people worldwide suffering from a range of genetic disorders and only a small number have shown any clinical benefit. The majority of current gene therapy clinical trials are involving the infective mechanisms of viruses, in particular, retroviruses. These vectors are able to integrate at random sites in the host's cell genome and can pose risks to patients due to random insertional mutagenesis and potential oncogenesis (cancer). Other approaches include direct injection of the gene into the cell, merging it into the cell with a fat particle called a liposome, or by antibody-like proteins that can recognise the cell surface.

The liposomes are able to encapsulate DNA molecules and act as vectors in the delivery of therapeutic genes. Much research is now in progress to develop efficient in vivo gene delivery systems. As an alternative to gene delivery there is also an active alternative strategy of gene repair. The natural regulatory elements of genes are retained and segments of synthetic

Table 11.6	Selected human genetic diseases for possible single gene therapy	
Disease	Target tissue	Incidence
Thalassaemia	Bone marrow	1:600 in some populations
Cystic fibrosis	Liver	1:500
Duchenne muscular dystrophy	Muscle/brain	1:300 males
Haemophilia A	Liver/	1:6000 males
Haemophilia B	Fibroblasts	1:30 000 males

Source: Johnson (1991) *Chemistry & Industry*, 644–66

DNA and RNA, to hopefully interact with malfunctioning genes and repair them, are delivered to cells.

It is, however, essential to distinguish between *germ cell gene therapy* and *somatic cell gene therapy*. In germ cell gene therapy changes are directed at the individual's genetic make-up, which can be passed onto the offspring. Should gene therapy be considered in humans for non-therapeutic purposes, e.g. genetic 'enhancement' to increase human physical and mental capabilities above what is considered normal? Should this technology be used to make a body better rather than making a bad body good? Ethics and practical wisdom ensures that this type of therapy will *not* be permitted in any country, in the foreseeable future. In contrast, in somatic cell therapy, functioning genes are introduced into body cells that lack them. The effects of the therapy are confined to the person undergoing the treatment and are *not* passed onto the offspring. Because only somatic cells are receiving the human DNA the treatment will probably have to be repeated for the person's lifetime.

The main thrust of gene therapy has been directed at correcting single-gene defects (mutations) that have been observed in families by their Mendelian pattern of inheritance, such as cystic fibrosis and haemophilia (Table 11.6). It is believed by some that many hundreds of such diseases could be treated by this process and the next decade should see significant progress if the many technical problems can be readily overcome. At present most genetic diseases have no effective treatment so gene therapy could offer hope for many people. Somatic cell gene therapy for complex multifactorial diseases, e.g. Parkinson's, cancer, etc., must be a long way off. In many of these diseases there can be many genes involved as well as an interaction with environmental factors.

Gene therapy has not yet lived up to its original promise, but some recent successes in the treatment of certain genetic blood diseases may herald a new era of success. The potential of this area of medical science could yet be realised in the near future.

Gene therapy is a complex series of events relying heavily on new biotechnological techniques. Therapy will require a full understanding of the mechanism by which the defective or unusual gene exerts its effect on the individual, and an ability to switch off the defective gene and to substitute a healthy gene copy (Fig. 11.4). It is truly a multidisciplinary activity

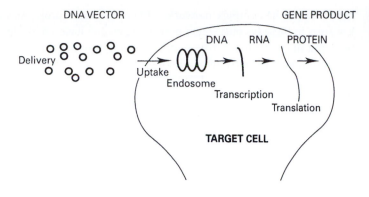

Fig. 11.4 Functional steps in gene transfer and expression. Gene therapy involves the delivery of DNA vectors to specific target cells within the body, uptake (commonly by endocytosis), transcription and translation of sequences within the DNA vector, and production of a therapeutic gene product.

involving skills in molecular biology, cell biology, virology, pharmacology, clinical application and patient interaction. Gene therapy products will present difficult challenges in development, manufacturing, testing and distribution. While safety problems have dogged gene therapy efficacy has been much harder to achieve. The challenge still is getting enough gene expression for a sufficient period of time. The USA is the undoubted world leader in gene therapy research and application. Some of the protocols are now proceeding through regulatory processes and already patent coverage for gene construction, delivery systems and supporting technology has been granted. Private medical systems internationally must see gene therapy as a very lucrative market in the affluent nations.

Gene therapy technologies are indeed part of the continuum of technologies that insert foreign genes into the human body.

Organ transplantation is a source of foreign genes, which can synthesise functional levels of enzymes and other substances that may be deficient because of genetic disease, e.g. lung transplantation for cystic fibrosis; bone marrow transplantation for severe immune deficiencies and leukaemia. Vaccination similarly leads to irreversible changes in white blood cell DNA leading to the synthesis of antibodies that mediate immunity to many viral and bacterial diseases.

Gene therapy technology is not without risk and following several high-profile events there continues to be considerable focus on the ethics and safety of gene therapy trials.

11.10 | Systems biology and medicine

The Human Genome Project has enhanced the view that biology is an information science with static and dynamic elements. The genome comprises all the instructions for the development and functioning of an organism. When genetic changes occur there will be functional loss or alteration of these instructions. Disease can result from genetic changes. From this perspective the treatment of the disease state could be the replacement of the information that is malfunctioning or the correction of the information that is erroneous in the form of DNA or protein. A systems biology approach will seek to elucidate the various hierarchies of biological information; the complex networks of genomics and proteonics are the key areas in these systems where perturbations can have a defining impact resulting in concomitant disease processes but also offering potential for medical intervention. Systems biology will ultimately develop predictive models for human diseases. Mainline drugs in the future will not simply target one system but will eventually target multiple systems at common interception points.

Chapter 12

Stem cell biotechnology

12.1 | The nature of stem cells

Within the mammalian body there is a ranking system of cells from the undifferentiated to the highly specialised cell types and tissues, e.g. liver, brain, lung, blood, skin, etc., which have arisen by the process of cellular differentiation. Cellular differentiation occurs by a variety of biological processes that involve the switching on and off of specific genes, of cell signalling and, especially, where the cell is situated in the body. When a cell achieves terminal differentiation it cannot reproduce itself. Yet, it has long been recognised that systems and tissues of the adult body must have some ability to replace cells such as cells of the blood system (haematopoietic cells) and skin cells (epidermal tissue). The body does, however, retain certain undifferentiated cells within tissues and such cells are termed tissue or adult stem cells (TS).

What are stem cells? Stem cells are undifferentiated cells that have the capacity to self-renew and to achieve multilineage differentiation. Within a particular cell population they can remain in an undifferentiated state and, as such, do not have any specialised function. However, when required they can be induced to differentiate into specific cell types. Stem cells have specific enzymes and cell-specific antigens and have the ability to express developmentally regulated genes. Stem cells have been characterised as totipotent, pluripotent and multipotent.

In order to fully appreciate the scientific and medical interest in stem cells it is necessary to understand the cellular details of early human development from the fertilised egg (the zygote) to an embryo and then a foetus. Within 24 hours after fertilisation mitotic cell division to form two cells will have occurred followed by four, eight, sixteen cells, etc. At this stage all of the cells retain the potential to form an embryo – they are 'totipotent'. By about four days after fertilisation, a sphere of specialised cells has been developed – the blastocyst (Fig. 12.1). The outer ring of cells of the blastocyst will later form the placenta and related tissues while the mass of cells – the epiblast or inner cell mass – will go on to form all of the cells and tissues of the embryo and the human body. However, while such cells are

Table 12.1	Sources of stem cells

- Surplus embryos discarded from in vitro fertilisation (IVF) or pre-implementation genetic diagnosis
- Cells from aborted foetuses
- Embryos created exclusively from stem cell research in a laboratory using IVF methods from donated eggs and sperm
- Blastocysts created exclusively from stem cell research in a laboratory by cell nuclear replacement using donated eggs and adult tissue
- Parthenogenetic embryos created exclusively for stem cell research by activating a human egg without a sperm
- Adult or foetal tissues containing tissue stem cells
- Umbilical cord blood containing tissue stem cells
- Amniotic fluid

Source: Barfoot (2005)

Fig. 12.1	The blastocyst.

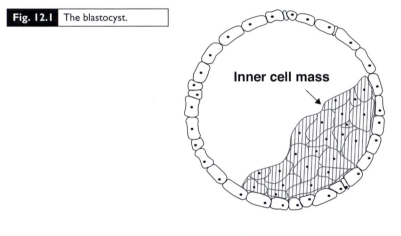

Inner cell mass

considered 'pluripotent' and more widely known as 'embryonic' stem cells (ES), they cannot individually form a foetus since they are unable to form the placenta. The ability of ES cells to differentiate into a wide range of cell and tissue types has created a huge interest in the possibilities of remedial medicine. At present embryo research studies cannot legally go beyond the 14-day stage of development. Multipotent cells are more likely to be tissue restricted, existing in specific foetal or adult tissues and can mostly give rise to differential cells of that tissue only (Table 12.1).

Human embryonic stem cells (hES) were first isolated in the University of Wisconsin in 1998 and have an undoubted potential to be a source of pluripotent cells for human cell replacement therapies, for screening drugs and toxins, and as a model for the early stages of human cellular development. Adult tissue stem cells (TS) have long been derived from blood, bone marrow, fat and several other tissues and now exist as established cell lines capable of continuous propagation. Human embryonic stem cells are the most flexible type of stem cells but have, for obvious reasons, generated the most controversy (Table 12.2).

Haematopoietic stem cell transplants to produce new blood cells are now routine clinical practice, and many hundreds of patients with type 1

Table 12.2	Defining properties of an embryonic cell

- Derived from the inner cell mass of the blastocyst
- Capable of undergoing an unlimited number of systematic divisions without differentiating (long-term self-renewal) in vitro
- Exhibit and maintain a stable, full (diploid), normal complement of chromosomes (karyotype) over extended culture
- Can give rise to differentiated cell types corresponding to endoderm, mesoderm and ectoderm derivatives of the embryo
- Capable of integrating into a foetal tissue during development
- Capable of colonising the germ line and giving rise to egg or sperm
- Able to give rise to a colony of genetically identical cells, which have the same properties as the original cell
- Show telomerase activity

Source: adapted from Barfoot (2005)

diabetes have now undergone transplants of islet cells, with a considerable proportion of patients staying off insulin injections for several years. The possibility of isolating and producing stem cells that can yield large numbers of islet-type cells is now being intensively researched. Stem cells may soon be used to replace damaged or dead heart muscle cells (cardiomyocytes) and also to replace vascular endothelial cells and smooth muscle cells, which form the blood vessels that transport the cardiomyocyte cells. Skin grafting of healthy skin to repair damaged tissue areas is now widely used. It is now possible to grow a patient's epidermal stem cells on artificial scaffolding and use them for grafting.

Recently, stem cells have been derived from amniotic fluid and have demonstrated a wide range of cell types representing the three primary embryonic cell lineages of mesoderm, ectoderm and definitive endoderm. Thus, amniotic fluid-derived stem (AFS) cells could become an important source of cells for regenerative medicine. They are easily accessible, are pluripotent and could well have advantages over hES and TS cells. In particular, such cells would not have the ethical complexities of hES cells!

12.2 | Stem cell cultivation

The principles of large-scale mammalian cell culture are discussed elsewhere (Chapter 4), and the main uses of mammalian cells have been for vaccine and recombinant protein production. Numerous cell lines for TS and hES cells have now been established and methods for large-scale production are now being extensively researched. Such cells will be required for fundamental studies on cell differentiation, reproducibility and stability prior to their anticipated use in remedial medicine.

The cultivation of stem cells requires suitable media and substratum on which the cells can be cultured and maintained in an undifferentiated state (Fig. 12.2). The substratum for hES cells can be lysed murine or human embryonic fibroblasts (termed 'feeders'), or conditioned medium

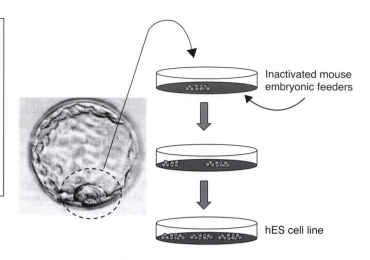

Fig. 12.2 Schematic of derivation of hES cell lines from a human blastocyst. The inner cell mass (ICM) is removed and placed upon inactivated mouse embryonic feeders. Serial passaging of these cells results in the formation of an hES cell line. (Reprinted with permission from Veeck, L. and Zaninovic, N. (eds) *An Atlas of Human Blastocysts*. Parthenon, Boca Raton, Florida 2003.)

Inactivated mouse embryonic feeders

hES cell line

containing basic fibroblast growth factor on Matrigel, laminarin or fibronectrin substrate for long-term growth. A uniform medium for all hES cell lines has yet to be agreed.

As the cells grow on the substratum they will adhere to each other. For passaging onto fresh media the cells must be disrupted or disaggregated. This is achieved in two ways: mechanical or enzymatic. Mechanical agitation disaggregates the colonies and allows the cells to move onto new tissue culture plates. Enzymatic passaging involves exposing the culture tissue to enzymes, e.g. collagenase IV, which allows the cells to dissociate. In both cases it is difficult to generate cultures with consistent cell density from passage to passage.

While it is one thing to produce large numbers of stem cells under axenic culture conditions will such cells be amenable to cell therapy experiments? Will cells produced under different culture regimes be similar to one another? Optimal culture conditions will most probably depend on the future use of the cells. If hES cells are to revolutionise regenerative medicine it is imperative to find the means of producing the desired differentiated cell type. For example, if the therapeutic target is Parkinson's disease, culture preparations of hES cells must generate large quantities of functional, transplantable and stable dopaminergic neurons.

Do stem cells need to be differentiated in vitro before transplantation to achieve optimum therapeutic outcome? The major challenge in stem cell regenerative medicine will be to understand the appropriate genetic, biochemical and environmental cues that will guide such pluripotent hES cells down appropriate developmental pathways – a challenge that will undoubtedly occupy developmental scientists for years and, indeed, decades (Table 12.3).

Remedial medicines involving stem cells will require large-scale production methods, which will be required to comply with international good manufacturing practice (GMP) regulations (Fig. 12.3). Such methods must guarantee purity and authenticity and freedom from human pathogens. Can transplanted cells always be relied upon to follow projected differentiation pathways? Renegade cells could possibly become uncontrolled leading to carcinogenesis! Could such cells be destroyed after transplantation?

Table 12.3	Stem cells and regenerative medicine: problems to be overcome

- Which stem cells will provide maximal tissue repair?
- What number of cells must be administered?
- Can stem cell therapy be delivered to ensure therapeutic benefit without causing side-effects?
- Which diseases are amenable to stem cell therapy?
- Can grafting and function of stem cell implants be enhanced with immunological or pharmacological therapy?
- Can the growth of implanted stem cells be controlled to avoid overgrowth and possible carcinogenesis?
- How safe is stem cell therapy?

Source: adapted from O'Donoghue and Fisk (2004b).

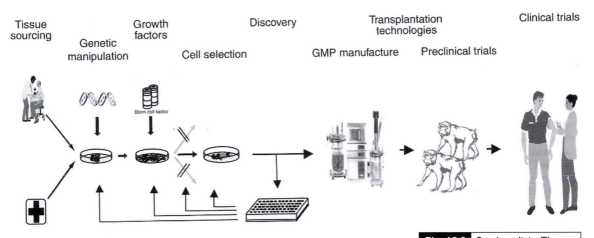

Fig. 12.3 Road to clinic. The steps to move cell-based therapies down the pathway from laboratory to clinic are similar whether they involve embryonic or adult stem cells. A source for cells is found (such as the patient), researchers coax the cells to differentiate and then to grow in a laboratory dish as well as in vivo, and the company scales-up cell production in order to guarantee a steady, pure and uniform supply, as well as bring the costs down. (*Source*: Stem Cell Sciences, Edinburgh.)

In separate studies from Japan and the USA researchers have exposed cultivated stem cells to four transcription factors, naturally occurring biochemicals that regulate genes. In each case viruses were used to incorporate the transcription factors into the cultured skin cells. Subsequently, the skin cells produced new cells that closely resembled embryonic stem cells. Each group were able to demonstrate that these cells could develop into brain, heart and other tissues.

Does this herald a new era for stem cells, removing the need to use ethically problematic hES cells? Not yet it would appear! The US FDA would not allow virally modified cells to be used in patients, as such cells may cause cancer. However, while further studies are continuing for possible use of these new cells in remedial medicine, there are no problems with using them in drug discovery and toxicological testing.

12.3 | Human–animal embryos

The potential of hES cells to develop into any of the differentiated cells of the human body has generated much scientific and public excitement over their possible use to reverse the effects of certain human degenerative diseases. However, human eggs are rarely obtained and are also difficult to work with. By contrast, many animal eggs can be obtained in high numbers and in good quality. There is now intense scientific interest in the possible use of human–animal hybrid eggs.

The proposal is to take animal eggs, e.g. rabbit, remove all the rabbit contents (genome) and replace these with a human nucleus or cell containing the human genome (nuclear transfer). The egg divides repeatedly to form the mass of cells that make up an early embryo, the components of the rabbit egg having been replaced by human components. The embryonic stem cells obtained from such embryos will be almost 100% human. Such hES cells will be used only for research and *never* used in patients. Human–animal eggs will never be allowed to grow into a developed hybrid animal *but* will allow research to improve embryonic stem cell production. In this way fundamental stem cell research can be carried out that would be almost impossible with the limited number of human embryos.

12.4 | Commercial potential for stem cell therapies

At present, there is a large unmet medical need for the treatment of human degenerative diseases and, consequently, there would be a considerable economic potential for successful therapies. Currently, the science underlying stem cell-based technologies has a high public profile with keen expectations for success in the future. Bone marrow transplants after leukaemia chemotherapy have already proved the success of adult stem cell replacement therapy.

Why, then, do the current stem cell companies experience difficulties in raising adequate funding from private equity sources, such as venture capital? In part, this is due to the poor commercial history of cell therapy, the considerable ethical and political uncertainties associated with hES cells and the confusing patenting situation. In general, stocks in stem cell companies are more volatile than the rest of biotechnology stocks. Most commercialised products that exist have not yet lived up fully to their market potential.

Most aspects of stem cell research should continue to be developed in academia or research establishments until a deeper scientific understanding and reproducibility are achieved, when they can graduate into a commercial operation. Sadly, desperate patients are travelling to countries with low medical standards for dubious stem cell therapies. Such operations could seriously damage the patient and the regulation of stem cell research.

Transforming stem cell technologies into routine clinical practice will require painstaking characterisation and purification of the donor cells, systematic elucidation of the developmental mechanisms by which cells interact, form new tissues and, above all, restore function at the site of engraftment. Human cells display immense levels of complexity, fragility and variability.

The potential of stem cells raises many scientific and ethical concerns all of which must be answered before they can be considered safe and suitable to be committed to clinical applications.

Chapter 13

Protection of biotechnological inventions

13.1 | Introduction

In the present climate of increasing globalisation, biotech companies must seek to acquire strong protection for their products and technologies in all the areas of the world where they wish to operate. It has been projected that the sales worldwide from new biotechnology alone could exceed £60 billion per annum by early this century. This will be derived from a wide range of biotechnology-based products and processes, which have evolved in most cases from many years of expensive research and development. How can such biotechnology products and processes, often referred to as intellectual property (IP), be protected and the due financial profits returned to the rightful inventors and industrial developers? Inventors in the area of biotechnology can be protected by way of different titles of protection including patents for invention, plant breeders' rights and trade secrets.

Intellectual property rights are designed to allow new technologies to be available, so that the originating scientist or company receives a reward for the initiative demonstrated. Intellectual property assets can be any codified knowledge, innovation or anything of actual or potential economic value that has arisen from basic research, analysis and manipulation of biological systems, biological property, industrial application or commercial use.

It is important to differentiate between invention and innovation. Because an invention may not always involve the commercialisation of a new idea, it follows that not all inventions result in innovation. Innovation should be seen as an interactive process of effectively creating, managing and leveraging an invention and successfully taking a new product through to the marketplace.

In the context of biotechnology, inventions can be in the form of products or processes.

- *Products*. These can be considered *either* as living entities of natural or artificial origin, e.g. animals, plants and microorganisms, cell lines, organelles, plasmids and DNA sequences, or as naturally occurring substances – primary or secondary – derived from living systems.

- *Processes*. These can include those of isolation, cultivation, multiplication, purification and bioconversion. Such processes can be involved in the isolation or the creation of the above products, e.g. antibiotic production; for the production of substances through bioconversion of products, e.g. enzymatic conversion of sugar to alcohol; or the use of the products for any purpose, e.g. monoclonal antibodies used for analysis or diagnosis; and of microbes for biocontrol of pathogens.

13.2 | Patent protection

What is a patent? A patent is a legal right, which owes its existence to a granting act by a governmental administrative authority, i.e. a Patent Office. The Patent Office must be certain that the patent meets three critical criteria.

(1) *Novelty*. It has not been done before or even talked about in public meetings.
(2) *Utility*. It has a useful purpose. For instance, a gene is not patentable in its own right but should be related to a product.
(3) *Enablement*. It can be repeated by someone.

With the granting of the patent, the holder or patentee is given the right to exclude, for a limited time period, all others within the territory of application of the patent for commercial utilisation of the patent invention. In return for this monopoly situation, the patentee discloses the details of the invention to the public so that at the end of the monopoly period, the invention may be worked freely by the public (i.e. other competitors). To obtain patent rights in, for example, Europe, the USA and Japan, the patent application must be made in each country. Such multiple applications can be very expensive and restricting. Some parts of the world still do not have legally installed patent systems and may attempt to exploit published patents without any financial return to the patentee.

After the patent application has been scrutinised and granted, the patent is in the form of a letter patent which *inter alia* contains the name of the inventor, the name of the patentee (if different), a description of the patent and the relevant claims. Patents can be granted for inventions that:

(1) are novel
(2) involve an inventive step
(3) can lead to industrial application
(4) are seen to be properly disclosed in the patent specification.

Unlike other fields of technology, inventions in biotechnology most often relate to living material, which can raise some unique difficulties in their legal protection. Problems can arise in how to describe an invention relating to living material for the purpose of obtaining patent protection, and most basically whether living matter *should* be protectable under traditional schemes of industrial property protection and, if so, what range of protection should be given to such material. For example, the National Institute of Health in the USA was refused patent rights on segments of DNA isolated from the human genome. In this context the difference between discovery (not patentable) and invention for a biotechnological substance has been highlighted by the European Patent Office:

> To find a substance freely occurring in nature is . . . mere discovery and therefore unpatentable. However, if a substance found in nature has first to be isolated from its surroundings and a process for obtaining it is developed, that process is patentable. Moreover, if the substance can be properly characterised, either by its chemical structure, by the process by which it is obtained or by other parameters and if it is 'new' in the absolute sense of having no previous recognised existence, then the substance *per se* may be patentable.

From a microorganism standpoint the claim that a human-made, genetically engineered *Pseudomonas* bacterium capable of breaking down multiple components of crude oil (developed by Chakrabarty in the USA for oil spill biodegradation) was 'not to a hitherto unknown natural phenomenon, but to a non-naturally occurring manufacture or composition of matter – a product of human ingenuity having distinctional name, character and use'. The patent claim was for a new bacterium, which had potential for significant industrial use and had different characteristics from any found in nature, thereby qualifying this bacterium as a patentable subject – it was *not* nature's handiwork but that of the patentee. This patent award has significantly improved future success for genetically engineered organisms, which are now coming forward in ever-increasing numbers for patent consideration.

Another interesting example for patent consideration was the *onco-mouse* – a mouse genetically manipulated so that it was more predisposed to detect carcinogens than an ordinary mouse. The European Patent Convention excludes inventions 'in respect of plant or animal varieties or essentially biological processes for the production of plants or animals; this provision does not apply to microbiological processes or the products thereof.' Much of biotechnology is, however, microbiological and, therefore, prima facie patentable. Macrobiological processes involving plants and animals are excluded. A patent was awarded for the onco-mouse on the narrowest of grounds, in part because the process of production could not occur in nature (as the mice would not have existed had it not been for the microbiological gene insertion process into the mouse DNA) and, therefore, the process was not essentially biological.

The onco-mouse is more susceptible to developing tumours, which makes it valuable for studying cancer and the potential therapeutic benefit from drugs that could be used to treat cancer.

In Europe, there continues to be much vocal opposition to animal and human gene patenting, and to biotechnology in general. The US legal system views the patenting of human cells and tissues differently from the rest of the world, and several patents covering human-derived cells and tissues have been granted (see Klein (2007) for the history of gene patenting in the USA). In sharp contrast, elsewhere there are deep reservations on the commoditisation of human body parts. In the USA the prospect for patenting animals is less daunting and several transgenic animals have, so far,

Table 13.1	Benefits and disadvantages of the patent system	
Benefits	Disadvantages
1. The patent holder retains an absolute monopoly on product or process for the period of patent (up to 20 years in some cases). **2.** Administration of patent maintenance once it has been obtained is relatively easy.	**1.** Knowledge is in the public domain following expiry and could be valuable to competitors. **2.** Litigation can be expensive. **3.** Problems of lack of harmonisation of patent laws and other trading blocks not covered by patent could tolerate misuse.

been patented. However, advancements in this area of biotechnology will continue to face strong opposition more often from religious coalitions who believe that altering or creating new life forms is 'a revolt against the sovereignty of God and an attempt to be God'. Since these currently approved animal patents are for medical benefits there should be a distinction made between 'playing God' and 'playing doctor'. The fundamental policy behind the granting of patents is not the ownership of property rights, rather the encouragement of the development of technology and innovations.

It is increasingly apparent that public trust and understanding has become an essential component in many biotechnological research activities, especially in relation to such controversial areas as human embryonic stem cells (hES), other areas of cell research, e.g. genomics and proteomics, and large-scale biobanking. The potential patenting possibilities in such areas could easily generate social controversy. Yet, again, the strategic use of race as a genetic category to obtain patent protection and drug approval will not go unquestioned!

Patent laws are remarkably complex and tend to vary between different parts of the world. It is a legal minefield, but necessary to ensure the just financial returns for those who invest heavily in biotechnological research and development without which there would be no forward advance in the many dimensions of biotechnology. The benefits and disadvantages of patents are shown in Table 13.1.

Deciding when is the right time to file a patent application can be a testing decision in any technical field, but is particularly demanding in the highly competitive and rapidly developing areas of new biotechnology, e.g. gene technology, monoclonal antibodies, etc. Should you wait until there is a substantial volume of data and risk being upstaged by a competitor, or do you file early to secure a filing date but then risk being rejected because not enough experimental data has been submitted? Whether an invention should be patented must be a commercial decision, assisted by legal advice and involving a good level of business and common sense, together with an awareness of the main alternative to patenting, namely, secrecy. Only a very small percentage of patents will be real winners achieving high financial returns.

Levels of public disclosure prior to patent filing are a hotly contested area. Publication prior to patent submission would normally discount a patent's validity. Historically, the term 'printed publication' included only books or other documents prepared by way of a printing press. Now the term publication has become the new standard for exclusivity. To make certain of the potential validity of a patent it is best to follow the rule that 'silence is golden'.

Patenting of a new effective drug allows the manufacturer to sell the drug at a good profit for the duration of the patent without competition. Once the drug comes 'off patent' it can then be manufactured by others as a 'generic' product and profit margins drop dramatically. The clinical potential of double-stranded RNA molecules, which exist naturally in the cells of many species, is sure to introduce a new complexity into patent laws!

Recent reports have shown that US academic institutions are better integrated with the commercial sphere and more effectively bring ideas from the laboratory to the real world. Europe's main institutions are not achieving similar commercialisation of their undoubted high level of skills, and a major part of Europe's poor performance can be attributed to the EU's disparate patent laws and costs. When small centres attempt to patent their IP the cost of patenting an idea in the US is equivalent to €12 000, whereas in Europe it is €45 000. In many ways academia can be considered as the real driver of innovation in biotechnology, while the industrial consortium takes it through to the marketplace.

13.3 | Trade secrets

Many biotechnology companies prefer to use trade secrets to protect their products or processes rather than to apply for patents. The forms of information that can be protected include, for example, hybridoma cell lines for monoclonal antibody production, ideas, formulas, production details, experimental procedures, etc. In the fermentation industry, production strains and details of medium design and formulation are highly confidential and full details are only known by a few employees.

Undoubtedly the best kept trade secret in the world is the formula for Coca-Cola. The formula is kept in a bank in Atlanta, USA and only five people in the world are said to know the formula. The formula has remained a secret for one hundred years and has allowed a huge commercial empire to develop and continue.

The high financial input involved in developing new technologies and products combined with the enormous potential value of viable innovations means that biotechnology companies are prime targets for trade secret theft.

Such trade secrets can only be protected if they are kept confidential, and a company needs to operate appropriate measures to retain confidential information within the company. Contracts of employment can include confidentiality clauses and may even restrict an employee from later working for a competitor. In many biotechnology companies, such as the whisky industry, this has long been common practice. Companies that rely on trade secrecy must focus on preventing the loss by implementing

Table 13.2	Benefits and disadvantages of the trade secret system	
Benefits	Disadvantages
1. Knowledge of the system is not public and so not available to competitors. **2.** No time limit on the available protection.	**1.** Someone else could have the same idea and exploit it. **2.** Some countries may not recognise the protection of confidential information. **3.** In-house procedures need to be elaborate, time consuming and tedious. **4.** Enforcement of confidentiality procedures can be problematic.

the greatest security measures that can be justified or afforded. The benefits and disadvantages of proceeding by the trade secrets route are shown in Table 13.2.

13.4 | Plant breeders' rights

Under various national and international agreements and acts plant varieties are protected by giving the plant breeders limited monopoly rights over the varieties they have created, by way of a registration system for plant varieties. Those who use the seeds or plants will, by right, pay a royalty to the breeder. However, there is an important provision that the farmers can retain a proportion of the seeds of a crop for re-planting. Purchasers can also use the variety to develop new varieties, which the purchaser will own the rights to – not the creator of the original variety. The advent of recombinant DNA technology that can permit the creation of large numbers of new varieties much more easily and quickly than traditional genetic methods will undoubtedly undermine the protection conferred by plant variety rights. Intensive legal discussions are now in progress in nations with high commitment to plant genetic engineering methodology (for a comprehensive explanation, see Byrne (1992)).

Chapter 14

Safety in biotechnology

14.1 | Introduction

In previous chapters the many applications of biotechnology can be divided into the traditional domains of fermentation for the production of various potable beverages, bread, cheese, organic acids, antibiotics and waste treatment, and the new biotechnologies. The new biotechnologies include production and use of genetically modified organisms for the large-scale production of vaccines and therapeutic proteins; their use in plant and animal agriculture and in environmental clean-up; the use of hybridomas for the production of monoclonal antibodies for diagnostic and therapeutic end-points; and, of course, the controversial embryonic stem cells. As such, biotechnology spans a vast range of activities, and considerations of biosafety can potentially encompass activities within the research laboratory, the process plant, the final product and in many cases the environment. The term 'biosafety' has evolved as a new area of corporate activity created as an inevitable response generated by an expanding biotechnology industry and its increasing influence upon many aspects of commercial and public life. In particular, the many public issues recently generated, especially in Europe, concerning genetically modified (GM) crop trials has done much to raise the profile of this subject.

In all biotechnology processes, however, safety is of paramount importance. Table 14.1 lists the main areas of consideration for safety aspects of biotechnology.

14.2 | Concepts of hazard and risk

Essential to the understanding of biosafety is the recognition and appreciation of the terms 'hazard' and 'risk'. In the context of health and safety, the hazard can be a substance, object or situation with a potential for an accident or damage, and the risk is the likelihood that this will occur (Table 14.2). Simply put, a hazard is something with the potential to cause harm, while risk defines the chance of an individual or the environment

Table 14.1 | Safety considerations in biotechnology

Pathogenicity: the potential ability of living organisms and viruses (natural and genetically engineered) to infect humans, animals and plants and to cause disease.

Toxicity and allergy associated with microbial production.

Other medically relevant effects, e.g. increasing the environmental pool of antibiotic-resistant microorganisms.

Problems associated with the disposal of spent microbial biomass and the purification of effluents from biotechnological processes.

Safety aspects associated with contamination, infection or mutation of process strains.

Safety aspects associated with the industrial use of microorganisms containing in vitro recombinant DNA.

Table 14.2 | Hazard and risk determination

Hazard	Risk
Qualitative	Quantitative, potentially
Concerned with identification of the hazard and causes	Concerned with consequences
Also called 'what-if?'	Also called risk analysis, risk assessment, quantitative risk assessment
Best identified by teams	Singly or small groups

being harmed by the hazard. Biosafety standards are now based on international technical state-of-the-art and relevant legislation, which aims to prevent risk to human health and the environment resulting from activities involving biological agents.

14.3 | Problems of organism pathogenicity

Many microorganisms can infect humans, animals and plants and cause disease. Successful establishment of disease results from interactions between the host and the causal organism. Many factors are involved, only a few of which are well understood.

Most microorganisms used by industry are harmless and many are indeed used directly for the production of human or animal foods. Many such examples have been discussed elsewhere in this book and include yeasts, filamentous fungi and many bacteria. Their safety is well documented from long associations lasting up to hundreds of years. Only a small number of potentially dangerous microorganisms have been used by industry in the manufacture of vaccines or diagnostic reagents, e.g. *Bordetella pertussis* (whooping cough), *Mycobacterium tuberculosis* (tuberculosis) and the virus of foot-and-mouth disease. Stringent containment practices have been the norm when these microorganisms are used.

Table 14.3	Risk assessment

Elucidate the capacity of the microorganism to have an adverse effect on humans, animals or the environment.

Establish the probability that microorganisms might escape, either accidentally or inadvertently, from the production process system.

Evaluate the safety of the desired products and the methods for handling by-products.

In recent years there have been many scientific advances permitting alterations to the genetic make-up of microorganisms. Recombinant DNA techniques have been the most successful, but have also been the cause of much concern to the public. However, this natural anxiety has been ameliorated by several compelling lines of evidence.

(1) Risk assessment studies have failed to demonstrate that host cells can acquire novel hazardous properties from DNA donor cells (Table 14.3).

(2) More rigorous evaluation of existing information concerning basic immunology, pathogenicity and infectious disease processes has led to relaxation of containment specifications previously set down.

(3) Considerable experimentation has shown no observable hazard.

However, care must always be adopted when using recombinant DNA molecules. There have been suggestions made of the need for international protocols for the testing and shipment of genetically modified organisms. Existing international mechanisms are already dealing effectively with such potential safety issues connected with genetic engineering. While there is a vast amount of evidence that the application of genetic engineering is safe and that the biotechnological developments with plants and animals are being applied responsibly and safely, there are still some bodies of opinion that seek draconian biosafety protocols based on conjectured potential consequences of genetic engineering. Never has a new technology been more thoroughly scientifically scrutinised than these new areas of biotechnology. Many of the opponents use inflammatory and totally unscientific reasoning in their attempts to derail this potentially valuable technology. Scientific research on safety aspects of this technology will continue to be an important issue.

A European Federation of Biotechnology Working Party on Biosafety has now been established to provide recommendations on safety aspects of biotechnology with respect to the environment, the public, personnel and product, to include:

- identifying and monitoring hazards associated with various applications in biotechnology
- assessing and quantifying risks
- providing an international platform for issues related to safety in biotechnology
- producing statements and recommendations (based on science and technology)

Table 14.4	Classification of microorganisms according to pathogenicity

Class 1
Microorganisms that have never been identified as causative agents of disease in humans and that offer no threat to the environment.

Class 2
Microorganisms that may cause human disease and that might therefore offer a hazard to laboratory workers. They are unlikely to spread in the environment. Prophylactics are available and treatment is effective.

Class 3
Microorganisms that offer a severe threat to the health of laboratory workers, but a comparatively small risk to the population at large. Prophylactics are available and treatment is effective.

Class 4
Microorganisms that cause severe illness in humans and offer a serious hazard to laboratory workers and to people at large. In general effective prophylactics are not available and no effective treatment is known.

Class 5
Microorganisms that offer a more severe threat to the environment, particularly to animals and plants, than to people. They may be responsible for heavy economic losses. National and international lists and regulations concerning these microorganisms are already in existence in contexts other than biotechnology (e.g. for phytosanitary purposes).

- identifying areas of insufficient knowledge and inadequate technology with respect to safety in biotechnology and to propose research and development in such areas
- assisting in the implementation of the recommendations and guidelines in biotechnology.

A classification of the degree of potential hazard of microorganisms has been drawn up by the European Federation of Biotechnology (Table 14.4).

14.4 | Problems of biologically active biotechnology products

Vaccines and antibiotics are obvious examples of biologically active products, and care must be taken to prevent their indiscriminate dispersal. Contaminants in otherwise safe processes may produce toxic molecules that could become incorporated into final products leading to food poisoning. Allergic reactions to product formulations must also be guarded against. Overuse of antibiotics in agriculture could lead to carry-over into human foods, resulting in possible development of antibiotic resistance in human disease organisms. Many countries now restrict the use of antibiotics in agriculture.

When properly practised, biotechnology is safe and the benefits deriving from biotechnological innovations will surely lead to major improvements in the health and well-being of the world's population. However, biotechnology must always be subjected to sound regulations for its successful application. The potential risks of biotechnology are manageable, and regulations have been constructed for that management.

14.5 | Biowarfare and bioterrorism

The use of biological weapons (i.e. disease causing microorganisms) in warfare has a long and disgraceful history, easily pre-dating gunpowder and nuclear warfare as instruments of mass destruction. In the mid fourteenth century the Black Death epidemic, most probably caused by bubonic plague, swept through Europe, the Near East and North Africa and was undoubtedly the most devastating health disaster in recorded history. At that time the Mongols, when attacking besieged cities, hurled plague-infected cadavers into such cities and the rapid and ensuing epidemic weakened and destroyed the population. A spectacular and destructive use of biological weapons. History abounds with similar acts.

Bioterrorism has been defined as the intentional or threatened use of viruses, bacteria, fungi or toxins from living organisms or agents to produce death or disease in humans, animals and plants (Center of Disease Control and Prevention, Atlanta, USA). Within the armoury of weapons of mass destruction, biological weapons are considered more destructive than chemical weapons, including nerve gases, since with a biological attack it is never known when the contaminants have been removed.

Potential biological agents have been assigned to three categories (Centre of Disease Control and Prevention, Atlanta, USA).

- *Category A*: agents include the most serious – smallpox, anthrax, plague, botulism, tularaemia and viral haemorrhagic fevers such as Ebola
- *Category B*: agents have a similar potential for large-scale dissemination but generally cause less serious illnesses – typhus, brucellosis and food poisoning agents such as *Salmonella* and *E. coli* 0157
- *Category C*: agents include novel infectious diseases, which could emerge in future threats.

The production of microorganisms and their products for a multitude of purposes is now a worldwide activity. The know-how, technology, equipment and materials are now routinely used for entirely legitimate, peaceful and creative purposes. Unfortunately, such methods can also be used for the production of biological weapons. Consequently, in biological warfare or bioterrorism specific microorganisms or derived toxins that can cause disease in humans, animals and plants can be used to achieve military and/or political objectives. Unlike nuclear and chemical weapons, biological weapons are relatively easy and cheap to produce and manufacture, and can also be used on a small scale. In this way small countries and terrorist organisations might easily acquire biological weapons.

In the relatively recent past many nations worldwide including Japan, Russia, Germany, the USA and the UK have devoted extensive research

Table 14.5	Biological agents associated with bioterrorism or biocrimes to humans	
Type	Traditional biological warfare agents	Agents of biocrimes and bioterrorism
Pathogens	Smallpox virus Viral encephalitides *Bacillus anthracis* *Brucella suis* *Yersina pestis*	*Bacillus anthracis* HIV *Rickettsia prowazekii* (typhus) *Salmonella* spp. *Vibrio cholerae* *Yersinia pestis* (plague)
Toxins	Botulin Ricin Staphylococcal Enteroxin B	Botulin Cholera endotoxin Diphtheria toxin Ricin Snake toxin

Source: adapted from the 2000 *NATO Handbook on the Medical Aspects of NBC Defense Operations*

facilities towards gaining a greater awareness of the potential use of such systems in warfare.

The Biological Weapons Convention (BWC) signed in 1972 was the first agreement among nations that declared an entire category of weapons to be off-limits and now has 154 state parties or treaty members. All those who have signed have agreed 'not to develop, produce, stockpile or acquire biological agents, toxins and weapons-delivery mechanisms of types and qualities that have no justification for prophylactic properties and other peaceful purposes'. If a nation should proceed to develop biological weapons it will be violating international law. The BWC has condemned biological weapons as an illegitimate and immoral way to wage war. However, it remains an extremely difficult task to police and verify a nation's adherence to the principles of the BWC. The recent international concerns of possible biological weapons in Iraq bear witness to this. It is clear that in recent wars throughout the world the adversaries have refrained from using biological weapons not for moral concerns but rather because they feared retaliation. Though nations may well abstain from the use of biological weapons this might not be the view of the bioterrorist who may function alone or in groups. The bioterrorist might not aim at causing deaths on a large scale but rather causing economic and political turmoil. This happened recently in Washington, USA when anthrax spores sent through the postal system to various establishments caused national alarm and the final cost of clean-up was estimated at US$500 000–1 billion.

Following on from the 9/11 bioterrorist acts in New York and elsewhere in the USA, their Government has set in motion extensive programmes to counteract bioterrorism. The US Food and Drug Administration (FDA) has been instructed to develop programmes for the development of vaccines, drugs and diagnostic products (all aspects of biotechnology) (Table 14.5) to safeguard the nation's food supply system (Table 14.6) and to respond to bioterrorism threats. There is an urgent need to develop rapid and

Table 14.6 | Selected biological pathogens that could be used in agroterrorism

Disease	Target/vector	Agent
Animal diseases		
Foot-and-mouth	Livestock	Foot-and-mouth disease virus
African swine fever	Pigs	African swine fever virus
Plant diseases		
Stem pest for cereals	Oats, barley, wheat	*Puccinia* spp. (fungus)
Southern corn leaf blight	Corn	*Bipolaris mayalis* (fungus)
Rice blast	Rice	*Pyricularia grisea* (fungus)
Potato blight	Potato	*Phytophthora infestans* (fungus)
Citrus canker	Citrus	*Xanthomonas axonopodis* (bacterium)
Zoonoses		
Brucellosis	Livestock	*Brucella melitensis* (bacterium)
Japanese encephalitis	Mosquitoes	Japanese encephalitis virus
Cutaneous anthrax	Livestock	*Bacillus anthracis* (bacterium)

Source: adapted from Gilmore (2004)

highly sensitive assays for the detection of dangerous microorganisms and toxins.

From an historical consideration vaccines have been the single most cost effective public health intervention that has shielded populations from so many deadly diseases, e.g. smallpox. While vaccination has been highly successful against so many microbially induced diseases there are still many diseases where success is limited or non-existent. Furthermore, the very high costs and difficulties involved in vaccinating large populations quickly make it practically impossible to use vaccinations to protect against bioterrorist attacks.

A new approach to biodefence is now emerging in the USA in that the emphasis is moving away from vaccination – the cornerstone of past defence strategies – towards developing broad-spectrum therapies and technology and gaining a better understanding of natural immunity. The recent outbreaks of new and deadly infective diseases and strains, such as severe acute respiratory syndrome (SARS) and avian flu, as well as the bioterrorist use of anthrax and ricin in the USA have made the authorities aware that it is impossible to predict what disease calamity could be used by the bioterrorist. Thus developing single-purpose vaccines could well be risky in that they might not be needed or could become obsolete before they come through production. However, identification of causal agents and the rapid initiation of an appropriate response will be imperative, and it is planned to achieve greater interaction of public services and agencies.

While much emphasis has been placed on potential bioterrorist attacks directly on human populations, agroterrorism – the use of biological agents against crops, livestock, poultry and fish – is now being given considerable attention (Table 14.6).

While there is no evidence for an agroterrorist attack on the food chain throughout the world, attention must be given to the consequences of natural disease outbreaks, which can aptly illustrate the potential damaging consequences when this happens. In the UK, the bovine spongiform encephalopathy (BSE) epidemic from 1996–2002 had devastating animal health and economic effects. Approximately 6 million head of cattle (30 months or older) were slaughtered with a cost of over £5 billion. The costs incurred in slaughtering birds in Asia suspected of contracting avian flu have so far been extensive.

The introduction of animal and plant pathogens is not difficult to envisage with widespread health, economic and political impacts. Disturbance in the food chain by agroterrorism attacks would create huge economic instability incurring massive financial losses due to dislocational trade and health effects.

In the USA, for instance, all large-scale agricultural commodities are involved in 'futures' with complex interactions with Europe, Asia and Latin America. Any serious disruption will incur massive losses and supply chaos worldwide.

What can be done to reduce the potential dangers of agroterrorism? In the long term there must be massive investment in creating pathogen resistant crops through genetic engineering, to identify genes associated with disease resistance. This will also require a greater acceptance of GM crops. How will the opponents of GM crops come to terms with this new requirement? The availability of large animal genomes could lead to the development of new animal varieties resistant to animal pathogens. Undoubtedly the use of genetic engineering to create disease resistance in plants and animals must be a major requirement of the twenty-first century.

In military terms a biological weapon (BW) is more than a pathogenic microorganism or toxin, and will be composed of four definite components: (a) the *payload* (the biological agents); (b) the *munition* (a container that ensures that the payload will be kept intact *and* virulent during delivery; (c) the *delivery system* (artillery shell, missile, aircraft, etc.); and finally (d) the *dispersal mechanism* (an explosive force or spray device to disperse the agent at the target population) (see Lederberg (1999) for fuller details).

While many nations had extensive programmes on the potential of biowarfare, NATO and the former USSR lost interest in BWs per se as weapons of mass destruction because of their inability to predict combat effectiveness and area containment. To date, their use as BWs has been confined to isolated episodes of bioterrorism or assassination.

Chapter 15

Public perception of biotechnology: genetic engineering – safety, social, moral and ethical considerations

15.1 | Introduction

The manner in which the public perceive any new technology, including biotechnology, will have important influences on the timing and direction of innovation, and in the rate of uptake or degree of discrimination against the technology, its products and services. Public perception will also be influenced by geographical location, which will reflect several variables, for example, economic affluence, level of education, cultural and religious values and tradition, together with social and institutional ways of participation.

In the industrialised world public policy-makers on biotechnology have been influenced by the concerted interests of governments, industries, academia and environmental groups. Nationally and internationally such policies are being developed within a climate of tension and conflicting aims.

At the early stages of recombinant DNA research, a small group of well recognised molecular biologists met in the early 1970s to express their concern over the safety of this new technology. In a well publicised meeting, the famous (or infamous) Asilomar Conference, in California, they focused on the potential, but highly speculative, risks associated with recombinant DNA (rDNA) technology and how they should be managed. Unfortunately, this generated huge public concern arising from the alarmist media coverage, e.g. Frankenstein foods, Andromeda strains, etc. Following on from this conference and the continued huge media hype, the National Institute of Health (NIH) in the USA published *Guidelines for Research Involving Recombinant DNA Molecules*, which sent out a powerful message to the scientific community and federal government departments that the NIH were seriously concerned about the speculative risk scenarios. Sadly, these guidelines were to become the standard text for most world regulations on rDNA. At a later date most of those scientists who expressed concern were to withdraw their support, but the damage was done!

In the 30 years since that meeting there has been a wealth of sound scientific peer-reviewed studies, which have refuted the risk concerns and stated that the fears propagated by the alarmist press are largely ground-less. This has been a salutary lesson on how new technologies should be thoroughly assessed before regulations are set in stone.

Over the past decade there have been numerous soundings of public opinion on biotechnology (Eurobarometers). The most recent Eurobarom-eter poll, *Europeans and Biotechnology in 2005*, confirmed that most Euro-peans supported medical application of biotechnology when there were clear benefits for human health and also industrial applications. How-ever, they were still expressing scepticism towards agricultural biotech-nology but would probably be more supportive if new crops and prod-ucts were more advantageous to consumers. Surprisingly, consumers were more supportive of the use of GM plants for the production of medicines and pharmaceutical products. Stem cell research was strongly supported. In general, there was a feeling of increased appreciation towards the contributions of biotechnology to improving society since 1999 (www.ec.europa.eu/research/press/2006/pv1906eu.cfm).

There are also many who view the organised debates and so-called public discussion groups on biotechnology, especially GM crops, with extreme scepticism. They have been seen as a unique experiment to find out what 'ordinary' people really think once they have heard all the arguments. Sadly, many such meetings were dominated by anti-technology zealots, the only faction that was well enough organised and cared enough about the issues to attend. Let us also hope that more 'science correspondents' in the popular media will have some scientific training.

Central to most of these debates is the single main issue – should regula-tion be dependent on the characteristics of the products modified by (rDNA) technology or on the use of the rDNA technology per se? The product versus process debate has continued for many years and exposes conflicting views on what should represent public policies on new technology development. What is public interest? Should this be left to the scientists and technolo-gists to decide, or should the 'public' become part of such decision-making processes? The many crucial decisions to be made will affect the future of humanity and the planet's natural resources. Such decisions should be based on the best scientific information in order to allow effective choices for policy options.

A dominant feature of public perception of biotechnology is the extraor-dinary low and naive public understanding of the genetic basis of life and evolution.

Does public concern really exist or is it largely the manifestation of a well orchestrated and genuine lobby of knowledgeable opponents? Does genetic engineering get a biased press coverage, i.e. 'Frankenstein foods'? Luddite activists who trample and destroy legitimate field experiments for controlled scientific research into the safety and potential of GM plants should be punished, not applauded, for their nonsensical and destructive behaviour.

It does appear that new biotechnology provokes a variety of views within the public that have not been apparent with many other new technolo-gies. Opinions are influenced by nationality, religion, ethics, morality and knowledge of the core sciences; risk assessment is seldom considered by opponents. Clearly, there is a plurality of views that must be accommodated if democratic decisions are to be made. The need for public education is paramount.

It is important to note that after hundreds of thousands of studies involving rDNA and the development of many medically useful products used in millions of patients a year, the safety of humans, animals and the environment has been maintained. This clearly demonstrates that high levels of safety and control are being practised by the exponents of new biotechnology.

A comprehensive regulatory framework is now in place within the EU and most Western nations, with the aim of protecting human health and the environment from adverse activities involving genetically modified organisms (GMOs).

Some of the main public issues concerning rDNA technology will be examined in some detail.

15.2 | Release of genetically manipulated organisms into the environment

In the 1970s, when genetic engineering experiments with microorganisms were first being developed, many molecular biologists believed that the process was unsafe and that manipulated microorganisms should be strictly contained and prevented from release to the environment. The fundamental fear was, and with many still is, that genetically engineered microorganisms could escape from the laboratory into the environment with unpredictable and perhaps catastrophic consequences. It was believed that such released microorganisms could 'upset the balance of nature' or that 'foreign DNA' in the new microorganism could alter its metabolic activity in unpredictable and undesirable ways.

In response to these concerns, guidelines were established to ensure safe working practices and levels of containment based on potential hazards. However, with time and increased technical awareness, many of these regulations have been progressively relaxed with recognised low-risk systems. Many important medical products, such as insulin and human growth hormone, and some industrial enzymes are manufactured in large-scale containment fermentation processes, involving specific genetically manipulated microorganisms. The final products from these processes are free of the genetically manipulated host organism and, therefore, do not constitute a release problem. Such systems work well and, to date, there have been no health or environmental problems resulting from their operation. Rennet (chymosin) for cheese manufacture has been produced from genetically manipulated microorganisms. An honest, open marketing strategy has shown no adverse public opposition to the final cheese product.

In the previous examples, the manipulated organism was not subject to release and remained within the manufacturing site to be correctly disposed of. However, recombinant microorganisms are now being considered for deliberate release into the environment where they cannot be contained, e.g. biological control, inoculants in agriculture, live vaccines, bioremediation, etc. In addition, we are now witnessing the moving out in increasing numbers of recombinant plants from research laboratories, containment greenhouses and test-plots, to the fields and greenhouses of the farmer and large commercial agricultural and horticultural growers.

What are the dangers associated with environmental release of recombinant organisms – are they real or mostly imagined? Science fiction writing abounds with stories of deadly microorganisms or plants (e.g. *The Andromeda Strain* and *The Day of the Triffids*) arriving from outer space, enveloping and destroying the human population or the biosphere. Those who oppose the use of recombinant techniques have grasped onto this fiction, and have passionately striven to draw comparisons with the release of genetically manipulated organisms.

Increased pathogenicity of microorganisms, or microbial ability to destroy essential raw materials, are often cited as potential problems of genetically manipulated microorganisms. Pathogenicity is in itself a complex multifactorial process and it is most unlikely that it will be introduced into a previously safe microorganism by a simple gene insertion. Organisms with any possibility of unusual pathogenicity will never be permitted to be used. Where microorganisms are released to be used for biocontrol of, for example, insects, care must be taken that they will not influence other life forms. The use of a recombinant rabies vaccine in baits in Belgium has significantly reduced the level of rabies in wild animals. The public were informed and in general approved of this worthwhile use of the technology.

All releases into the environment are being carefully monitored and recorded. A major aspect will be to understand how recombinant microorganisms survive and multiply in the environment. Will the recombinant microorganism remain stable or revert back to the original form, and will there be exchange of the recombinant genetic material with other microorganisms? Soil microorganisms are very promiscuous, but there is little firm evidence on how much genetic exchange takes place. Much ecological monitoring of microorganisms is now taking place and new methods are being developed. Ecological microbial communities are dynamic systems neither closed to invasion nor robust in the face of all perturbations. How newly released organisms react to and interact with such complex microbial communities will be a major challenge to the microbial ecologist. At present all new releases of genetically modified microorganisms are considered by expert committees in a case-by-case evaluation. As the information base builds up it becomes more easy to judge new applications. It must be noted that there have been no adverse effects recorded from the examples so far of genetically modified microorganisms released into the environment.

Recombinant DNA technology is now being extensively used to improve specific characteristics of plants used for commercial food production. Most of these crops consequently must be grown on a large scale in the open environment to achieve commercial success. A foreseen impediment on the development of manipulated plants for commercial purposes will be the public attitude to such foodstuffs. What are the main concerns that must be addressed to ensure the correct development of this technology to plant agriculture?

The development of transgenic crop varieties is routinely conducted over two to five years of field trials to evaluate the performance of the new plants under field conditions. The tasks are normally conducted under strict conditions that prevent the movement of plants and pollen from the test sites. In the USA, since 1987, there have been thousands of field trials with transgenic plants and much valuable information acquired. In general, it would appear that transgenic plants do not look or behave wildly differently from ordinary crop plants. However, there has been some concern expressed that the contained conditions of the field trials do not adequately mirror the real field situations and some potential environmental hazards could be missed, which will only show up after release.

Could transgenic crops move out of the field of cultivation and become weeds? When all commercial crop plants are considered there are vanishingly few examples where this has happened, since such crops require special cultivation practices and are unable to compete with the indigenous wild plant populations. The possibility of gene transfer to compatible wild relatives has been given serious examination. Is it possible that herbicide and pest resistance incorporated into transgenic plants could find its way into other species and increase their 'weediness'? Under normal conditions gene transfer between close relatives is a very rare and unusual phenomenon, and there is little evidence that this will change with transgenic organisms. While such events are theoretically possible, their occurrence would be at such a low frequency that in practice the results are of virtually no consequence or concern. However, released transgenic plants will continue to be monitored to validate these conclusions. Some recombinant genes for pest resistance produce in the plant a product toxic to the pest. The possible toxicity of this to humans must always be considered and will be regularly assessed by standard techniques for testing the safety of foods.

15.3 | Genetic modification and food uses

Modern biotechnology has its ancestral roots in the early fermentations of foods and beverages, which span almost all societies. Since these early times, humans have progressively applied selection procedures to encourage beneficial improvements in the individual microorganisms, plants or animals used for food production. While early methods were mainly empirical, the expanding knowledge of genetics allowed a new approach to selective breeding between like species. These, now conventional genetic techniques, have become accepted worldwide and have not caused any public concern. Genetic engineering is increasingly being applied to many breeding programmes to achieve the same aims as the traditional methods, but offering two main advantages:

(1) the introduction of genes can be controlled with greater prediction and precision than by previous methods
(2) the introduction of genes into unrelated species, which is not possible to achieve by traditional methods.

The application of genetic engineering to food production is intended to enhance the useful and desirable characteristics of the organisms and to eliminate the undesirable. The overall aim of the food industry, with respect to genetic engineering, will be to improve the quantity and to increase the quality and properties of existing food production, to produce new products and, of course, to improve financial returns. The consumer has always shown a willingness to pay more for better and more convenient products and to reject products that do not achieve their expectations. New biotechnology now offers a major opportunity to tailor food products to public and individual demand.

Previous chapters have highlighted the many *benefits* that genetic engineering might give the producer including: disease and pest resistance, weed control, animal growth hormones, improved food microorganisms, novel products, improved keeping quality, 'tailored' products with improved qualities, etc. In contrast, some would consider that there are many potential *risks* associated with these new approaches including: unintentional transfer of genes into other crops, creation of herbicide resistant weeds, infringement of plant breeders' rights, increased monoculture and the undermining of traditional economies. Some believe that it is a technology out of control.

However, a strong prima facie case is increasingly being achieved by the further use of genetic engineering in the manipulation of food organisms for the purpose of improved food production. While the scientific case is strong and persuasive, public perception is somewhat ambivalent. While the public have readily accepted medical products produced from GMOs they are much less willing to accept such procedures with food. Genetic engineering is seen as 'unnatural' and unnecessary in food production. While scientific opinion is well respected in medical matters by the public, it is often perceived in matters of food as purely commercially driven (Table 15.1). People will influence decision-making by governments through the ballot box and through the presence of public opinion. Public confidence must be achieved for the success of any new technology.

Particularly in the EU, there are many forums ideologically opposed to transgenic crops and by various means they have been able to exploit the popular media, frighten the public, and exaggerate myths and conspiracy theories about genetic engineering. They have also made extensive use of the unregulated internet! Their Luddite convictions have regrettably influenced certain government attitudes to GM food, curtailing plant molecular biology and forcing young plant scientists to move to more enlightened countries, e.g. the USA. In a similar manner, animal rights activists with tactics of violence against individuals and research sites may well force certain pharmaceutical research centres to abandon the EU.

Also, when European governments show antipathy to agricultural biotechnology this view is adopted by government officials in many developing countries to the detriment of their own countries, which desperately need so many aspects of agricultural biotechnology (Table 15.2). Should Europeans' 'fear' of GM crops dictate the choice of action in Africa?

However, committed scientists must also have a responsibility to participate, where possible, in public dialogue about the implications of their

Table 15.1 | Public attitudes (in % responses) to applications of genetic manipulation in Europe

	Comfortable	Neutral	Uncomfortable
Microbial production of bioplastics	91	6	3
Cell fusion to improve crops	81	10	10
Curing diseases such as cancer	71	17	9.5
Extension of shelf life of tomatoes	71	11	19
Cleaning-up oil slicks	65	20	13
Detoxifying industrial waste	65	20	13
Anti-blood-clotting enzymes produced by rats	65	14	22
Medical research	59	23	15
Making medicines	57	26	13
Making crops to grow in the Third World	54	15	19
Mastitis-resistant cows by genetic modification of cows	52	16	31
Producing disease-resistant crops	46	29	23
Chymosin production by microorganisms	43	30	27
Improving crop yields	39	31	29
Using viruses to attack crop pests	32	26	49
Improving milk yields	22	30	47
Cloning prize cattle	7.2	18	72
Changing human physical appearance	4.5	9.5	84
Producing hybrid animals	4.5	12	82
Biological warfare	1.9	2.7	95

Table 15.2 | GM crops agreed by farmers, consumers and agriculturists in African Countries

Insect-resistant African maize varieties
Crops resistant to African viruses
Biofortified African crops
Drought tolerant crops
Maize resistant to parasitic weed *Strige*

Source: adapted from Thomson (2007)

science and how it will impact on society; so often such meetings are dominated by the anti lobby. In the longer term, let us hope that the public will receive more scientific awareness through education and also that science graduates should study the social implications of their respective sciences.

The safety of the human food supply is based on the concept that there should be a reasonable certainty that no harm will result from its consumption. Foods or food ingredients derived from GMOs must be considered to be as safe as, or safer than, their traditional counterparts before they can be recommended as safe. The most practical approach to the determination of safety is to consider whether the new foods are *substantially equivalent* to analogous conventional food products where they exist, and that their intended use and exposure are relatively similar. Where substantial equivalence is established, no additional safety concerns will normally be expected. Where substantial equivalence is more difficult to establish, then the identified differences or the new characteristics should be subjected to further safety considerations.

In many countries there are now specialist government-supported committees to check on the safety of GMOs in food production, which examine the technical details for their use or their products destined for the public. In the UK, this is the Advisory Committee on Novel Foods and Processes with a wide complement of independent, unpaid experts whose opinions and decisions are passed to the government food minister, who *then* makes the final official judgement and announcement. The committee is only influenced by the scientific facts and the ultimate safety of the product. Such committees now have, in addition to relevant scientific expertise, strong consumer guidance and expertise on ethics.

While the original concerns about genetically engineered foods were perceived mainly on safety issues, in recent years social, moral and ethical issues have come more to the forefront in decision-making processes (see Straughan and Reiss, 1996, for an expansive discussion).

There is obvious concern that the control of genetically engineered crop plants and their seeds by multinational agrochemical companies, and their need to recoup the high research and investment costs incurred in their development, will imply that only high-technology farmers will be able to carry the cost burden. This will not be true of the farmer in the Third World. Also, herbicide resistant crops may lead to dependence by farmers on such specific herbicides and hence their producing companies.

The concept of *substitutability* will also have dramatic effects on some developing countries. Thus, the development of novel sweeteners is already reducing the traditional sugar market for sugar cane and sugar beet, disrupting these economies. In this area developing countries will most certainly suffer more than the industrialised nations. Increased milk production from fewer cows by the injection of genetically engineered hormones will result in many small farmers in the USA and EEC being put out of business.

Thus, for many aspects of new biotechnology, there will be a social price to pay, and particularly in the developing countries the number of jobs in agriculture will decrease. Different value judgements must be made to reconcile the advantages to society against the disadvantages. The judgements will vary depending on which side of the poverty line you reside. However, it is encouraging to note that many developing nations are endeavouring to make substantial investments and progress in relevant biotechnology. Technical and financial aid *must* continue to flow to them from the advanced agricultural nations to ensure that they too can have the obvious benefits of this technology.

Transgenesis is seen by some as a fundamental breach in natural breeding barriers that nature set up through the process of evolution to prevent genetic interplay between unlike species. In this way the species is seen as 'sacred'. However, in the reductionist viewpoint of many molecular biologists the gene has become the ultimate unit of life − and that the gene is merely a unique aggregation of organic molecules (common to all types of cells) available for manipulation. Consequently, they see no ethical problem in transferring genes between species and genera.

It is undoubtedly in the genetic engineering of animals that the 'unnaturalness' of this technology is creating much public unease – for instance, the transfer of a 'human' gene into an animal, which reflects the fact that the new transgenic organism contains copies of the gene originally obtained from this source. While the transgene has human origin *and* structure, it is not its immediate source. Genes cannot be directly transported from one organism to another but must go through a complicated series of in vitro clonings. This is a series of amplification steps in which the original gene is copied many times during the overall process so that the original genetic material is diluted by about 10^{55}. The chance of the original human gene being in the final organism is infinitesimal or 'the chances of recovering the original human gene from the transgenic embryo are much less than the chances of recovering a specific drop of water released into the oceans of the world'. Since the transgenic organism does not contain the actual human gene but rather an artificially created copy of the gene, some would consider that the status of the transgene should be considered that of the new organism. Genes fulfil their biological role only by their activity within the cell of an organism.

An early UK report (by the Committee on the Ethics of Genetic Modification and Food Use, 1993) identified some of the main ethical concerns relating to the food use of certain transgenic organisms:

(1) transfer of human genes to food animals (e.g. transfer of the human gene for Factor IX, a protein involved in blood clotting, into sheep)
(2) transfer of genes from animals whose flesh is forbidden for use as food by certain religious groups to animals that they normally eat (e.g. pig genes into sheep) would offend Jews and Muslims
(3) transfer of animal genes into food plants, which may be of particular concern to some vegetarians (especially vegans)
(4) use of organisms containing human genes as animal feed (e.g. yeast modified to produce human proteins of pharmaceutical value and the spent yeast then used as animal feed).

Following consultations covering a wide range of religious beliefs, it was concluded that there were no overriding ethical objections to insist on an absolute prohibition of the use of food products containing copy genes of human origin. However, the report strongly recommended that the use of all ethically sensitive genes in food organisms should be discouraged when alternatives could be found. Products from transgenic organisms containing copy genes that are ethically unacceptable to some groups of the population subject to dietary restriction for their religion should be so labelled to ensure choice. The whole aspect of labelling GMO-derived foods is subject to much debate and may eventually be different in different parts of the world. In the not too distant future it is highly possible that all major food organisms will have had some form of genetic engineering in their development and this could lead to complex labelling criteria.

Current discussions between government bodies, industry and consumer organisations will decide the ultimate or realistic extent of labelling required to meet ethical requirements.

Genetic engineering of animals may also arouse severe moral opposition if there are instances of animals suffering as a result of this process. Already there is evidence of animals suffering severe arthritis following application of transgenic growth hormones to improve their meat quality.

While some religious groups exercise strong discrimination of the type of animal that can be eaten, the position can be quite different when considered from a medically derived product (insulin from a pig pancreas) or the transplant of an animal organ. Almost all faiths take the view that preservation of human life is the first priority. Thus pig-derived insulin can be accepted by a Jew and by a Muslim only with special religious permission. Similarly, a Jew could accept a pig organ transplant if absolutely essential. These contrary positions are supported by the view that the human body can only be violated by oral intake, and not by other methods of introduction such as by injection or surgery. A fuller appreciation of ethics and morality of animal biotechnology can be found in Straughan (1999).

A recent US Institute of Food Technologists Expert Panel concluded that continued development and use of food rDNA biotechnology could provide a number of important benefits to society:

- a more abundant and economical food supply for the world
- continued improvements in nutritional quality, including foods of unique composition for populations whose diets lack essential nutrients
- fresh fruit and vegetables with improved shelf life
- the development of functional foods, vaccines and similar products that may provide health and medical benefits
- further improvements in production agriculture through more efficient production practices and increased yields
- the conversion of non-productive toxic soils in developing countries to productive arable land
- more environmentally friendly agricultural practices through improved pesticides and pesticide usage practices; less hazardous animal wastes; improved utilisation of land; and reduced need to develop ecologically sensitive areas such as rain forests.

Furthermore, with respect to a range of environmental and economic concerns about rDNA biotechnology-derived food products, the panel also reached the following conclusions.

- New rDNA biotechnology-derived foods and food products do not inherently present any more serious environmental concerns or unintended toxic properties than those already presented by conventional breeding practices.
- Appropriate testing by technology developers, producers and processors, regulatory agencies and others should be continued for new foods and food products derived from all technologies, including rDNA biotechnology.

Table 15.3	Areas of public concern on human genome research

Confidentiality of testing and screening results
Scope of genetic testing and screening
Discrimination and stigmatisation
Commercial exploitation of human genome data
Eugenic pressures
Effects of germ line gene therapies on later generations

Source: from European Federation of Biotechnology (1995)

- Programmes should be developed to provide the benefits of safe and economical rDNA biotechnology-derived food products worldwide, including in less-developed countries.

15.4 | The applications of human genetic research

Several thousand genetic disorders of humans would appear to result from a mutation in a single gene, while many others have more complex genetic explanations and even possible interactions with environmental factors. Results from the Human Genome Project, discussed earlier, are now considered to offer an increased understanding of these fundamental genetic malfunctions and to give, in some cases, hope for alleviation and perhaps cure of the defect. However, paralleling the scientific breakthroughs and deeper understandings of gene mechanisms have come many areas of public concern (Table 15.3).

The major nations now committed to genome projects are also supporting research into the many ethical, legal and social issues that these studies are uncovering. Numerous committees now foster public debate and understanding of these highly complex issues. On the one hand the scientific discoveries could possibly bring much relief to millions of sufferers of genetic diseases, but on the other they give rise to questions of mind-bending implications to the way forward for the human race.

Genetic testing and screening

Where genetic disorders have previously been observed in families it is now possible in some cases to carry out prenatal testing to discover if the foetus carries the defect. The parents may then be able to sanction an abortion or be better prepared for the needs of the full-term baby. There are obvious concerns that this could result in a wide range of other conditions being selected for termination, e.g. gender and diseases of a minor nature. Soon it may be possible to have a much fuller awareness of an individual's 'genetic portfolio' and to possibly diagnose future medical problems, e.g. heart disease, cancer, etc., and advise treatment well in advance of the onset of the disease. However, would an individual wish to know that they would develop Huntington disease (presently an untreatable, debilitating and often fatal disease) in 30–40 years time? It has been suggested that genetic testing and screening should only occur with disorders where treatment is available.

The collection and long-term storage of biological material (blood samples, DNA, etc.) raises special ethical and policy issues about access and possible uses of the samples, which reflect around informed consent. Consensus opinion is that individuals should be made aware of policies for sample ownership, possible IP rights and the protection of privacy and confidentiality of genetic information.

Perhaps the most worrying aspect of such genetic testing is the use such information could be put to by insurance and mortgage institutions. While undoubtedly such financial systems would reduce the risk aspect of their investments, the effects on the individual would be devastating. It is increasingly viewed by ethics committees that insurance companies should not require or be allowed access to an individual's genetic information as a prerequisite for insurance. This may well prove to be an impossible task to monitor and control. It is becoming increasingly apparent that the course of an individual's future is not 'in the stars' but in reality in their own genes!

Human gene therapy

Gene therapy can be considered from either a somatic or germ-line approach. From an ethical viewpoint somatic gene therapy involving the insertion of single genes into a patient is really no different from the long accepted practice of transplants, e.g. hearts, lungs, etc., from other individuals. It is considered that such treatments should be used only to alleviate serious medical disorders and not for non-therapeutic applications. The application of gene therapy could be important to the pharmaceutical industry, but it is not yet clear whether it could be sold as an injectable 'product' or be dispensed as a service. Part of the confusion comes from the vast diversity of potential disease applications, ranging from immunotherapeutics to genetic diseases. In either case it will not be a cheap therapy. Somatic gene therapy must remain under close supervision to satisfy medical safety, legal implications and public concerns.

Germ-line gene therapy is presently not being pursued because it is technically extremely difficult and is ethically and socially unacceptable. Interfering with germ cells raises huge problems of eugenics, and there must be extensive public debate if it is ever to be used as a meaningful medical technique. The mood in society would appear to be supportive towards gene therapy at the present limited and mostly experimental level, with the proviso that safeguards are kept and are effective. Unscrupulous 'pioneer' surgeons should be carefully monitored.

Stem cell technology, while offering huge potential for therapeutic remedies for some of the world's worst debilitating diseases, has also generated major religious and moral concerns. While adult stem cells derived from various human tissues are relatively free from controversy this is not the case for hES cells derived from human blastocysts.

At one side of the argument it can be considered that the moral status of the hES cells is no different from that of other cells from the human body, and it could be deemed unethical to hold back research with such cells that could offer potential relief to millions of sufferers. In stark contrast, the religious view is that from the moment of conception the embryo cell should receive full moral standing as a person and, thus, it would be unethical to sacrifice the life of an individual for the benefit of others! Is it possible that science can avoid the moral dilemmas raised by this controversial line of research?

It is misleading to label hES cell study as immoral and to avoid the ever-increasing tangled ethical division and loss of valuable research progress; scientists and religious philosophers must enlighten the public on the true nature of this technology.

The debate revolves around the embryo or quasi-embryo. When does human life begin? Human development categorically requires implantation of the embryonic cell into the wall of the uterus, otherwise the embryo cannot develop into a new individual. Laboratory development of the embryo to a body is *not* possible.

Reference should be made to the papers listed in the 'Further reading' for a critical examination of this most contentious area of modern biotechnology.

Some general conclusions are now appearing from the increased level of discussion of these issues. The public does not accept or reject gene technology as a whole. Parts of it will be welcomed and utilised while others will have less or no support at all. The biotechnology community must aim to inform, not indoctrinate, the public. The consumers and patients of biotechnology products must be given clear and unequivocable information: a recent EEC Public Perception of Biotechnology meeting ended with the following message to biotechnology companies: 'Provide the information and listen to the public'.

When taking into consideration the scientific complexity of most new biotechnology products and processes, companies must use public relations effectively to provide consumers with adequate information about the advantages and benefits of their products. In this way the public will be able to make informed decisions about them. Similarly, scientists must learn to communicate with the public, be willing to do so and consider it a duty to do so! The most significant obstacles to the full creative resolution of new biotechnology are not expected to be scientific, economic or indeed environmental, but rather cultural!

Chapter 16

Looking to the future

Biotechnology is increasingly being viewed as a Promethean science, because in so many ways it is transforming the relationship between humans and the planet.

Biotechnology has been shown to be a spectrum of enabling technologies, which are increasingly being applied in many aspects of modern society. The applied use of biological systems, especially microorganisms, in such processes as brewing, wine making and cheese production was primarily accomplished in an empirical manner with the management of these processes seen more as an art rather than a science. In recent times, these ancient biotechnological processes have been subjected to rigorous scientific study and analysis, which has largely led to the replacement of traditional empiricism. Better understanding of microbial strain selection, molecular biology and genetics, together with improved bioprocess technology, have yielded major advances in all of the traditional biotechnology industries and will continue to achieve improved quality and safety together with cost effectiveness.

A central feature of new biotechnological advances derives from an increasing understanding of the mechanisms of life and how these will eventually transform human lives, as well as giving a deeper appreciation of agriculture, aquaculture, forestry and the biological environment. The ability to select and manipulate genetic material within and outside species has permitted unprecedented opportunities to alter life forms for the benefit of society. The successful sequencing of the human and other genomes is the beginning of a new scientific period of discovery. However, rather than genomic sequences being an end in themselves, they are at the beginning of scientific study to put the information into context with regard to the biological significance to the organism. Currently, sequence data have been utilised to identify species, to derive evolutionary linkages and to study the basis of organism diversity.

Many molecular biologists have postulated that a genetic or DNA sequence analysis of an individual could be predictive of future disease occurrence, e.g. cardiovascular, cancer, Alzheimer's, etc. This has generated much interest, especially with insurance companies. However, to rely on sequence analysis alone would be insufficient, as this would not take into consideration all the multivarious adaptive systems of the living organism as well as the environmental input threshold on an individual's lifespan. However, new microarray technology, where thousands of single nucleotide polymorphisms can be analysed, together with advances in proteomics may well give a meaningful patient read-out on potential susceptibility and early diagnosis of an impending problem allowing much earlier medical or lifestyle intervention. Recombinant DNA technology of mammalian cell cultures has produced many recombinant proteins, e.g. insulin and recombinant vaccines, that are now bringing considerable medical benefit to a wide range of human diseases. Undoubtedly, there will be continued research and application in this area.

The present applications of genetic engineering technology to the life sciences, through apparently revolutionary techniques, are indeed nothing to what will evolve in the future. The further implementation of genomics and proteomics will allow a much deeper understanding of the biology of molecules, cells and whole organisms. Doctors and patients will have much to gain from the outcome of these studies. Much will be learned about human individuality and how these findings could influence individual health and disease susceptibility.

Molecular genetic testing is increasingly being incorporated into clinical medicine, and this trend is likely to accelerate in the near future. However, there could well be problems with patent holders that claim ownership of correlations between human genetic variants and predisposition to disease, response to therapeutic drugs and susceptibility to pharmacological side-effects.

Plant-based genetic engineering did not really start until the early 1980s with the development of the Ti plasmid of *Agrobacterium tumifaciens*, which has allowed the introduction of simple genetic constructs into most of the important crop plants. These processes are now relatively routine and the changes made within the plants have been so slight that it requires highly sophisticated biochemical assays to distinguish GM varieties from their predecessors. Notwithstanding the large and growing body of evidence that the application of plant genetic engineering is safe and that development has always been applied responsibly and safely, there has been a small but highly organised and vociferous opposition to the application of the technology.

The application of any new technology is often fraught with public misconception and mistrust of scientific opinion. No technology can ever be free of risk and in our present affluent developed world perfection is now the expectation. Irrresponsible media 'experts' (often with no scientific experience) lead the public to expect zero impact and risk from the new technological innovations of plant genetic engineering, and if any slight deficiency, real or imagined, is detected they will propose the complete condemnation of the practice. The demands for moratoria or outright banning of GM food products, particularly in Europe, have their origins in inflammatory and unscientific phrases such as 'biological pollution' and 'Frankenstein food' and erroneous comparisons made with BSE, foot-and-mouth disease and nuclear power plants. The scientific community involved in GM food studies has shown a level of caution that has been lacking in most other new technologies. The basic work is routine and well established. There are few if any real risks associated with genetic engineering of crop plants that could in any way compete with the hazards that society presently accepts in order to uphold current ways of life, e.g. transport, smoking, alcohol and many others.

In 2001, the estimated global commitment to GM crops was 53 million hectares being grown by 5.5 million farmers (since that date there has been at least a doubling of planted acreage). The USA grew 68% of the total followed by Argentina (22%), Canada (6%) and China (3%). Many other countries including Bulgaria, Uruguay, Indonesia, Brazil and Mexico are now in early stages of growing transgenic crops. There is increasing evidence that GM crops are giving significant yield increases, savings for growers and pesticide use reductions in both developed and developing countries. Yet another important feature of certain GM plants is that they use less water, and undoubtedly in many parts of the world water availability will be the determining factor for successful food production by both animals and plants. Desertification has already overtaken millions of hectares of low altitude areas depriving communities of essential food production. Lack of water could result in mass population migrations and even hostilities. There is no doubt that this will happen. Unfortunately, Europe will continue to suffer bureaucratic/political constraints on the legislation of GM crops. There is clearly no scientific basis or thinking that can justify this Luddite approach.

At present single gene transfers are the basis of current plant genetic engineering. However, current studies on plant genomes are now identifying sets of genes that influence plant architecture such as root thickness and area, leaf size and shape, which will be of great value to plant breeders to increase yields without increasing acreage. At the present time many of the applications of plant GM technology have benefited the farmer rather than the consumer. However, in the near future this trend will change with more emphasis being given to human and animal nutrition.

Our present knowledge of human nutrition is now well defined at a population level, and food processors can now compensate for most nutrient imbalances in staple foods by adding supplements such as essential amino acids and vitamins. In the future the plant breeder and the farmer may well be able to manipulate crop plants to much more exact nutritional requirements. Rice is deficient in vitamin A, resulting in blindness in children in many developing communities where it is a dietary staple. The development of GM rice strains with raised levels of vitamin A and iron has now been achieved and will be of immense nutritional value, especially to populations in developing countries. All patent rights on this production in the developing world have been waived by the scientists and companies involved. Future GM plant technology will facilitate in-plant formulation of nutrients for human consumption.

Since plant crops such as cereals are the basis of most farmed animal diets it can be anticipated that most crops will be engineered to suit the exact nutritional requirements of individual animal species, e.g. cattle, pigs and poultry.

The new aspects of biotechnology such as transgenic plants and animals, recombinant proteins and vaccines will bring huge benefits to humankind but not without generating concern in some sections of the population. Biotechnologists, in general, stand accused of not communicating with the lay public, largely because the scientists have mostly been unable or unwilling to take the time to explain in simple understandable language the basic principles of the science involved. They must be more circumspect in the claims made for the future outcome of their studies. There are still vast areas of biological knowledge that must be deciphered before most speculative projects can be achieved. Also the time-scale for accomplishment must be more realistic.

The future role of stem cell technology with respect to therapeutic replacement therapy is a subject of much public interest. This whole subject is now being researched extensively throughout the world, and it is hoped that answers will be found to overcome not only the moral and ethical issues that have been expressed but also the many technical problems that must be solved before such cells can meaningfully be incorporated into human systems.

The ethical and moral issues raised by some aspects of new biotechnology must be addressed by continued open discussion and informed communication. Scare stories generate more public interest than honest reassuring facts. Furthermore, and a direct criticism of the present educational system, most of the population are ignorant of even simple biological facts and naturally find the complexity of genetic engineering bewildering and threatening.

In practice, the majority of products to be derived from biotechnology will be recognisable extensions of existing ones, or stem from improvements in production. Minor improvements in processes by many of these new technologies may not be highly newsworthy, but will help to give producer companies a competitive edge. The history of biotechnology shows how intimate must be the interplay between industry and academia to maintain the creative effort to generate new products and to expand its scope, profitability and social benefits.

Although there is now a vast reservoir of relevant biological and engineering knowledge and expertise waiting to be put into productive biotechnological use, the eventual rate of application will be determined not primarily by science and technology, but rather by many other equally important factors such as industrial investment policies, the establishment of market needs, economics of the marketing skills needed to introduce new products into commercial use and above all how the public perceive this new range of innovative technologies.

Climate change is now a worldwide recognised concern. A number of approaches are now being considered to counter the effects of global warming. From a biotechnological consideration biofuel development has gained international recognition and a wide range of options are being progressed to ascertain which biofuels can become cost-effective alternatives to fossil fuels. Choice and availability of substrates for biofuel generation will continue to be debated. Cultivations for biofuels should not replace food products. Is there enough agricultural land to allow for significant biofuel development without impacting food productivity adversely? In 2007, the amount of US farmland devoted to biofuel generation grew by nearly half, with only a negligible net increase in acreage under plough! There can be no doubt that within the next decade biotechnology will be the dominant global paradigm in world agriculture.

The potential of aspects of biotechnology to be used in biowarfare have been well highlighted. However, other aspects of biotechnology, for example, vaccine and drug developments, could well counteract many such acts of terrorism. What will be the role of the biotechnology industry in the war against bioterrorism? In the USA there have been huge research and commercial programmes planned but, as yet, unfulfilled. 'Bioshield, a biodefense procurement programme is synonymous with bureaucratic backtracking, political opportunism, poor accountability, cronyism and fiscal mismanagement' (editor, *Nature Biotechnology* 2007, 23, 603). It's not surprising that many biotechnology companies are not rushing to get involved. Sadly, six years since 9/11 there is yet to be a coherent plan!

Biotechnology will play a major role in the continued search for solutions to the many problems that will affect the society of tomorrow: health, food supply and a safe biological environment. Continued scientific research will be paramount to achieving these ends. However, as Louis Pasteur commented on the inexorable nature of scientific studies: 'As the circle of light increases, so too does the circumference of darkness'.

Glossary

Activated sludge process Aerobic sewage treatment process using aerobic microorganisms present in sewage sludge to break down organic matter in sewage.

Aerated pile Microbial composition of organic waste matter where the wastes are heaped in piles and forced aeration supplies oxygen.

Aerobic Living or acting only in the presence of oxygen.

Amino acids The building blocks of proteins.

Anaerobe Microorganisms that can grow and multiply in the absence of oxygen.

Anaerobic digestion A microbial fermentation of organic matter to methane and carbon dioxide, which occurs in near absence of air; a sewage treatment process.

Antibiotic A specific type of chemical substance that is used to fight microbial infections usually in humans or animals. Most antibiotics are produced by microorganisms. Semi-synthetic antibiotics are natural antibiotics modified chemically.

Antibody A protein produced by the immune system on exposure to a specific antigen, characterised by specific reactivity with its complementary antigen.

Antigen A molecule introduced into an organism and recognised as a foreign material, resulting in the elicitation of antibody production (immune response) directed specifically against the foreign molecule.

Antisense genes Genes in which the mirror image of the normal nucleotide base sequences are inserted, preventing expression of the natural genes.

Ascites Liquid accumulation in the peritoneal cavity, widely used as a method for propagating hybridoma cells for monoclonal antibody formation.

Bacteriophage A virus that multiples in bacteria.

Biodiesel A biofuel intended as a substitute for diesel.

Bioethanol Ethanol formed by microbiological activity.

Bioethics The ethics of medical and biological research.

Biofuel Fuel derived directly from living systems.

Biohazard A risk to human health or the environment arising from biological research.

Biological oxygen demand (BOD) The oxygen used in meeting the metabolic needs of aerobic organisms in water containing organic compounds.

Biomass All organic matter that derives from the photosynthetic conversion of solar energy; the total quantity of organisms in a given area or volume.

Biopharmaceutical A biological macromolecule used as a pharmaceutical.

Bioreactor (fermenter) Containment system for fermentation purposes.

Bioremediation The use of either naturally occurring or deliberately introduced microorganisms to consume or break down environmental pollutants.

Biosensor An electronic device that uses biological molecules to detect specific compounds.

Bioterrorism The intended use by any human agents, other than uniformed military personnel, of organisms (or their products) to cause harm or death to humans, animals or plants.

Bioweapon A harmful biological agent used as a weapon of war.

Blastocyst A cluster of around 250 cells formed about five days after fertilisation.

Bovine somatotropin Growth hormone that can be produced by recombinant DNA technology and used to increase the milk yield of cows.

Callus Plant cells capable of repeated cell division and growth.

Cell line Cells that acquire the ability to multiply indefinitely in vitro.

Chimera An organism containing a mixture of genetically different tissues.

Chromosome A discrete unit of DNA (containing many genes) and protein that carries genetic inheritance. Different species have different numbers of chromosomes.

Chromosomes The threads of DNA in the nucleus that carry genetic inheritance.

Chymosin An enzyme used to clot milk, which is used in the manufacture of cheese.

Clone A collection of genetically identical cells or organisms derived from a common ancestor; all members of the clone have identical genetic composition.

Cloning The process of making a genetically identical copy (a clone) by propagation, embryo splitting or by nuclear replacement.

Composting A process for decaying organic material.

Conjugation The transfer of genetic material from one cell to another by cell-to-cell contact.

Continuous fermentation A fermentation process that can run for long periods, in which raw materials are supplied and products and microorganisms are removed continuously.

Diagnostics The process or techniques of diagnosis.

DNA Abbreviation for deoxyribonucleic acid, which makes up genes.

DNA probes Isolated single DNA strands used to detect the presence of the complementary (opposite) strands, and used as very sensitive biological detectors.

Downstream processing Separation and purification of product(s) from a fermentation process.

Electroporation Introducing DNA or chromosomes into cells using an electric pulse to create temporary pores in the cell membrane.

Embryo transfer Implantation of embryos from donor animals or generated by in vitro fertilisation into the uteri of recipient animals.

Embryonic stem cells (ESs) Stem cells from the inner cell mass of the blastocyst, which will go on to produce every cell in the adult human body.

Enzyme A class of proteins that controls biological reactions.

Enzyme bioreactor A reactor in which a chemical conversion reaction is catalysed by an enzyme.

Fermentation The process by which microorganisms turn raw materials such as glucose into products such as alcohol.

Gene A unit of heredity; a segment of DNA coding for a specific protein.

Gene transfer The use of genetic or physical manipulations to introduce foreign genes into host cells to achieve desired characteristics in progeny.

Genetic engineering Technologies, including DNA technologies, used to isolate genes from an organism, manipulate them in the laboratory and insert them into another cell system.

Genome The genetic endowment of an organism or individual, which resides with the nucleic acids of the chromosomes.

Hybridoma A unique fused cell that produces quantities of a specific antibody and reproduces endlessly.

Immobilised enzyme An enzyme that is physically defined or localised in a defined region, enabling it to be re-used in a continuous process.

Immunoassay A procedure for detecting or measuring substances through their properties as antigens.

Intellectual property Intangible property that is the result of creativity, e.g. patents or copyrights.

Landfill The disposal of waste material by burying it.

Ligase enzyme Enzyme used by genetic engineers to join cut ends of DNA strands.

Lignocellulose The composition of woody biomass, including lignin and cellulose.

Metabolite Product of biochemical activity.

Microarray Miniaturised solid support (typically a glass slide) containing a grid of single-stranded DNA fragments that can represent all, or a sub-population of, the genes from the organism.

Micropropagation Use of small pieces of tissue, such as meristem, grown in culture to produce large numbers of plants.

Monoclonal antibody An antibody derived from a single source or clone of cells, which recognises only one kind of antigen.

Multipotent cells Stem cells able to give rise to a subset of fully differentiated cells.

Mutagen A substance that causes genetic mutations.

Mutation Stable changes of a gene inherited on reproduction.

Mycelium Collective term for a network of fungal hyphae.

Mycoprotein Protein derived from fungi for human consumption.

Particle gun bombardment This is a method to introduce DNA into a host plant cell. It involves precipitating DNA onto microscopic particles or projectiles. The particles are then accelerated and penetrate the plant cells depositing DNA.

Patent A legal right that owes its existence to a granting act by a government administrative authority, i.e. a patent office.

Phenotype Properties (e.g. biochemical or physiological) of an organism that are determined by the genotype.

Plasmid Loop of DNA found in bacteria and some other organisms, e.g. yeasts, that carries non-essential genes and replicates independently of the chromosomes.

Pluripotent cell Cell capable of giving rise to all the cell types of a mature organism, but not able to support development into an embryo.

Polymerase chain reaction (PCR) The action of an enzyme (polymerase) to produce many copies of a polynucleotide sequence of DNA.

Promoter sequence A regulatory DNA sequence that initiates the expression of a gene.

Protein engineering Generating proteins with subtly modified structures, conferring properties such as higher catalytic specificity or thermal stability.

Proteins Large molecules consisting of amino acids, and the products of genes.

Proteome The collective body of proteins made within an organism's cells and tissues.

Proteomics The branch of molecular biology concerned with determining the proteome.

Protoplast Microbial or plant cell whose wall has been removed so that the cell assumes a spherical shape.

Recombinant DNA The hybrid DNA produced by joining pieces of DNA from different organisms.

Restriction enzymes Enzymes used by molecular biologists to cut through DNA at specific points.

Restriction fragment length polymorphism (RFLP) Fragments of differing lengths of DNA that are produced by cutting DNA with restriction enzymes.

Scale-up Expansion of laboratory experiments to full-sized industrial processes.

Single-cell protein Cells or protein extracts of microorganisms grown in large quantities for use as human or animal protein supplements.

Somaclonal variation Genetic variation produced from the culture of plant cells from a pure breeding strain.

Somatic cells Cells of the body other than the germ line (e.g. sperm or egg) cells.

Splicing Gene splicing, manipulation, the object of which is to attach one DNA molecule to another.

Stem cells Cells that can divide indefinitely (are never terminally differentiated) and can give rise to specialised cells.

Systems biology Aims to describe and to understand the operation of complex biological systems and to develop predictive mathematical models; sometimes also referred to as metabolic engineering.

Tissue culture A process where individual cells, or clumps of plant or animal tissue, are grown artificially.

Transduction The transfer of bacterial genes from one bacterium to another by a virus (bacteriophage).

Transformation The acquisition of new genetic markers by the incorporation of added DNA.

Transgenic organism Animals, plants or microorganisms where hereditary DNA has been augmented by the addition of DNA from a source other than parental germ plasm.

Vectors Vehicles for transferring DNA from one cell to another.

Vaccine An antigenic preparation used to stimulate the production of antibodies and provide immunity against disease.

Further reading

New developments in biotechnology are covered in many journals. In particular reference should be made regularly to *Nature Biotechnology* (ISSN 1087-0156), Nature Publishing Group (www.nature.com/nbt/index.html).

Chapter 1: The nature of biotechnology

Acharya, T., Daao, A. S. and Singer, P. A. (2003). Biotechnology and the UN's Millennium Developmental Goals. *Nature Biotechnology* **21**, 1434–6.

Advisory Committee on Science and Technology (1990). *Developments in Biotechnology*. London: HMSO.

BIOTOL (Biotechnology by Open Learning). A series of books. Oxford: Butterworth (Heinemann Ltd).

Budd, R. (1993). *The Uses of Life: A History of Biotechnology*. New York: Cambridge University Press.

European Federation of Biotechnology (1998). *Dialogue in Biotechnology*. Briefing Paper 7. Task Group on Public Perceptions of Biotechnology. Holland: EFB.

Fumento, M. (2003). *Bioevolution: How Biotechnology is Changing our World*. USA: Encounter Books.

McCormick, D. K. (1996). First words, last words. *Biotechnology* **14**, 224.

Pisano, G. P. (2006). *Science Business: the Promise, the Reality and the Future of Biotech*. Harvard: Harvard Business School Press.

Chapter 2: Biomass: a biotechnology substrate?

Hacking, A. J. (1986). *Economic Aspects of Biotechnology*. Cambridge Studies in Biotechnology 3. Cambridge: Cambridge University Press.

Organisation for Economic Co-operation and Development (1992). *Biotechnology, Agriculture and Food*. Paris: OECD.

Chapter 3: Genetics and biotechnology

Clark, M. (2006). Immunochemical applications. In *Basic Biotechnology*, 3rd edn, eds. Ratledge, C. and Kristiansen, B. Cambridge: Cambridge University Press, pp. 625–55.

Graham, A. (1994). A haystack of needles: applying the polymerase chain reaction. *Chemistry & Industry* **October**, 718–20.

Harwood, C. R. and Wipat, A. (2006). Genome management and analysis: prokaryotes. In *Basic Biotechnology*, 3rd edn, eds. Ratledge, C. and Kristiansen, B. Cambridge: Cambridge University Press, pp. 73–118.

Wells, D. A. and Herron, L. L. (2002). Automated sample preparation for genomics. *Pharma Genomics* **2**, 52–5.

Chapter 4: Bioprocess/fermentation technology

Archer, R. and Williams, D. J. (2005). Why tissue engineering needs process engineering. *Nature Biotechnology* **23**, 1353–5.

Chisti, Y. (2006). Bioreactor design. In *Basic Biotechnology*, 3rd edn, eds. Ratledge, C. and Kristiansen, B. Cambridge: Cambridge University Press, pp. 181–200.

Davies, J. E. and Demain, A. L. (1999). *Manual of Industrial Microbiology and Biotechnology*, 2nd edn. Washington, DC: American Society for Microbiology.

Herrera, S. (2005). Struggling to see the forest through the trees. *Nature Biotechnology* **23**, 165–7.

Kamarck, M. F. (2006). Building biomanufacturing capacity – the chapter and verse. *Nature Biotechnology* **24**, 503–5.

Kristiansen, B. and Chamberlain, H. (1983). Fermenter systems. In *The Filamentous Fungi*, Vol. 4. eds. Smith, J. E., Berry, D. R. and Kristiansen, B. London: Edward Arnold, pp. 48–81.

McNeil, B. and Harvey, L. M. (eds.) (1990). *Fermentation: A Practical Approach*. Oxford, New York: Oxford University Press.

Ottens, M. and Wesselingh, J. A. (2006). Downstream processing. In *Basic Biotechnology*, 3rd edn, eds. Ratledge, C. and Kristiansen, B. Cambridge: Cambridge University Press, pp. 219–49.

Stanbury, P. F. and Whitaker, A. (1984). *Principles of Fermentation Technology*. New York: Pergamon Press.

Wurm, F. M. (2004). Production of recombinant protein therapeutics in cultivated mammalian cells. *Nature Biotechnology* **22**, 1393–8.

Chapter 5: Enzyme technology

Berka, R. M. and Cherry, J. R. (2006). Enzyme biotechnology. In *Basic Biotechnology*, 3rd edn, eds. C. Ratledge and B. Kristiansen. Cambridge: Cambridge University Press, pp. 477–98.

Godfrey, T. and West, S. (eds.). (1966). *Industrial Enzymology*, 2nd edn. New York: Stockholm Press; London: MacMillan.

Gray, J. (1990). *The Genetic Engineer and Biotechnologist*. Swansea: GB Biotechnology Ltd.

Kirk, O., Borchest, T. V. and Fuglsang, C. C. (2002). Industrial enzyme applications. *Current Opinions in Biotechnology* **13**, 345–51.

Smith, J. E. (1985). *Biotechnology Principles*. Aspects of Microbiology II. Holland: Van Nostrand Reinhold.

Van Beilan, J. B. and Li, Z. (2002). Enzyme technology: an overview. *Current Opinions in Biotechnology* **13**, 338–44.

Wymer, P. (1990). Making sense of biosensors. NCBE Newsletter. Reading, UK: Reading University.

Chapter 6: Biological fuel generation

Bellamy, D. and Barrett, J. (2007). Climate stability: an inconvenient proof. *Civil Engineering* **160**, 66–72.

Bevan, M. W. and Franssen, M. C. R. (2006). Investing in green and white biotechnology. *Nature Biotechnology* **24**, 765–7.

Burke, D. (2007). Biofuels – is there a role for GM? *Biologist* **54**, 52–6.

Herrera, S. (2006). Bonkers about biofuels. *Nature Biotechnology* **24**, 755–60.

House of Lords (2006). The EU strategy on biofuels: from field to fuel. www.publications.parliament.uk/pa/ld200506/lets-elect/ldeu.com/

Loewrier, A. (1998). Biodiesel: tomorrow's liquid gold. *Biologist* **45**, 17–21.

Morton, O. (2006). Biofuelling the future. *Nature* **444**, 669–78.

Schubert, C. (2006). Can biofuels finally take center stage? *Nature Biotechnology* **24**, 777–84.

Smith, P. (2006). Bioenergy: not a new sports drink but a way to tackle climate change. *Biologist* **53**, 23–9.

Stewart, Jr C. N. (2007). Biofuel and biocontainment. *Nature Biotechnology* **25**, 283–4.

The Economist (2007). Iowa's ethanol economy: the craze for maize, 12 May.

The Economist (2007). Really new advances – briefing RNA. 16 June, pp. 91–3.

Vertres, A. A., Innis, M. and Yukawa, H. (2006). Implementing biofuels on a global scale. *Nature Biotechnology* **24**, 761–4.

Webster, B. (2006). Home-grown crops accelerate drive towards biofuels. *The Times*, 23 August. http://business.timesonline.co.uk

Wooley, T. (2006). Biomass and the UK's energy future. *Biologist* **53**, 118–19.

Chapter 7: Environmental biotechnology

Bio-Wise (2001). *Industrial Solid Waste Treatment. A Review of Composting Technology.* Bio-wise, PO Box 83, Didcot, Oxfordshire OX11 0BR.

Bull, A. T. (2003). Clean technology: industry and environment, a viable partnership. *Biologist* **47**, 61–4.

Burke, M. (2004). Prosecuting the polluters. *Chemistry World* **May**, 44–9.

deLorenzo, V. (2006). Blueprint of an oil-eating bacterium. *Nature Biotechnology* **24**, 952–3.

European Federation of Biotechnology (1995). *Environmental Biotechnology.* Briefing paper 4. Task Group on Public Perceptions of Biotechnology. Holland: EFB.

Forster, C. F. (1985). *Biotechnology and Waste-Water Treatment.* Cambridge Studies in Biotechnology 2. Cambridge: Cambridge University Press.

Glick, B. R. (2004). Teamwork in phytoremediation. *Nature Biotechnology* **22**, 526–7.

Meagher, R. B. (2006). Plants tackle explosive contamination. *Nature Biotechnology* **24**, 101–63.

Moser, A. (1994). Sustainable biotechnology development: from high-tech to eco-tech. *Acta Biotechnology* **12**, 2–6.

Organisation for Economic Co-operation and Development (1998). *Biotechnology for Clean Industrial Products and Processes Towards Industrial Sustainability.* Paris: OECD.

Rawlings, D. E. and Silver, S. (1995). Mining with microbes. *Biotechnology* **13**, 773–8.

Seshadri, R. and Heidelberg, R. (2005). Bacteria to the rescue. *Nature Biotechnology* **23**, 1236–7.

Vandevivere, P. and Verstaete, W. (2006). Environmental applications. In *Basic Biotechnology*, 3rd edn, eds. C. Ratledge and B. Kristiansen. Cambridge: Cambridge University Press, pp. 403–31.

Verstraete, W. (2002). Environmental biotechnology for sustainability. *Journal of Biotechnology* **94**, 93–100.

Chapter 8: Plant and forest biotechnology

Bates, S. I., Zhao, J.-Z., Roush, R. T. and Shelton, A. M. (2005). Insect resistance management in GM crops: past, present and future. *Nature Biotechnology* **23**, 57–62.

Bevan, M. W. and Franssen, M. C. R. (2006). Investing in green and white biotechnology. *Nature Biotechnology* **24**, 765–7.

Cohen, J. I. (2005). Poorer nations turn to publicly developed GM crops. *Nature Biotechnology* **23**, 27–33.

Dale, P. J. (2000). The GM debate: science or scaremongering. *Biologist* **47**, 7–10.

Editorial (2004). Drugs in crops – the unpalatable truth. *Nature Biotechnology* **22**, 133.

Editorial (2005). Reburnishing Golden Rice. *Nature Biotechnology* **23**, 395.

Fox, J. L. (2006). Turning plants into protein factories. *Nature Biotechnology* **24**, 1191–3.

Hellwig, S., Drossard, J., Turyman, R. M. and Fischer, R. (2004). Plant cell cultures for the production of recombinant proteins. *Nature Biotechnology* **22**, 1415–22.

Herrera, S. (2005). Struggling to see the forest through the trees. *Nature Biotechnology* **23**, 165–7.

Johnson-Green, P. (2002). *Introduction to Food Biotechnology*. Boca Raton, USA: CRC Press.

Marrier, M. (2005). Pharmaceutical crops. In *McGraw Hill Year Book of Science and Technology*, pp. 257–9.

Paine, J. A., Shipton, C. A., Chaggar, S. *et al.* (2005). Improving the nutritional value of Golden Rice through increased pro-vitamin A content. *Nature Biotechnology* **23**, 482–7.

Parry, B. (2005). Ode to energy crops. *Biologist* **53**, 11–12.

Patera, C. (2007). Blooming biotech. *Nature Biotechnology* **25**, 963–5.

Powell, W. and Hillman, J. R. (eds.) (1992). *Opportunities and Problems in Plant Biotechnology*. Edinburgh: The Royal Society of Edinburgh.

Robinson, C. (1999). Making forest biotechnology a commercial reality. *Nature Biotechnology* **17**, 27–30.

Shelton, A. M., Zhao, J. Z. and Roush, R. T. (2002). Economic, ecological, food safety and social consequences of the deployment of *Bt* transgenic plants. *Annual Review of Entomology* **47**, 845–81.

Smith, P. (2006). Bioenergy: not a new sports drink but a way to tackle climate change. *Biologist* **53**, 23–9.

Stewart, C. N. (2003). *Transgenic Plants: Current Innovations and Future Trends*. Norfolk: Horizon Press.

Straughan, R. and Reiss, M. (1996). *Ethics, Morality and Crop Biotechnology*. Biotechnology and Biological Sciences Research Council. www.bbsrc.ac.uk.

Strauss, J. M. and Bradshaw, H. D. (eds.) (2005). *The Bioengineered Forest: Challenges to Science and Society*. Washington, DC: Resources for the Future Press.

The Economist (2005). The story of wheat: ears of plenty, 24 December, pp. 26–30. [An essential read].

The Royal Society (2000). *Transgenic Plants and World Agriculture*. London: The Royal Society.

The Royal Society (2002). *Genetically Modified Plants for Food Use and Human Health – An Update*. London: The Royal Society. www.royalsoc.ac.uk

Williams, C. G. (2005). Framing the issues on transgenic forests. *Nature Biotechnology* **23**, 530–2.

Chapter 9: Animal and insect biotechnology

Barrett, T. and Rossiter, P. (1999). Rinderpest: the disease and its impact on humans and animals. *Advances in Virus Research* **53**, 89–110.

Church, S. L. (2006). Nuclear transfer saddles up. *Nature Biotechnology* **24**, 605–7.

Dove, A. (2005). Clone on the range: what animal biotech is bringing to the table. *Nature Biotechnology* **23**, 283–5.

Fulka, J., Miyashita, N., Nagai, T. and Ogura, A. (2006). Do cloned mammals skip a reprogramming step? *Nature Biotechnology* **22**, 25–6.

Hammer, R. E., Pursel, V. G., Rexroad Jr, C. E., Wall, R. J. and Bolt, D. J. (1995). Production of rabbits, sheep and pigs by microinjection. *Nature* **315**, 680–3.

Handler, A. M. and James, A. A. (eds.) (2000). *Insect Transgenesis Methods and Applications*. Boca Raton, USA: CRC Press.

Holland, A. and Johnson, A. (eds.) (1998). *Animal Biotechnology and Ethics*. London: Chapman and Hall.

Johnson-Green, P. (2002). *Introduction to Food Biotechnology*. Boca Raton, USA: CRC Press.

Liangxue, L., Lai, L., Kang, J. X. *et al.* (2006). Generation of cloned transgenic pigs rich in omega-3 fatty acids. *Nature Biotechnology* **24**, 435–9.

Powell, A. M., Talbot, N. C., Wells, K. D. *et al.* (2004). Cell donor influences success of producing cattle by somatic nuclear transfer. *Biology and Reproduction* **71**, 210–16.

Rudenko, L., Matheson, J. C. and Sundlof, S. F. (2007). Animal cloning and the FDA – the risk assessment paradigm under public scrutiny. *Nature Biotechnology* **25**, 39–43.

Straughan, R. (1999). *Ethics, Morality and Animal Biotechnology*. Biotechnology and Biological Sciences Research Council. www.bbsrc.ac.uk.

Suk, J., Bruce, A., Gert, R. *et al.* (2007). Dolly for dinner? Assessing commercial and regulatory trends in cloned livestock. *Nature Biotechnology* **25**, 47–53.

Wall, R. J., Powell, A. N., Paapa, M. J. *et al.* (2005). Genetically enhanced cows resist intra-mammary *Staphylococcus aureus* infection. *Nature Biotechnology* **23**, 445–50.

Wilmut, I. (2004). Derivation of human embryo stem cells by nuclear replacement for technology development and the study of motor neuron disease. www.hfea.gov.uk

Wimmer, E. A. (2005). Eco-friendly insect management. *Nature Biotechnology* **23**, 432–3.

Chapter 10: Food and beverage biotechnology

Angold, R., Beech, G. and Taggart, J. (1989). *Food Biotechnology*. Cambridge: Cambridge University Press.

Berka, R. M. and Cherry, J. R. (2006). Enzyme biotechnology. In *Basic Biotechnology*, 3rd edn, eds. C. Ratledge and B. Kristiansen. Cambridge: Cambridge University Press, pp. 477–98.

Campbell-Platt, G. (1989). *Fermented Foods of the World: A Dictionary and Guide*. London: Butterworth.

Chang, S.-T. (1999). World production of cultivated edible and medicinal mushrooms in 1997. *International Journal of Medicinal Mushrooms* **1**, 291–300.

European Federation of Biotechnology (1994). *Biotechnology in Foods and Drinks*. Briefing Paper 2. Task Group on Public Perceptions of Biotechnology. Holland: EFB.

Eggeling, L., Pfefferle, W. and Sahm, H. (2001). Amino acids. In *Basic Biotechnology*, eds, C. Ratledge and B. Kristiansen. Cambridge: Cambridge University Press, pp. 281–304.

Fuller, R. (2004). What is a probiotic? *Biologist* **51**, 232.

Gibson, G. (2005). The rise and rise of probiotics. *Biologist* **52**, 95–8.

Godfrey, T. and West, S. (eds.). (1966). *Industrial Enzymology*, 2nd edn. New York: Stockholm Press; London: MacMillan.

Gray, J. (1990). *The Genetic Engineer and Biotechnologist*. Swansea: GB Biotechnology Ltd.

Johnson-Green, P. (2002). *Introduction to Food Biotechnology*. Boca Raton, USA: CRC Press.

Kirk, O., Borchest, T. V. and Fuglsang, C. C. (2002). Industrial enzyme applications. *Current Opinions in Biotechnology* **13**, 345–51.

McCarthy, K. C. and Rastall, R. A. (2003). Sticking your 'ose in it: prebiotics. *Biologist* **50**, 259–62.

Ratledge, C. and Kristiansen, B. (2006). *Basic Biotechnology*, 3rd edn. Chapter 14: Amino acids; Chapter 15: Organic acids; Chapter 16: Microbial polysaccharides and single cell oils. Cambridge: Cambridge University Press.

Rodger, G. (2001). Production and properties of mycoprotein as a meat alternative. *Food Technology* **85**, 36–41.

Scotch Whisky Association. *Scotch Whisky: Questions and Answers*. www.scotch_whisky.org.uk.

Smith, J. E. (1985). *Biotechnology Principles*. Aspects of Microbiology II. Holland: Van Nostrand Reinhold.

Sullivan, R., Smith, J. E. and Rowan, N. J. (2006). Medicinal mushrooms and cancer therapy. *Perspectives in Biology and Medicine* **49**, 159–70.

Trinci, A. P. J. (1992). Myco-protein: a twenty year overnight success story. *Mycological Research* **96**, 1–13.

Van Beilan, J. B. and Li, Z. (2002). Enzyme technology: an overview. *Current Opinions in Biotechnology* **13**, 338–44.

Wiebe, H. G. (2004). Quorn™ myco-proteins – overview of a successful fungal product. *Mycologist* **18**, 17–20.

Wood, B. J. B. (ed.) (1998). *The Microbiology of Fermented Foods*, Vols. 1 & 2, 2nd edn. London: Elsevier Applied Science Publishers. [A brilliant comprehensive coverage.]

Wymer, P. (1990). Making sense of biosensors. NCBE Newsletter. Reading, UK: Reading University.

Yokotsuka, T. (1985). Fermented protein foods in the Orient, with emphasis on shoyu and miso in Japan. In *Microbiology of Fermented Foods*, Vol. 1. ed. B. J. B. Wood. London: Elsevier, pp. 351–415.

Chapter 11: Biotechnology and medicine

Bains, W. and Evans, C. (2001). The business of biotechnology. In *Basic Biotechnology*, 2nd edn, eds. C. Ratledge and B. Kristiansen. Cambridge: Cambridge University Press, pp. 255–79.

Clark, M. (2006). Immunochemical applications. In *Basic Biotechnology*, 3rd edn, eds. Ratledge, C. and Kristiansen, B. Cambridge: Cambridge University Press, pp. 625–55.

Focus on Diagnostics (2006). *Nature Biotechnology* **24**(8). [A comprehensive series of papers covering all aspects of molecular diagnostics.]

Forde, G. M. (2005). Rapid-response vaccines – does DNA offer a solution? *Nature Biotechnology* **23**, 1059–62.

Golub, E. (1994). *The Limits of Medicine: How Science Shapes Our Hope for the Cure*. New York: Time Books.

Groundsmith, J. (2004). *Viral Fitness. The Next SARS and West Nile in the Making.* Oxford: Oxford University Press.

Hockley, D., Robinson, T. and Fleck, R. (2004). Biological standards: measuring the potency of biological medicines. *Biologist* **51**, 150–4.

Hook, D. J. (2006). Production of antibiotics by fermentation. In *Basic Biotechnology*, 3rd edn, eds. Ratledge, C. and Kristiansen, B. Cambridge: Cambridge University Press, pp. 433–55.

Kresse, G. B. (2006). Recombinant proteins of high value. In *Basic Biotechnology*, 3rd edn, eds. Ratledge, C. and Kristiansen, B. Cambridge: Cambridge University Press, pp. 499–21.

Schellekens, H. (2004). How similar do 'biosimilars' need to be. *Nature Biotechnology* **22**, 1357–9.

Sheridan, C. (2005). The business of making vaccines. *Nature Biotechnology* **23**, 1359–66.

Chapter 12: Stem cell biotechnology

Barfoot, J., Mauelshagen, C., Bruce, D., Henderson, C. and Bowness, M. (ed). (2005). *Stem Cells: Science and Ethics.* Edinburgh: The Scottish Institute for Biotechnology Education.

Department of Health and Human Services (2001). *Stem Cells: Scientific Progress and Future Research Directions.* http://stemcells.nih.gov/info/scireport

Hoffman, L. M. and Carpenter, M. K. (2005). Characterisation and culture of human embryonic stem cells. *Nature Biotechnology* **23**, 699–708.

O'Donoghue, K. and Fisk, N. M. (2004a). Potential application of stem cells. Part 1. *Biologist* **51**, 125–9.

O'Donoghue, K. and Fisk, N. M. (2004b). Potential application of stem cells. Part 2. *Biologist* **51**, 185–8.

Veeck, L. and Zanimovic, N. (eds). (2003). *An Atlas of Human Blastocysts.* Boca Raton, USA: Parthenon.

Verfaillie, C. M. (2002). Adult stem cells: assessing the case for pluripotency. *Trends in Cell Biology* **12**, 502–9.

Wilan, K. M., Scott, C. T. and Harris, S. (2005). Chasing a cellular fountain of youth. *Nature Biotechnology* **23**, 807–15.

Wilmut, I. (2004). Derivation of human embryo stem cells by nuclear replacement for technology development and the study of motor neuron disease. www.hfea.gov.uk

Chapter 13: Protection of biotechnological inventions

Byrne, N. (1992). Patents for plants and genes under the European Patent Convention. *Proceedings of the Royal Society of Edinburgh* **99b**(3/4), 141–52.

Elliott, S. M. (2007). The threat from within: trade secrets' theft by employees. *Nature Biotechnology* **25**, 293–5.

European Federation of Biotechnology (1996). *Patenting in Biotechnology.* Briefing Paper 1. Task Group on Public Perceptions of Biotechnology. Holland: EFB.

Kahn, J. (2006). Patenting race. *Nature Biotechnology* **24**, 1349–50.

Klein, R. D. (2007). Gene patents and genetic testing in the United States. *Nature Biotechnology* **25**, 989–90.

Teitelbaum, R. and Cohen, M. S. (2004). Publish and perish: what constitutes a bar under the patent law. *Nature Biotechnology* **22**, 1449–51.

White, N. I. (2007). Time waits for no man: deciding when to file a patent application in Europe. *Nature Biotechnology* **25**, 639–41.

Chapter 14: Safety in biotechnology

Block, S. M. (2001). The growing threat of biological weapons. *American Scientist* **89**, 28–37.

Gilmore, R. (2004). US food safety under siege. *Nature Biotechnology* **22**, 1503–5.

Gorka, S. and Sullivan R. (2002). Biological toxins: a weapon threat in the 21st Century. *Security Dialogue* **33**, 141–56.

Grönwall, G. K. (2005). A new role for scientists in the Biological Weapons Convention. *Nature Biotechnology* **23**, 1213–15.

Guillemin, J. (2006). *Biological Weapons: From the Invention of State Sponsored Programs to Contemporary Bioterrorism*. New York: Columbia University Press.

Harley, J. P. (2005). Bioterrorism. *McGraw-Hill Year Book of Science and Technology*. New York: McGraw-Hill, pp. 32–4.

Küenzi, M., Assi, F., Chmiel, A., Collins, C. H. and Donikian, M. (1985). Safe biotechnology: general considerations. *Applied Microbiology and Biotechnology* **21**, 1–6.

Lederberg, J. (ed.) (1999). *Biological Weapons: Limiting the Threat*. Cambridge, Massachusetts: MIT Press.

Lelieveld, H. L. M., Bachmayer, H., Boon, B. and Brunius, G. (1995). Safe biotechnology. Part 6. Safety assessment, in respect of human health of microorganisms used in biotechnology. *Applied Microbiology and Biotechnology* **43**, 389–93.

Madden, L. V. and Wheelis, M. (2003). The threat of plant pathogens as weapons against US crops. *Annual Review of Plant Pathology* **41**, 155–76.

The Royal Society (1994). *Scientific Aspects of Control of Biological Weapons*. London: The Royal Society.

Wheelis, M., Rozsa, L. and Dando, M. (eds.) (2006). *Deadly Cultures: Biological Weapons since 1945*. Harvard: Harvard University Press.

Chapter 15: Public perception of biotechnology: genetic engineering – safety, social, moral and ethical considerations

Bruce, D. M. (2006). Moral and ethical issues in gene therapy. *Human Reproduction and Genetic Ethics* **12**, 10–23.

Durant, J. R., Evans, G. A. and Thomas, G. P. (1989). The public understanding of science. *Nature* **340**, 11–14.

Hutton, P. (2006). GM foods: what Europeans really think. www.brandenergyresearch.co.uk

Maschke, K. J. (2005). Navigating an ethical patchwork: human gene banks. *Nature Biotechnology* **23**, 539–44.

Millar, H. I. and Conko, G. (2004). *The Frankenfood Myth: How Protest and Politics Threaten the Biotech Revolution*. New York: Praeger Publishers.

Miller, H. I. (2006). *Vox populi* and public policy: why should we care? *Nature Biotechnology* **21**, 1431–2.

Scott, C. T. (2005). *Stem Cell Now: From the Experiment That Shook the World to the New Politics of Life*. Pi Press.

Scottish Council on Human Bioethics (2006). Embryonics fetal and post-natal human mixtures: an ethical discussion. *Human Reproduction and Genetic Ethics* **12**, 36–60.

Straughan, R. (1999). *Ethics, Morality and Animal Biotechnology*. Biotechnology and Biological Sciences Research Council. www.bbsrc.ac.uk.

Straughan, R. and Reiss, M. (1996). *Ethics, Morality and Crop Biotechnology*. Biotechnology and Biological Sciences Research Council. www.bbsrc.ac.uk.

Suyder, E. J., Hinman, L. M. and Kalichman, M. W. (2006). Can science resolve the ethical impasse in stem cell research? *Nature Biotechnology* **24**, 397–400.

Thompson, J. (2007). Genetically modified crops – good or bad for Africa? *Biologist* **54**, 129–33.

Turnpenny, L. (2005). Public perception of cloning and embryonic stem cells. *Biologist* **52**, 310–12.

Val Giddings, J. L. (2006). Whither agbiotechnology? *Nature Biotechnology* **24**, 274–6.

Chapter 16: Looking to the future

Taverne, D. (2005). The new fundamentalism. *Nature Biotechnology* **23**, 415–16.

Index